Nursing
and
Healthcare
Research
at a Glance

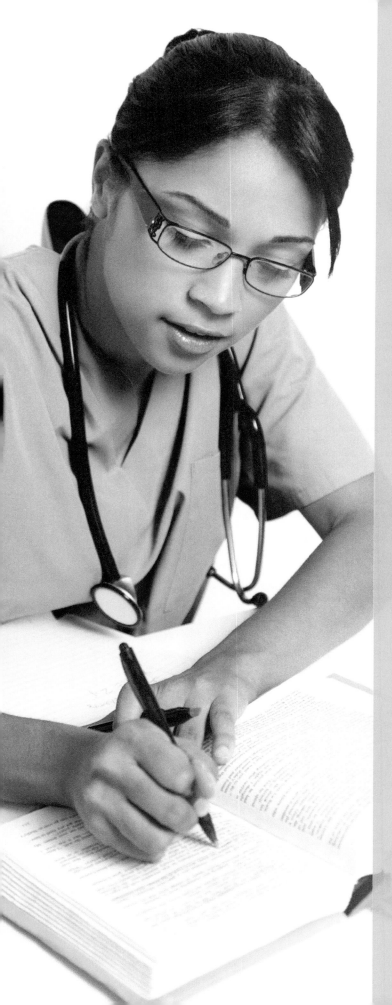

Nursing and Healthcare Research
at a Glance

Edited by

Alan Glasper

Professor Emeritus
Faculty of Health Sciences
University of Southampton
Southampton, UK

Colin Rees

Lecturer (retired)
School of Health Care Sciences
Cardiff University
Cardiff, UK

Series Editor: Ian Peate

WILEY Blackwell

This edition first published 2017 © 2017 by John Wiley & Sons, Ltd

Registered office: John Wiley & Sons, Ltd, The Atrium, Southern Gate, Chichester, West Sussex, PO19 8SQ, UK

Editorial offices: 9600 Garsington Road, Oxford, OX4 2DQ, UK
The Atrium, Southern Gate, Chichester, West Sussex, PO19 8SQ, UK
111 River Street, Hoboken, NJ 07030-5774, USA

For details of our global editorial offices, for customer services and for information about how to apply for permission to reuse the copyright material in this book please see our website at www.wiley .com/wiley-blackwell

Library of Congress Cataloging-in-Publication Data

Names: Glasper, Edward Alan, editor. | Rees, Colin, editor.
Title: Nursing and healthcare research at a glance / Alan Glasper, Colin Rees.
Other titles: At a glance series (Oxford, England)
Description: Chichester, West Sussex ; Hoboken, NJ : John Wiley & Sons, Inc.,
   2017. | Series: At a glance series | Includes bibliographical references and index.
Identifiers: LCCN 2016002851 (print) | LCCN 2016003461 (ebook) | ISBN
   9781118778791 (pbk.) | ISBN 9781118778753 (pdf) | ISBN 9781119267140 (epub)
Subjects: | MESH: Nursing Research | Health Services Research | Delivery of Health Care
Classification: LCC RT81.5 (print) | LCC RT81.5 (ebook) | NLM WY 20.5 | DDC
   610.73072—dc23
LC record available at http://lccn.loc.gov/2016002851
Library of Congress LCCN Permalink for 2016002851
lccn.loc.gov
LCCN Permalink provides persistent links to metadata records in the LC Online Catalog.
   LCCN: 2016002851

A catalogue record for this book is available from the British Library.

Wiley also publishes its books in a variety of electronic formats. Some content that appears in print may not be available in electronic books.

Cover image: [Production Editor to insert]
Image credit: ©Getty/Alejandro Rivera

Set in Minion Pro 9.5/11.5 by Aptara

1   2017

Contents

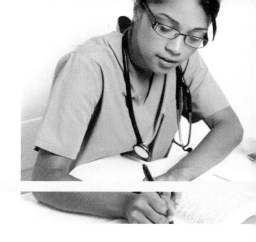

Part 7 — Educational research 171

Part 8 — Appendices 185

Contributors

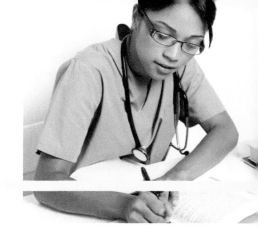

Parveen Ali
Lecturer
The School of Nursing and Midwifery
University of Sheffield
Sheffield, UK

Palo Almond
Former Senior Lecturer, Public Health
School of Health Sciences
University of Brighton
Brighton, UK

Tom Andrews
Lecturer in School of Nursing and Midwifery
University College Cork
Cork, Ireland

Naomi Barnes
Postdoctoral Fellow
Griffith Institute of Educational Research
Queensland, Australia

Cliodhna Ni Bhuachalla
Clinical Microbiology Specialist Registrar (SpR)
Department of Clinical Microbiology
Cork University Hospital
Cork, Ireland

Alan Bleakley
Emeritus Professor of Medical Education
Plymouth University Peninsula School of Medicine
Plymouth, UK

Maria Brenner
Lecturer and Programme Coordinator Critical Care
Nursing (Children)
School of Nursing, Midwifery and Health Systems
University College Dublin
Dublin, Ireland

Sarah Brien
Senior Research Fellow
University of Southampton
Southampton, UK

Claire Mary Buckley
Department of General Practice
University College Cork
Cork, Ireland

Diane Carpenter
Lecturer, MSc Health Sciences
Faculty of Health Sciences
University of Southampton
Southampton, UK

Bernie Carter
Professor of Children's Nursing
Edge Hill University
Ormskirk, UK

Jane Coad
Professor in Children and Family Nursing
Faculty of Health and Life Sciences
Coventry University
Coventry, UK

Reinie Cordier
Associate Professor
Faculty of Health Sciences
Curtin University
Perth, Australia

Fiona Cowdell
Reader in Wellbeing in Long-Term Conditions
Faculty of Health and Social Care
University of Hull
Hull, UK

Imelda Coyne
Professor in Children and Young People's Nursing
School of Nursing and Midwifery
Trinity College Dublin
Dublin, Ireland

Maria Cozens
Nurse Lecturer – Learning Disabilities
College of Midwifery and Healthcare
University of West London
Brentford, UK

Ruth Davies
Associate Professor, Child and Family Health
Swansea University
Swansea, UK

Yvonne Dexter
Senior Lecturer Child Health Nursing
College of Nursing, Midwifery and Healthcare
University of West London
Brentford, UK

Julie Dix
Research Student
School of Health
University of Central Lancashire
Preston, UK

Judith Dyson
Senior Lecturer Mental Health
University of Hull
Hull, UK

Maria Edwards
Research Sister
Sheffield Teaching Hospitals NHS Foundation Trust
Sheffield, UK

Alys Einion
Assistant Professor of Midwifery
College of Human and Health Science
University of Swansea
Swansea, UK

Terri Fletcher
Lecturer in Children's Nursing
Faculty of Health Sciences
University of Southampton
Southampton, UK

Bob Gates
Professor of Learning Disabilities
University of West London;
Visiting Professor of Learning Disabilities
Derby University;
Emeritus Professor
Centre for Learning Disability Studies
University of Hertfordshire
Hatfield, UK

Steve George
Emeritus Fellow
University of Southampton
Southampton, UK

Richard Giordano
Senior Lecturer
Faculty of Health Sciences
University of Southampton
Southampton, UK

Alan Glasper
Professor Emeritus
Faculty of Health Sciences
University of Southampton
Southampton, UK

Mary Gobbi
Professorial Fellow (Healthcare Education)
Faculty of Health Sciences
University of Southampton
Southampton, UK

Lesley Goldsmith
Research Fellow
Plymouth University
Plymouth, UK

Mary Hughes
Lecturer in Children's Nursing
University College Dublin
Dublin, Ireland

Sarah Adrienne Hughes
Senior Lecturer
Pre-qualifying Nursing
Buckinghamshire New University
Uxbridge, UK

Mahnaz Ilkhani
Former doctoral student
University of Southampton
Southampton, UK

Neil James
Senior Lecturer
Unit for Development in Intellectual Disabilities
Faculty of Life Sciences and Education
University of South Wales
Pontypridd, UK

Nikki Jarrett
Lecturer in Nursing
Faculty of Health Sciences
University of Southampton
Southampton, UK

Judith Lathlean
Visiting Professor
Faculty of Health Sciences
University of Southampton
Southampton, UK

Kah Wai Lee
General Practitioner
Park View Surgery
Hessle, UK

Rachel Lennon
Lecturer in Nursing
Faculty of Health Sciences
University of Southampton
Southampton, UK

Joan Livesley
Senior Lecturer Post Graduate Studies
CYP@Salford
University of Salford
Salford, UK

Jennifer Loke
Lecturer, Faculty of Health and Social Care
University of Hull
Hull, UK

Tony Long
Professor of Child and Family Health
University of Salford
Salford, UK

Sandy Mackinnon
IT Business Relationship Manager
iSolutions
University of Southampton
Southampton, UK

Carl May
Professor of Healthcare Innovation
Faculty of Health Sciences
University of Southampton
Southampton, UK

Eloise Monger
Lecturer in Nursing
Faculty of Health Sciences
University of Southampton
Southampton, UK

Gary Mountain
Associate Professor in Child and Family Health
School of Healthcare
University of Leeds
Leeds, UK

Peter Nicholls
Visiting Lecturer, Statistics
Faculty of Health Sciences
University of Southampton
Southampton, UK

Ruth Northway
Professor of Learning Disability Nursing
Unit for Development in Intellectual Disability
Faculty of Life Sciences and Education
University of South Wales
Pontypridd, UK

Anja K. Peters
Medical Historian and Nursing Scientist
Neubrandenburg
Germany

Gill Prudhoe
Lecturer in Children's Nursing
Faculty of Health Sciences
University of Southampton
Southampton, UK

Edward Purssell
Senior Lecturer
Florence Nightingale Faculty of Nursing and Midwifery
King's College London
London, UK

Lavinia Raeside
Advanced Neonatal Nurse Practitioner
NICU, Royal Hospital for Children
Queen Elizabeth University Hospital
Glasgow, UK

Colin Rees
Lecturer (retired)
School of Health Care Sciences
Cardiff University
Cardiff, UK

Salma Rehman
PhD Student
Faculty of Health and Social Care
University of Hull
Hull, UK

Lisa Rudgley
Senior Systemic Psychotherapist and
    Clinical Nurse Specialist
CAMHS
Berkshire Healthcare NHS Foundation Trust
Bracknell, UK

Julie Santy-Tomlinson
Senior Lecturer
Faculty of Health and Social Care
University of Hull
Hull, UK

Linda Shields
Professor of Nursing
Charles Sturt University
Bathurst, New South Wales;
Honorary Professor of Medicine
The University of Queensland
Queensland, Australia

Michael Simon
Tenure-Track Assistant Professor
Institute of Nursing Science
University of Basel
Basel, Switzerland;
Head of Nursing Research Unit
University Hospital Inselspital
Bern, Switzerland

Carol Sinnott
Academic Research Fellow in General Practice
University College Cork
Cork, Ireland

Grahame Smith
Principal Lecturer and Subject Head (Allied Health)
Liverpool John Moores University
Liverpool, UK

Sherrill Snelgrove
Senior Lecturer in Nursing and Psychology Applied to
    Healthcare
Swansea University
Swansea, UK

Nicky Spence
Programme Leader for the MSc in Advanced
    Physiotherapy
School of Health Sciences
University of Salford
Salford, UK

Phitthaya Srimuang
Senior Lecturer
Department of Community Health
Sirindhorn College of Public Health
Khonkaen, Thailand

David Stanley
Associate Professor, Nursing
Charles Sturt University
Bathurst
NSW, Australia

Laurence Taggart
Reader
School of Nursing
University of Ulster
Coleraine, UK

Joanne Turnbull
Lecturer in Health Services Research
Faculty of Health Sciences
University of Southampton
Southampton, UK

Sharmila Vaz
Senior Research Fellow
Faculty of Health Sciences
Curtin University
Perth, Australia

Roger Watson
Professor of Nursing
University of Hull
Hull, UK

Robin Watts
Emeritus Professor
School of Nursing, Midwifery and Paramedicine
Curtin University
Perth, Australia

Tessa Watts
Associate Professor, Nursing
Department of Nursing
Swansea University
Swansea, UK

Mark Weal
Associate Professor in Web Science
University of Southampton
Southampton, UK

Seth A. Wiafe
Assistant Professor
Loma Linda University
Loma Linda
California, USA

Christopher Wibberley
Principal Lecturer
Faculty of Health, Psychology and Social Care
Manchester Metropolitan University
Manchester, UK

Kristin Wicking
Lecturer
Nursing, Midwifery and Nutrition
James Cook University
Townsville
Queensland, Australia

Tracey Williamson
Reader (Public Involvement, Engagement and
    Experience)
University of Salford
Salford, UK

Preface

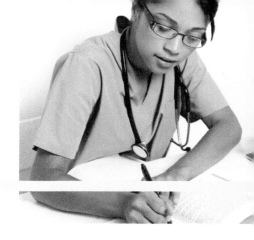

Despite the pleasures and satisfaction of being a health professional, healthcare continues to be a difficult and pressurised activity. Complexities in illness and service provision have increased, along with the obligation to ensure that clinical decisions provide best patient outcomes. To some extent, improvements have been made through the introduction of evidence-based practice. However, this requires all health professionals to have some understanding of the nature and quality of the evidence used in decision-making, often when there are competing demands on time to deal with an increasing workload.

This innovative book is designed to reduce some of these challenges by increasing your knowledge of key research issues, and developing your skills in locating and critically analysing research studies and reviews of the literature. It brings together a large number of well-known experts in the field to provide you with clear, brief information, along with strong visual reminders of essential points and skills.

As research is a wide and often complex academic activity, we have divided the content into a number of logical sections. These focus on both variations in research approaches, and the varying complexities of reviews of the literature. This makes it easier for you to place ideas in context and rapidly understand relevant features of research, its utilisation and implementation.

We hope that three types of reader will benefit from this new format for a research book. Firstly, undergraduate nursing and other healthcare students who are undertaking perhaps their first modules in healthcare research and evidence-based practice. Secondly, postgraduate healthcare students who are undertaking masters and taught clinical doctorate programmes, who will find this book a quick and easy reference for exploring differing research paradigms and methodologies. Thirdly, it will support qualified staff in their role of applying the research evidence in the clinical area, as well as helping students apply the theory of evidence-based care to practice.

All three groups can find themselves faced with assessing published studies that assume knowledge of the methodologies used in research. Although such papers are designed to illuminate and build the evidence base of contemporary practice, sometimes the unfamiliar principles, language and conventions of research can act as barriers to understanding and, as a consequence, affect judgements on a study's contributions to clinical success. In whichever group you find yourself, we sincerely believe that this book will provide you with rapid access to knowledge and understanding that will allow you to overcome many of these challenges in the use of research evidence, and provide you with the knowledge to benefit patients in a multitude of clinical settings and situations.

Alan Glasper
Colin Rees

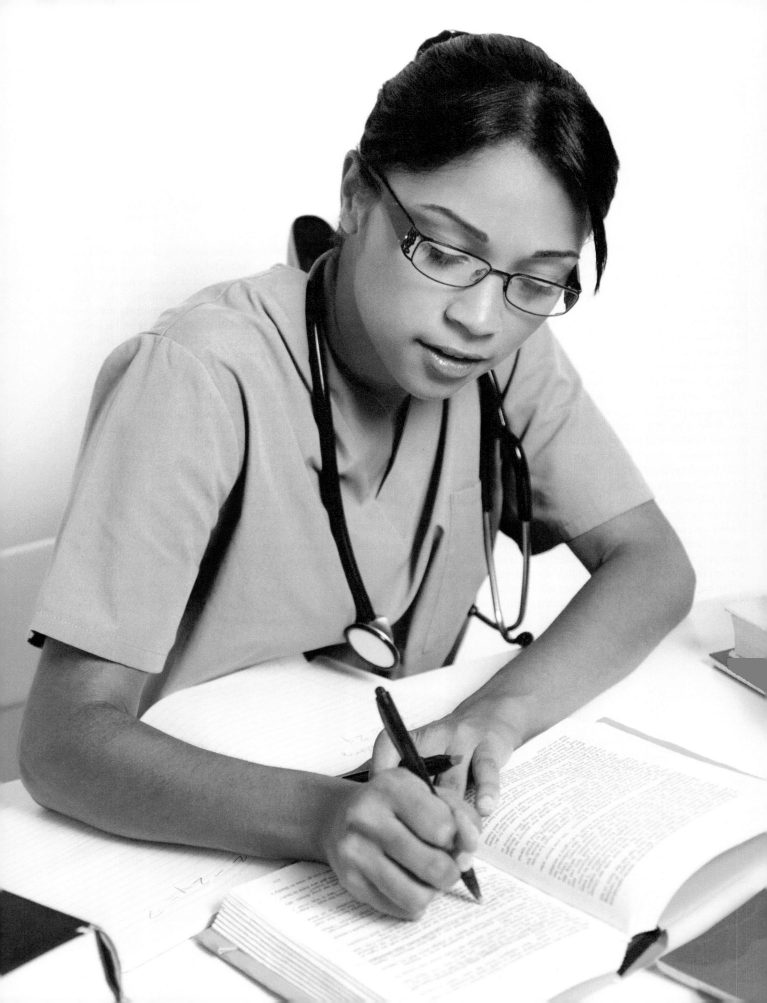

What is healthcare research?

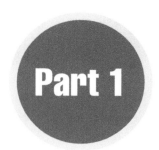

Part 1

Chapters

The research journey

Figure 1.1 The steps of the nursing research journey: it begins and ends with nursing practice.

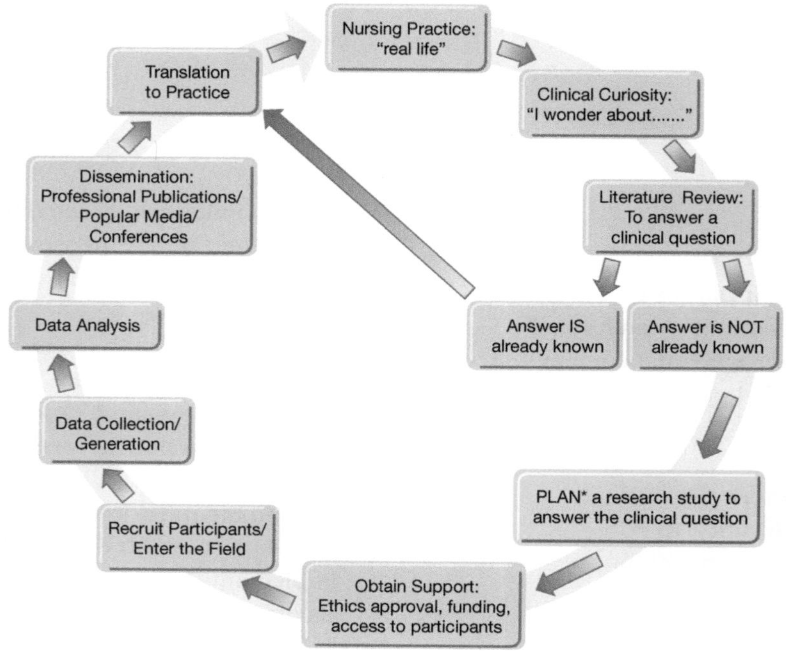

Nursing Practice:
"real life"

Clinical Curiosity:
"I wonder about......."

Literature Review:
To answer a
clinical question

Answer IS
already known

Answer is NOT
already known

PLAN* a research study to
answer the clinical question

Obtain Support:
Ethics approval, funding,
access to participants

Recruit Participants/
Enter the Field

Data Collection/
Generation

Data Analysis

Dissemination:
Professional Publications/
Popular Media/
Conferences

Translation
to Practice

Figure 1.2 Planning: the pivotal step.

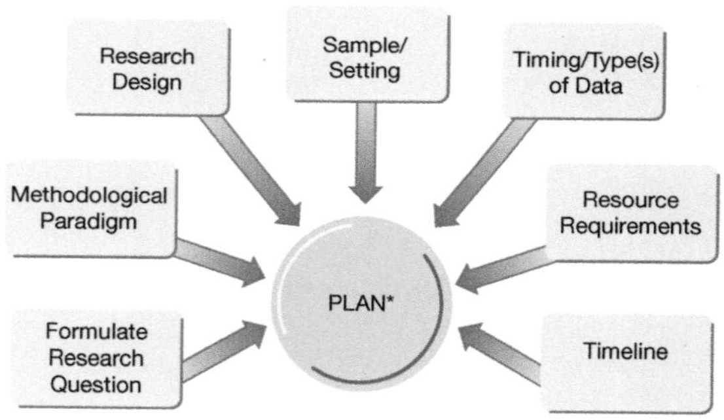

Research
Design

Sample/
Setting

Timing/Type(s)
of Data

Methodological
Paradigm

Resource
Requirements

Formulate
Research
Question

PLAN*

Timeline

Clinical curiosity

The first step in the research journey is to begin to wonder about something. A vibrant research culture will foster this clinical curiosity. If the patient or client's best interests are truly at the heart of a healthcare organisation, then its employees will always be on the lookout for how things might be done better, for how some vexing recurring problem might finally be solved. The first step of research is to observe, to notice, to look around, to wonder why things are happening the way they are, and to envision how they might be improved (Figure 1.1).

Literature searching

The next step is to see if our curiosity can be immediately satisfied by what is already known in the existing body of research evidence available at our fingertips. This step includes finding the research literature, then appraising it both for quality and for applicability to our own practice context. If there have already been a number of rigorously conducted studies and they concur on the best approach after studying populations that are similar to our own clients, then we can immediately apply that evidence to our own practice without the need to conduct further research. This process of translation of research evidence into the practice setting requires excellent leadership and change management skills, as well as project management. Evidence must be presented, appraised and discussed before any change can, or indeed should, occur.

Planning a research study

However, an exhaustive search of the current body of research evidence may fail to unearth a compelling, congruent body of work. The clinician may still be left wondering how best to care for their client. Once such a gap in the literature has been identified, this gap may justify the expenditure of human and

Nursing and Healthcare Research at a Glance, First Edition. Alan Glasper and Colin Rees. © 2017 by John Wiley & Sons, Ltd. Published 2017 by John Wiley & Sons, Ltd.

material resources to conduct a study to answer the clinical question. This is where the fun really begins!

Research question

It is vital to carefully delineate exactly what it is that you are trying to discover in any research project, as that research question will drive all the other decisions you will need to make as you devise your research plan (Leedy & Ormrod, 2013) (Figure 1.2).

Methodological paradigm

Once you know your question, you can begin to select the best methodological paradigm to use to frame your research plan (Schneider & Whitehead, 2013). If you are trying to test an intervention for effectiveness, the 'gold standard' is to conduct a randomised controlled trial (RCT) in the positivist paradigm, by gathering quantitative data to use in statistical comparisons. However, there are many other types of research questions you may be wondering about, and if you choose the wrong paradigm you are still going to get an answer, but not to *your* question.

Research design/methods

Once you have chosen the most appropriate and relevant methodological paradigm, you can begin to plan the 'nuts and bolts' of your study (Leedy & Ormrod, 2013). Who will be your participants – your sample? Where will you recruit your participants? What kind of data will you collect from them: numbers, words or both kinds of data? Will it come from interviews, chart audits, questionnaires, focus groups, observations, document analysis? Will the data be collected once or a number of times, and how far apart? Who will collect the data and how will they be hired and trained? How much time and money will you need to conduct the study? Are there ethical or legal considerations that you need to address in your research plan?

Obtain support

Ethical approval

Most research requires the oversight and approval of a human research ethics committee (HREC), which evaluates all your carefully considered plans to ensure two things. First, that you are conducting research properly, so that it will have merit and usefulness, and not be trivial and a waste of everyone's time. Second, that you have included safeguards to ensure that the ethical rights of the participants in your study are maintained. You will need to prepare a participant information sheet and an informed consent form for the HREC to review and approve. The committee will also wish to see any questionnaire you want participants to complete, or the questions you may ask during an interview or focus group, or the kinds of biological or other measurements you may be planning on obtaining (e.g. blood pressure, waist circumference, serum glucose level).

Funding

A number of sources, both public and private, are available to fund research, but nearly all require the project to be fully described in a proposal that includes all the components and decisions we have been discussing thus far, including a detailed budget. Interim and final reporting will be required, stating how the budget was followed and what the research findings revealed.

Access to participants

It is important to ensure that you are able to reach the participants who can tell you what you want to know. If they are patients (or staff) within a healthcare facility, you will need the permission of that facility to recruit there. You need to show the HREC that you have a letter of support from the facility, which indicates that the management of that facility agree that your research is useful and appropriate, and that they will help you find and connect with the participants you need to recruit.

Recruit participants/enter the field

A recruitment plan needs to be included in the overall research plan. You need to 'sell' your study to potential participants, so that they will donate the time and attention needed to collect data from them, or in qualitative studies to generate data with them (Birks & Mills, 2015).

Data collection/generation

Once you have attracted participants, you need to administer a questionnaire, draw a blood sample, conduct an interview or in some way obtain the data you need in order to answer your research question. It is important to have considered and decided on as many details as possible in advance, but this level of preparation will vary according to research design. In an RCT, a strict protocol must be folowed (Schneider & Whitehead, 2013); in a qualitative study, some of the decisions about when, where, how and who will provide data will evolve based on earlier data gathered and analysed (Birks & Mills, 2015).

Data analysis

This stage can occur after all data has been collected, or occur concurrently with data collection. It may consist of statistical analysis of quantitative data using computerised software such as SPSS, or thematic analysis of qualitative data using computerised software such as NVivo, or both kinds of data analysis in a mixed methods study.

Dissemination

Once you have analysed your data, it is time to tell the world what you have found. Research left gathering dust on a shelf in a university library is a paradise lost. Research that is not disseminated widely cannot possibly be translated into practice, and it is beholden on every responsible researcher to share their findings, both locally and globally (Schneider & Whitehead, 2013). This sharing is done through professional conferences, peer-reviewed professional journals and textbooks, and speaking to the popular press to ensure lay people (future or current clients) also become aware of the findings.

Translation into practice

This final stage can be the most challenging, and is more than just dissemination. Changing the practice of experienced clinicians in established healthcare settings can be an uphill battle, and one that requires education, motivation and perspiration. However, if we know better and do not do better, then we have failed our patients and also failed our past, present and future researchers. The legacy of research must be concrete improvements in the care of our clients, our clinicians, our clinical contexts and our communities.

References

Birks, M. & Mills, J. (2015) *Grounded Theory: A Practical Guide*, 2nd edn. Los Angeles: Sage.

Leedy, P.D. & Ormrod, J.E. (2013) *Practical Research: Planning and Design*, 10th edn. Boston: Pearson.

Schneider, Z. & Whitehead, D. (2013) *Nursing and Midwifery Research: Methods and Appraisal for Evidence-based Practice*, 4th edn. Sydney: Mosby Elsevier.

2 Types of review and their purpose

Figure 2.1 Conducting a literature review.

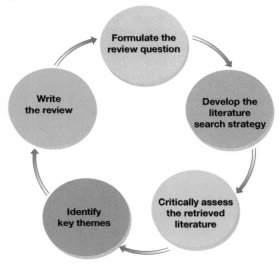

Review tips

- Consider seeking help, for example from university librarians.

- Maintain a clear and detailed record of your searches.

- Learn how to use a bibliographic referencing system such as EndNote to make the work easier and quicker.

- Talk to experienced researchers in the field about your interpretations and impact of the research methods employed.

- Read other published reviews/literature reviews in postgraduate dissertations/theses.

- Do not underestimate the time it takes to complete a high-quality review.

- Take care to ensure your review is accurate and complete.

Formulate the review question

Develop the literature search strategy

The precise nature of the search strategy will be shaped by the type of review being undertaken and its overall purpose. However, there are a number of common elements to be considered.

- Identify potential sources of literature: databases (it is not sufficient to focus on CINAHL or Medline alone); relevant journals; article reference lists; grey literature; websites ; conference proceedings; government reports and strategies; citation indexes; direct contact with academics or professionals.
- Decide whether search terms should include everyday language and/or synonyms? Check that databases feature facility for wild cards and Boolean operators (e.g. AND, OR, NOT).
- Inclusion and exclusion criteria: language, timeline, research methodology.

Critically assess the literature retrieved and identify key themes

This stage of the review process necessitates focused reading in order to:
- Establish the current state of knowledge: what has been written; why it has been written; what research has been undertaken; what research methods have been used and the methodological quality of the research.
- Identify emergent themes which incorporate theoretical and empirical literature and which will be used to structure the overall 'findings' section.

Write the review and draw conclusions

Although tables will be used in certain review types, in writing the review it is important to be analytical, balanced and not overly descriptive. A review is not meant to be a descriptive list of published papers or summaries of individual research studies. Ideally the review should be a logically structured synthesis of material which is related to the review question. Finally, it is important to be aware of and state the limitations of the review.

Literature reviews have a long history in health research. A literature review is an analysis of existing published works on a particular subject and is both a process and an outcome. In recent decades, escalating emphasis on evidence-based practice and policy-making, coupled with the drive to enhance methodological rigour, has given rise to a proliferation of diverse types of reviews, each with its own unique systematic method, or process. Methods continue to evolve.

The type of review employed is contingent upon the question the review seeks to answer. However, the different review genres all share common defining attributes, namely gathering, analysing, synthesising and presenting available theoretical and research literature (Figure 2.1). Thus, regardless of type, the outcome of the review process is a structured analytic synthesis of a potentially vast array of existing knowledge and ideas on a subject.

A significant strength of literature reviews is that they bring together a body of literature on a particular subject. However, they can be at risk of subjectivity, bias and insufficient analysis and synthesis.

Types of reviews

Narrative review

The narrative review is often referred to as the 'traditional' review. The narrative review serves to provide a comprehensive overview of a broad range of recent and current literature, including research, on a given subject. Baumeister and Leary (1997) identify five key purposes of a narrative review: to develop theory, evaluate theory, summarise the state of knowledge about a subject in terms of what is known and unknown, identify problems in a field of knowledge, and present a historical account of theory and research development within a field. Yet despite its breadth of focus which serves its intrinsic purpose, a frequent criticism of the narrative review is that it is unsystematic, subject to bias and thus unscientific.

Systematic review

Systematic reviews synthesise the findings from several primary quantitative studies to summarise best available research on a very specific, clearly defined question. Systematic reviews have become increasingly popular as a means by which primary research evidence is gathered, evaluated and synthesised.

The systematic review process is characterised by an explicit predefined protocol and a well-developed, comprehensive, specific, rigorous and reproducible method. Guidance for conducting systematic reviews is available from the Cochrane Collaboration and the NHS Centre for Reviews and Dissemination. However, the systematic review privileges the hierarchy of evidence where the randomised controlled trial is perceived as the gold standard. Moreover, publication bias threatens the validity of systematic reviews and the review process is extremely labour-intensive.

Qualitative evidence synthesis

Sometimes referred to as qualitative systematic reviews, this evolving complex review genre systematically identifies and draws together findings from individual qualitative studies. There are two broad categories of qualitative evidence synthesis: thematic integrated reviews and interpretive synthesis. A number of different methods of synthesis have been identified, including meta-ethnography, grounded theory, thematic synthesis and meta-narrative. The method selected will be influenced by the nature of the research question and the precise purpose of the review.

The broad purpose of qualitative evidence synthesis is to arrive at an understanding of a phenomenon or aspects such as need, appropriateness, acceptability, experiences, preferences and influencing factors relating to interventions or models of service delivery and from the perspective of individuals or groups.

Integrative review

The integrative review is a comprehensive type of review which combines diverse research methodologies and may also incorporate theoretical literature. In an important paper, Whittemore and Knafl (2005) suggested that the integrative review served several purposes, including definition of concepts and review of theories and evidence with the broad aim of generating new perspectives on the subject reviewed. Combining a diverse body of literature with multiple methodological perspectives is challenging and complex. However, a number of criticisms have been levelled at this type of review, including lack of rigorous method and poorly formulated methods of analysis and synthesis.

Scoping review

Scoping reviews seek to swiftly identify and assess the main concepts underpinning a research area and the nature and extent of available evidence in a particular field. Scoping reviews are often undertaken as preliminary work in order to systematically establish the feasibility of or necessity for a full systematic review. They are also conducted to precis and distribute findings from empirical studies, to identify what is known and what is not known in extant literature and to determine future research needs. The focus is on breadth of knowledge rather than depth. In methodological terms, scoping reviews are restricted by limitations of rigour, specifically the lack of attention to quality assessment. Moreover, there is no clear definition of scoping.

References and further reading

Baumeister, R. & Leary, M. (1997) Writing narrative literature reviews. *Review of General Psychology* **1**, 311–320.

Higgins, J.P.T. & Green, S. (eds) (2011) *Cochrane Handbook for Systematic Reviews of Interventions*. Available at http://handbook.cochrane.org/ (accessed 9 March 2014).

NHS Centre for Reviews and Dissemination (2009) *Systematic Reviews*. Available at http://www.york.ac.uk/inst/crd/pdf/Systematic_Reviews.pdf (accessed 9 March 2014).

Whittemore, R. & Knafl, K. (2005) The integrative review: updated methodology. *Journal of Advanced Nursing* **52**, 546–553.

3 Using databases to search the literature

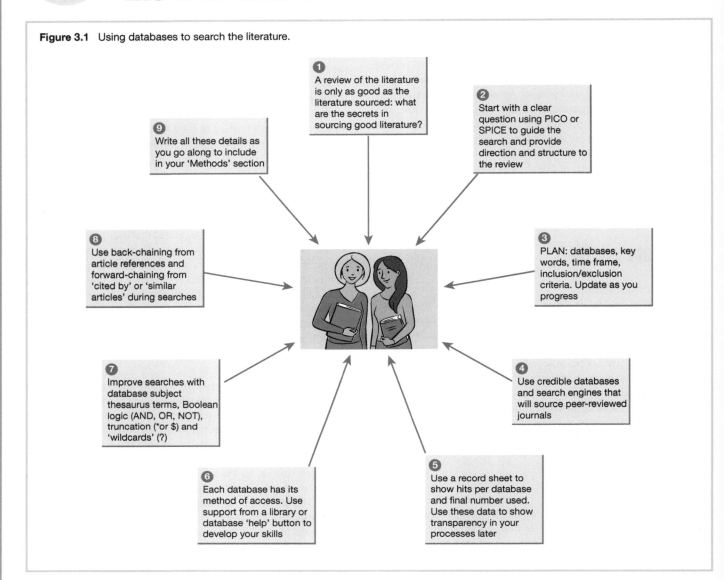

Figure 3.1 Using databases to search the literature.

1 A review of the literature is only as good as the literature sourced: what are the secrets in sourcing good literature?

2 Start with a clear question using PICO or SPICE to guide the search and provide direction and structure to the review

3 PLAN: databases, key words, time frame, inclusion/exclusion criteria. Update as you progress

4 Use credible databases and search engines that will source peer-reviewed journals

5 Use a record sheet to show hits per database and final number used. Use these data to show transparency in your processes later

6 Each database has its method of access. Use support from a library or database 'help' button to develop your skills

7 Improve searches with database subject thesaurus terms, Boolean logic (AND, OR, NOT), truncation (*or $) and 'wildcards' (?)

8 Use back-chaining from article references and forward-chaining from 'cited by' or 'similar articles' during searches

9 Write all these details as you go along to include in your 'Methods' section

Nursing and Healthcare Research at a Glance, First Edition. Alan Glasper and Colin Rees. © 2017 by John Wiley & Sons, Ltd. Published 2017 by John Wiley & Sons, Ltd.

The foundation of a good literature review is finding or 'sourcing' good-quality recent literature. The purpose of a review is to add to professional knowledge and take practice and knowledge forward. This means using literature that can be trusted. The main source of this information lies in *peer-reviewed* journals where someone has carefully examined the articles before publication. However, it does not mean the articles are perfect but they have been judged to be of a high standard.

A successful search of the literature requires forethought and planning, so before looking for literature it is important to write your 'search strategy', i.e. the plan you will follow to find relevant literature. This plan and some of the later decisions and experiences will be included in writing up your review.

These are the essential ingredients you will need for your search strategy (Figure 3.1).
• A carefully worded question where possible using a PICO or SPICE format.
• A list of key words and synonyms and alternative spellings.
• A list of likely databases.
• Clear inclusion and exclusion criteria that will identify the kind of material you need.
• A time frame, i.e. the years between which your literature should be published.
• A recording system to keep track of progress including likely articles.
• A clear and methodical way of working and recording your progress.

Method for developing your search strategy

The most important advice that will help you includes the following.
1 Open an electronic or paper file marked 'Search information' ready to include your literature search experiences. As most assignments and reports require you to include much of this information, it is better to start recording it right from the start.
2 A review cannot start without an aim or review question. Successful aims are usually structured using the PICO or SPICE format. Write this clearly.
3 Make a list of the databases you intend to search. Useful databases include Cumulative Index Nursing and Allied Health Literature (CINAHL), British Nursing Index (BNI), Scopus, and the Cochrane database of systematic reviews. You can add to these where there may be specialist databases for the particular topic you are exploring. You can also list the time frame, i.e. how far back you intend to search. Normally, this will be between 5 and 10 years. There is a greater risk that the information may be out of date the further back in time you explore.
4 List key words to search the databases. What are the key words in your question? If you are using PICO or SPICE, this will be easy to answer as the main terms under each part of PICO/SPICE will provide you with your search terms. Write these terms in a

row across a page with a space between each word, and room below them. Underneath each word write synonyms and alternative spellings (remember when using UK and US databases that some English words are spelt differently; include both spellings where this happens). Add to this list as you work through the process, especially when you look at the key words section in any articles you find. When you have developed the list, think how you may reduce the number of 'hits' by combining the terms using *Boolean logic*. This includes words such as 'and', 'or' and 'not'. Your librarian will give you advice on this.
5 There are also a number of shortcuts that will help you make the most of your time. These include the use of truncation, whereby a word is shortened and the missing part replaced by an asterisk (*); for example 'nurs*' will search for words such as 'nurse', 'nursing' and 'nurses'. The other option is the use of a 'wildcard', indicated by a question mark, which enables the identification of variant spellings of the same word; for example 'lab?r' searches for 'labour' and 'labor'.
6 List your inclusion and exclusion criteria at the start of the review, as this will help you when you are undecided whether an article should be included. Do this in much the same way as the key words by starting with your own ideas of the kind of articles you definitely do want to include in your work and those you definitely do not want to include. Then look at those listed in similar articles and add any applicable to your search to either list.
7 Start searching for articles. For each database you will need to record your key words, number of hits and final number included in your work. Set up a table to record this information and start recording the results right at the start.
8 Capture further possible articles while following your search strategy. As you go through your search strategy look at the reference list of articles (the more recent the better) and see if there are any titles that can be added to your search list (*back-chaining*). When using some databases you may be offered a list of more recent articles that the article you are currently searching for is 'cited in'. Other databases may offer 'similar articles' and both of these may lead you to more recent articles (*forward-chaining*).
9 When you have completed a list of titles identified by your search, check through for multiple citations and delete the repeated mentions.
10 Your next stage will be to critically evaluate each article captured in your search.

Further reading

Aveyard, H. (2014) *Doing a Literature Review in Health and Social Care: A Practical Guide*, 3rd edn. Maidenhead: Open University Press.

Glasper, A. & Rees, C. (2013) *How to Write Your Nursing Dissertation*. Chichester: Wiley-Blackwell.

Holland, K. & Rees, C. (2010) *Nursing: Evidence-based Practice Skills*. Oxford: Oxford University Press.

4 Undertaking a Cochrane systematic review

Figure 4.1 Undertaking a systematic review.

> **Always start with your research question**

The protocol (proposal) describes what you are going to do. When you write the review, say what you have done.

Write a proposal (protocol)

Say what you are going to do (for Cochrane and JBI reviews, these will be publications by themselves: they are peer-reviewed and edited). Include:

- Background information to inform the topic
- Significance: why do the review
- Aims
- Research question
- Methods
  - Describe your search strategy
  - Define inclusion and exclusion criteria
  - How you are going to analyse what you include
  - Who is going to do what job

No ethics approval is needed as you are using publicly available data and you are not investigating anything about live people or animals.
Make sure you have enough people on your team: six is probably a good number, as the jobs mount up and include sorting through a lot of papers. Always have a librarian and a statistician/epidemiologist on your team. Do not try to do either the searches or the statistical analysis (unless you are very, very good at them). They are very complex.
Allocate jobs.
Work out at the start the order of names for the publication (this can save a lot of grief later).

Generate review

To produce the review, follow the protocol.
Use the PRISMA diagram to help with sorting.

Use your tools to assess:
- the topic in studies
- quality of included studies.

Assessment of the risk of bias is extremely important (for further information, see http://handbook.cochrane.org/chapter_8/8_assessing_risk_of_bias_in_included_studies.htm). This consists of:

- Rigour
- Blinding of participants
- Blinding of researchers
- Blinding of outcome assessment
- Sequence generation
- Allocation concealment
- Incomplete data
- Selective outcome reporting

Use the PRISMA checklist to make sure you have covered everything (available at http://www.prisma-statement.org).

Writing up

Your review paper consists of:

1 **Introduction**
2 **Lay summary**
3 **Background**
4 **Significance**
5 **Methods**
   (a) Aims
   (b) Research question
   (c) Design
   (d) Search strategy
   (e) Search terms
   (f) Participants and settings
   (g) Inclusion and exclusion criteria
   (h) Types of studies
   (i) Quality assessment
   (j) Data collection and synthesis

6 **Results**
   (a) Search outcomes (different to review outcomes)
   (b) Descriptions of participants
   (c) Outcomes
       (i) Meta-analyses
       (ii) Descriptions of studies

7 **Discussion**
   (a) Limitations:
       (i) of review
       (ii) of topic
   (b) Recommendations
   (c) Implications for practice
   (d) Implications for further research

8 **Conclusions**

Identification
- Records identified through database searching (n =)
- Additional records identified through other sources (n =)

Records after duplicates removed (n =)

Screening
- Records screened (n =)
- Records excluded (n =)

Eligibility
- Full-text articles assessed for eligibility (n =)
- Full-text articles excluded with reasons (n =)

Included
- Studies included in qualitative analysis (n=)
- Studies included in qualitative synthesis (meta-analysis) (n=)

Source: Moher D et al., The PRISMA Group (2009). The PRISMA Statement. PLoS Med 6(6): e1000097. doi:10.1371/journal.pmed1000097

HAVE FUN!

Any literature review gathers what has been written, said, created about a particular topic, and synthesises it. What makes a systematic review so important is that it is, well, systematic. The Cochrane Collaboration clarifies its role by saying:

> A systematic review attempts to identify, appraise and synthesize all the empirical evidence that meets pre-specified eligibility criteria to answer a given research question. Researchers conducting systematic reviews use explicit methods aimed at minimizing bias, in order to produce more reliable findings that can be used to inform decision making.
>
> (http://www.thecochranelibrary.com/view/0/About CochraneSystematicReviews.html)

Reviews take a number of forms, for example a *narrative* review will tell a story when existing work is synthesised. A *scoping* review will examine what is out there on a topic. A *descriptive* review will describe what exists in literature about a topic, while an *opinion piece* (the commonly used term for an essay) uses literature to form and back up an argument or opinion. No one type of review is more valuable than another: each has a function and fulfils a specific need. Authors need to work out what sort of literature review is required to best serve their purpose.

A rigorous and well-conducted *systematic* literature review provides Level I evidence, and offers the best and most reliable information available about a topic. The National Health and Medical Research Council of Australia, in common with similar bodies, has categorised evidence within the following hierarchy (Coleman *et al.* 2009, p. 6).

- Level I: a systematic review of Level II studies.
- Level II: a randomised controlled trial.
- Level III-1: a pseudo-randomised controlled trial (i.e. alternate allocation or some other method).
- Level III-2: a comparative study with concurrent controls:
  - Non-randomised experimental trial.
  - Cohort study.
  - Case–control study.
  - Interrupted time.
- Level III-3: a comparative study without concurrent controls:
  - Historical control study.
  - Two or more single arm study.
  - Interrupted time series without a parallel control group.
- Level IV: case series with either post-test or pre-test/post-test outcomes.

Naturally, Level I evidence is the best and most reliable. This categorisation is important when clinicians are trying to determine if a particular intervention is safe to use on patients/clients, for example the use of paracetamol versus ibuprofen in febrile children. A Cochrane systematic review by Wong *et al.* (2013) to evaluate whether giving both paracetamol and ibuprofen treatments together for febrile children is more effective than giving paracetamol or ibuprofen alone found only low-level evidence and so the findings were not as strong as if they had found several randomised controlled trials (Level II evidence). In contrast, a well-written systematic review of randomised controlled trials constitutes Level I evidence.

Specialist sources of systematic reviews

The Cochrane Collaboration (http://www.cochrane.org/) was set up to collect, appraise and collate evidence about interventions so that users (health professionals and the general public) could efficiently use their time to implement the best way to do something, for example a treatment of some kind. Like all systematic reviews, Cochrane reviews synthesise existing studies and create easily accessed and read conclusions on a topic, so the busy clinician and interested health consumer need read only one paper rather than a large number of single studies. Cochrane reviews are trusted as they follow rigorous processes in their production and include an intense and lengthy peer review and editorial system. These safeguards mean that the conclusions in a review are as safe as they can be.

The Joanna Briggs Institute (JBI) (http://joannabriggs.org/) began in Adelaide, Australia, and has established a reputation for systematic reviews of evidence other than randomised controlled trials (though it does do some), and was keenly welcomed by health professions, including nursing, that rely on psychosocial outcomes. Its systematic reviews are also the result of a rigorous peer review and editorial process, providing Level I evidence on a range of health-related topics.

The Campbell Collaboration (http://www.campbell collaboration.org/) is very similar to the Cochrane Collaboration. However, it reviews evidence generated by disciplines outside health, for example education and the social sciences. Nurses and midwives may find relevant evidence on its website and it is worth checking if evidence from outside the health disciplines is required.

Finally, many journals carry reviews produced from authors such as students who publish systematic reviews as part of their theses. These are also valuable additions to the body of knowledge, if done well and judged to fit with the levels of evidence scale above.

Some systematic reviews find no studies to include, usually because they do not meet the pre-set inclusion criteria or their quality is poor. These so-called *empty reviews* can be valuable in that they show where gaps in research exist.

For those producing a review, two really useful documents shown in Figure 4.1 are the PRISMA diagram, which provides a framework for sorting out the studies that can be included, and the PRISMA checklist, which ensures that everything is covered before the review is completed. As the figure emphasises, a systematic review of the literature is the same as any research project: everything hangs on the research question and the clear identification of the answer to the following. What are you looking for? What question is being answered?

References

Coleman, K., Norris S., Weston, A. *et al.* (2009) NHMRC additional levels of evidence and grades for recommendations for developers of guidelines: stage 2 consultation, early 2008 to end June 2009. Available at http://www.nhmrc.gov.au/_files_nhmrc/file/guidelines/stage_2_consultation_levels_and_grades.pdf (accessed 17 June 2014).

Wong, T., Stang, A.S., Ganshorn, H. *et al.* (2013) Combined and alternating paracetamol and ibuprofen therapy for febrile children. *Cochrane Database of Systematic Reviews* (10), CD009572.

5 Undertaking a Joanna Briggs Institute systematic review

Figure 5.1 Conducting a JBI systematic review.

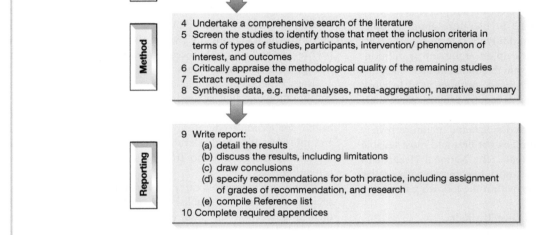

A systematic review is a type of literature review that uses pre-specified, explicit and rigorous methods to identify, critical appraise and synthesise research and other related sources of evidence relevant to a selected topic.

Preparation

1. Identify topic or question of interest
2. Develop a focused, answerable question – PICO
3. Develop a protocol as a guide for the systematic review

Method

4. Undertake a comprehensive search of the literature
5. Screen the studies to identify those that meet the inclusion criteria in terms of types of studies, participants, intervention/ phenomenon of interest, and outcomes
6. Critically appraise the methodological quality of the remaining studies
7. Extract required data
8. Synthesise data, e.g. meta-analyses, meta-aggregation, narrative summary

Reporting

9. Write report:
   (a) detail the results
   (b) discuss the results, including limitations
   (c) draw conclusions
   (d) specify recommendations for both practice, including assignment of grades of recommendation, and research
   (e) compile Reference list
10. Complete required appendices

Nursing and Healthcare Research at a Glance, First Edition. Alan Glasper and Colin Rees. © 2017 by John Wiley & Sons, Ltd. Published 2017 by John Wiley & Sons, Ltd.

A systematic review (SR) is a type of literature review that employs a specific methodology. An SR uses pre-specified, explicit and rigorous methods to identify, critically appraise and synthesise research and other related sources of evidence relevant to a selected topic. This type of research is sometimes referred to as secondary research as it synthesises primary/original research studies on the same topic. The purpose of an SR is to pull together the currently available evidence related, in this case, to a clinical question. Recommendations for practice and research flow from this evidence to improve patient care. The Joanna Briggs Institute (JBI) focuses on reviewing evidence related to effectiveness, appropriateness, meaningfulness and feasibility.

The nature of the question the SR aims to answer indicates what type of evidence should be sought to best answer that question. For example, studies addressing the question of the effectiveness of a treatment or procedure focus on quantitative studies. In contrast, if the topic of interest is the experiences of people with a particular diagnosis, studies collecting qualitative data would be appropriate. The JBI has developed a number of methodologies for synthesising evidence for this purpose. In addition to quantitative and qualitative evidence, there are methodologies for evidence related to economic aspects of healthcare, diagnosis, prognosis, prevalence and incidence.

A JBI SR (Figure 5.1) can be confined to just one type of evidence (e.g. qualitative) or two or more types of evidence (e.g. qualitative and quantitative). The latter type is referred to as a comprehensive SR.

Process for undertaking a systematic review

Although there are differences in the various methodologies mentioned above, the stages worked through when undertaking the review are similar. The process is systematic and can generate large amounts of information and data which must be carefully recorded. There are specially designed templates and software programs to assist with record-keeping and analysis, and to ensure the final report meets the publication criteria specified in the Preferred Reporting Items for Systematic Reviews and Meta-analyses (PRISMA) statement. Two reviewers are required to independently undertake steps 6 and 7, with a third reviewer to adjudicate if assessments differ.

1 Identify topic or question of interest. A preliminary search of the literature should be undertaken to see if a systematic review has already addressed this topic or is currently in progress, and also whether sufficient studies or other sources of evidence are available to make the effort of completing an SR worthwhile.

2 If these questions are satisfactorily answered, the next step is to develop a focused, answerable question using the mnemonic PICO, which stands for Population, Intervention, Comparator, Outcome; alternatively, in the case of a qualitative SR, the 'I' refers to the phenomenon of interest and the 'C' to context.

3 Then a protocol is drafted which will guide the SR process. The protocol details the focus of the SR; the background to the topic; and the methods that will be employed including literature searching, data collection and synthesis. Any deviation from this protocol must be detailed in the final report.

4 Once the protocol is approved, work on the SR can commence. Using the strategies and databases identified in the protocol, a literature search is conducted to identify studies or other documents that might be relevant to the SR. It is important to include databases that list 'grey' literature (e.g. theses or conference papers) and to hand-search recent issues of journals that might not yet be indexed in databases.

5 This process can generate large numbers of papers that need to be culled down to those that are specifically relevant to the review question. This step includes several sub-steps to eliminate irrelevant papers. Working from titles, abstracts and, if necessary, the full article, the papers that are eligible for consideration for inclusion in the SR are identified based on their meeting the criteria for the type of study, population, intervention and outcomes specified in the protocol.

6 The remaining studies are then critically appraised for quality using the appropriate standardised form. Those that pass this assessment are then included in the SR.

7 Standardised forms are also used for data extraction. The type of data extracted will vary with the type of SR, for example for qualitative studies the findings and linked participant quotes are extracted, while for quantitative studies dichotomous and continuous data are recorded, together with details about the study.

8 Data synthesis. A meta-aggregative approach to data synthesis is adopted for qualitative SRs, while meta-analyses may be possible for quantitative data. If the included quantitative studies vary (e.g. they use different methods to measure outcomes), a narrative summary is developed.

9 The final step is writing up the SR. All the above steps and their outcomes are reported along with the results of the data synthesis, the discussion and the conclusion as for any other study report. In addition, specific recommendations for clinical practice and research are formulated. The clinical practice recommendations are assigned a grade (A or B) depending on the type of evidence provided by the SR to support the recommendation.

10 Numerous appendices are also included. These detail aspects such as literature search strategies and their results, the included studies, and reasons for excluding studies. These enable readers to assess the quality of the SR.

Further reading

Joanna Briggs Institute. *Reviewers' Manual 2014 Edition*. Joanna Briggs Institute, University of Adelaide, South Australia. Available at http://joannabriggs.org/assets/docs/sumari/ReviewersManual-2014.pdf

6 Using EndNote

Figure 6.1 The EndNote window.

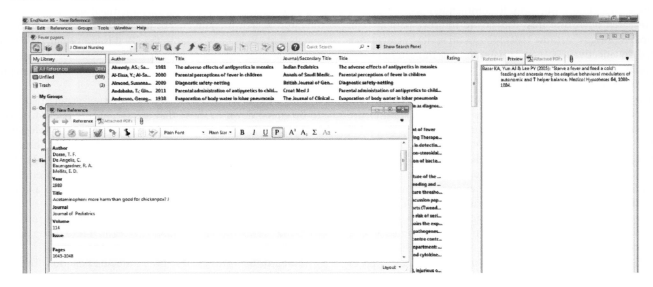

Figure 6.2 The EndNote toolbar.

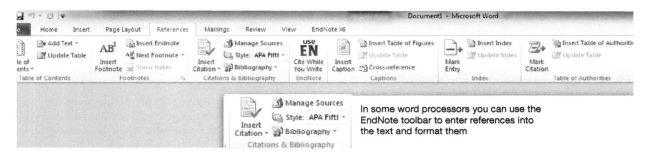

In some word processors you can use the EndNote toolbar to enter references into the text and format them

Nursing and Healthcare Research at a Glance, First Edition. Alan Glasper and Colin Rees. © 2017 by John Wiley & Sons, Ltd. Published 2017 by John Wiley & Sons, Ltd.

Using EndNote reference management software

Reference management software packages such as EndNote are designed to help with managing references and bibliographies. They do this by providing facilities that allow the user to search databases directly and share references with others, as well as the more familiar tasks of importing and organising references, and producing and formatting references lists.

EndNote

EndNote is just one of the many software packages that can be used for this purpose. It works with the Windows and Macintosh operating systems, but not with Linux, for which alternatives such as Bibus and Zotero exist. Zotero also works with the other operating systems.

The EndNote window

The main window that is used with EndNote is shown in Figure 6.1. The main part of the window shows the current *library*, i.e. the list of references that are in the file. You may have a number of such files or libraries for different subjects or projects. To the right of this is the *preview pane* (it may be in another position depending on how EndNote is set up), which shows how the currently selected reference will look in the reference list. To the left is the *New Reference window*, which allows you to manually add a reference to the library or to change details. This will not normally be there, but appears when you want to add a reference.

Importing references

EndNote allows references to be imported directly, either by searching databases directly or through importing individual references from journal websites. This saves users from having to type all the details into the program themselves, although it is necessary to check that the reference is correct as not all publishers' websites do this equally well. Look for a link that says something like 'Export reference' or 'Send to reference manager'; make sure that the appropriate library is open and follow the instructions as they appear. This facility can save a lot of time.

The alternative is to enter the details of the reference manually. To do this you need to click on 'Reference' in the toolbar and then select 'New reference'. This will bring up the new reference box described earlier. After selecting the reference type (book, book chapter, journal paper, etc.), enter the details; when this window is closed, the reference will be added to the library.

When entering references either manually or by direct import, make sure that the *URL* of the paper is included as this provides a direct link to the online version of the paper or book, making it much easier to find the paper in the future.

Inserting references into a paper

This is the feature of any reference management software that most people will use most often. EndNote as a facility known as Cite While You Write™, which allows you to highlight a reference in the library window by clicking on it, and then by pressing the appropriate button, either in EndNote or the word processor, inserting the reference in the current position of the document on which you are working. This feature is available for both Microsoft Word and OpenOffice (but not the Linux versions of OpenOffice). If you are using these programs and your word processor does not have this button, you need to ensure that the EndNote toolbar is activated (Figure 6.2). Remember that you can always check what the reference will look like by looking in the preview window before inserting it.

Output styles

Because academic institutions and journals require references to be formatted differently, EndNote is able to reformat the information from each entry in the library into the appropriate style. While some journals use generic styles such as the Vancouver or APA styles, others are more specific and in many such cases output style files can be downloaded from the EndNote website. Remember when you change the output style that you can always preview what the resulting reference will look like by highlighting it in the main library window and looking in the preview pane.

Reformatting the paper

When you make changes to the format of your references, you may need to reformat the paper to change those that you have already inserted. To do this, just click on the format bibliography button, and when the dialogue box appears select the style you require in the output style box and click 'OK'. This should result in the references in both the paper and the reference list being updated to the new style.

Finding a reference

If you can't find a reference (it happens to us all), you can reorder the references either by author or any of the other details of the reference by clicking on the appropriate header for that column in the library window. If you cannot remember that, you can try to find it by putting a term into the *quick search box* and clicking on the magnifying glass.

Advanced features

This chapter has introduced a number of the many features that EndNote and similar programs have to offer, but EndNote has many other advanced features including directly searching databases and removing duplicates, which is very useful when conducting a systematic review using more than one database. In addition, it also allows you to move between full journal names, which are often needed for assignment, and abbreviated titles which is necessary for some journals.

7 Using the PICO framework

Figure 7.1 Using the PICO framework to formulate an answerable question.

PICO is the first step in evidence-based healthcare and is used to appropriately search the bibliographical databases. There are four elements to the posing of a PICO question. These four common features of the PICO format are helpful in allowing healthcare practitioners to carefully consider the questions they wish the literature they interrogate to answer. The four components are:

P = Patient/problem

I = Intervention

C = Comparison (control)

O = Outcome

This formula facilitates the posing of focused, answerable questions that will allow a more efficient literature search and eventual retrieval of scholarly empirical journal papers.

Nursing and Healthcare Research at a Glance, First Edition. Alan Glasper and Colin Rees. © 2017 by John Wiley & Sons, Ltd. Published 2017 by John Wiley & Sons, Ltd.

What is the PICO model?

The creation of a precise and answerable question facilitates a more efficient literature search and eventual retrieval of empirical journal papers. There are four elements to the PICO question (Figure 7.1). These four common features of the PICO format are helpful in allowing healthcare practitioners to carefully consider the questions they wish the literature to answer. Melnyk and Fineout-Overholt (2005) believe each aspect of the PICO format should be considered in depth to generate a clearly articulated question. The four elements are:

P   Population
I   Intervention
C   Comparison (control)
O   Outcome

Booth (2006) outlines each element of the PICO model as follows.

Population

These are the recipients or potential beneficiaries of a health service or intervention. The population could include the following.
• Patients/clients with a disease or condition (e.g. gastrointestinal disease).
• Patients/clients with a stage of disease (e.g. advanced Crohn's disease).
• A specific gender/ethnicity (e.g. Afro-Caribbean women with postnatal depression).
• A specific age group (e.g. children with congenital talipes equinovarus).
• A specific socioeconomic group (e.g. semi-skilled and unskilled manual workers with alcohol-related disease).
• A specific healthcare setting (e.g. mental healthcare patients attending an outpatient department).

Intervention

The service or planned action that is being delivered to the population. This could include a number of interventions.
• A type of drug therapy for renal disease, or surgical procedures used in renal disease, or types of radiotherapy used in treating malignancies.
• A level of intervention, for example the frequency of administration of a particular medication or the dosage of a particular drug, or radiotherapy treatment.
• The stage of intervention expressed as, for example, prevention, secondary or advanced.
• The delivery of an intervention, for example intravenous infusion or self-medication.

Comparison

This represents an alternative service or action that may or may not achieve similar outcomes. For example, the use of peritoneal dialysis compared with haemodialysis in managing renal failure, or the use of antibiotic drug A compared with antibiotic drug B. In some cases the comparison may be the usual named interventions (sometimes called the control) or no specific intervention.

Outcomes

This is the way in which the service or action can be measured to establish whether it has had the desired effect. This can be expressed as what happened to the population being studied as a direct result of the intervention. This can be measured in a number of ways.
• Specifically patient-oriented: for example, an improvement in quality of life, or a reduction in the severity of symptoms, or a reduction in adverse events such as drug errors. However, these outcomes should be expressed in measurable ways, such as 'lower pain scores', 'fewer episodes of nausea and vomiting', anything that shows there has been a clear and measurable difference as a result of the intervention.
• Organisation-oriented: for example, cost-effectiveness, less days in hospital or reduction in the number of personal injury claims or complaints by patients.

Example of a PICO question

P   Older women with varicose leg ulcers
I   Application of larvae therapy to the ulcerating wound
C   Traditional silver-impregnated wound dressings
O   Improved wound healing measured by time

References and further reading

Booth, A. (2006) Clear and present questions: formulating questions for evidence-based practice. *Library Hi Tech* **24**, 355–368. Available at www.emeraldinsight.com/0737-8831.htm

Glasper, A. & Rees, C. (2013) *How to Write Your Nursing Dissertation*. Chichester: Wiley-Blackwell.

Melnyk, B.M. & Fineout-Overholt, E. (2005) *Evidence-based Practice in Nursing and Health Care. A Guide to Best Practice.* Philadelphia: Lippincott Williams & Wilkins.

8 Using the SPICE framework

Figure 8.1 Using the SPICE framework to formulate an answerable question.

The SPICE model is an alternative to the PICO framework used in evidence-based healthcare to appropriately search the bibliographical databases.

There are five elements to the posing of a SPICE literature search question. These five common features of the SPICE format are helpful in allowing healthcare practitioners to carefully consider the questions they wish the literature they interrogate to answer. The five components are:

S = Setting, i.e. where and what context

P = Perspective, i.e. for whom? Who are users/potential users of the service?

I = intervention, i.e. what is being done to them/for them

C = Comparison, i.e. compared with what. What are alternatives?

E = Evaluation, i.e. with what result and how will you measure whether the intervention will succeed?

This facilitates the posing of focused, answerable questions which will allow a more efficient literature search and eventual retrieval of scholarly empirical journal papers

What is the SPICE model?

The creation of a precise and answerable question facilitates a more efficient literature search and eventual retrieval of empirical journal papers. SPICE is an alternative to the use of PICO. There are five elements to the posing of a SPICE literature search question (Figure 8.1). These five common features of the SPICE format are helpful in allowing healthcare practitioners to carefully consider the questions they wish the literature they interrogate to answer. The SPICE model has been proposed by Booth (2006) and is a derivation of the PICO model. It was designed originally for use primarily by librarians to help more clearly focus some types of literature search enquiry that did not always fit the PICO framework. The SPICE model framework has five components and is helpful for students who are not asking a specific clinically focused question. The five elements are:

S   Setting: where and what is context?

P   Perspective: for whom? Who are users/potential users of service?

I   Intervention: what is being done to them/for them?

C   Comparison: compared with what? What are alternatives?

E   Evaluation: with what result and how will you measure whether the intervention will succeed?

Although the SPICE structure is similar to that of PICO, Booth (2006) points out that by separating the traditional medical-type population aspect of the PICO model into firstly a setting and secondly a perspective that this enables SPICE to be used for posing non-medical-type questions, i.e. more of a social scientific approach. Similarly, by substituting the term 'outcome' with the term 'evaluation' the SPICE model facilitates other elements of research that are broader and incorporate concepts such as outputs or impacts.

SPICE question example 1

'What is the impact of an increase in the level of cost-sharing on access to health services for the chronically ill in European countries?'

Setting: (a selection of) European countries
Perspective: chronically ill patients
Intervention: increased cost-sharing (from among the European community)
Comparison: no increase in current funding arrangements
Evaluation: access to health services

This example is from the Belgian Health Care Knowledge Centre (http://www.kce.fgov.be/index_en.aspx?SGREF=5225). This is a semi-governmental institution that analyses healthcare data from various research studies with the aim of improving evidence-based practice.

SPICE question example 2

'How does it feel to wait for your relative (child, spouse/partner or parent) to return to the ward after emergency surgery and await the results?"

Setting: hospital surgical wards
Perspective: relatives of patients requiring emergency surgery
Intervention: dedicated waiting area with refreshments and tangible levels of distraction such as flat screen televisions or contemporary topical magazines
Comparison: no special area or levels of distraction
Evaluation: satisfaction measured by questionnaire given to relatives when leaving the hospital or on return home

Reference and further reading

Booth, A. (2006) Clear and present questions: formulating questions for evidence-based practice. *Library Hi Tech* **24**, 355–368. Available at www.emeraldinsight.com/0737-8831.htm
Glasper, A. & Rees, C. (2013) *How to Write Your Nursing Dissertation*. Chichester: Wiley-Blackwell.
Melnyk, B.M. & Fineout-Overholt, E. (2005) *Evidence-based Practice in Nursing and Health Care. A Guide to Best Practice*. Philadelphia: Lippincott Williams & Wilkins.

Nursing and Healthcare Research at a Glance, First Edition. Alan Glasper and Colin Rees. © 2017 by John Wiley & Sons, Ltd. Published 2017 by John Wiley & Sons, Ltd.

9 Using grey literature in the quest for evidence

Figure 9.1 Using grey literature in the quest for evidence.

What does grey literature include? There are many sources but principally:
- Government documents such as healthcare policies
- PhD theses and other dissertations
- Academic conference proceedings
- Research reports
- Clinical protocols and guidelines
- Reports from esteemed bodies such as the Royal College of Nursing

Grey literature is not grey!
It comes in a variety of colours and sizes, some good, some bad and some just ugly

What is the definition of grey literature?
Grey literature stands for manifold document types produced on all levels of government, academics, business and industry in print and electronic formats that are protected by intellectual property rights of sufficient quality to be collected and preserved by library holdings or institutional repositories, but not controlled by commercial publishers, i.e., where publishing is not the primary activity of the producing body.'
(Gelfand and Tsang, 2015)

Try these sources:
The Healthcare Management Information Consortium (HMIC) database contains records from the Library and Information Services Department of the Department of Health (DH) in England and the King's Fund Information and Library Service

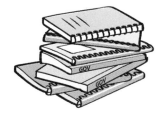

Where can I find grey literature?
It is not easy to find recent and original literature through conventional channels. There are many websites that can help in locating and exploring this useful body of information. The World Wide Web has become the portal for grey literature in the 21st century

What is grey literature?

Despite its name, grey literature comes in a variety of colours and sizes, some good, some bad and some just ugly. Although the term 'grey literature' has been used for at least 40 years and such literature included in healthcare systematic reviews of the literature, its definition has been frequently debated. For example, Gelfand and Tsang (2015) follow the development of one of the most frequently cited definitions built up through discussions at a number of international grey literature conferences and end with the following, known as the Prague definition, which states:

> Grey literature stands for manifold document types produced on all levels of government, academics, business and industry in print and electronic formats that are protected by intellectual property rights of sufficient quality to be collected and preserved by library holdings or institutional repositories, but not controlled by commercial publishers, i.e., where publishing is not the primary activity of the producing body.

From this we can see that grey literature is composed of any literature that is not formally published in usual publishing formats such as textbooks or scholarly journals (Figure 9.1). The important aspect of the definition that helps to separate it from other sources is that those producing it do not do so for their commercial value as with many other forms of publication.

Importantly, Alberani *et al.* (1990) have explored the importance of grey literature as a means of primary but non-conventionally published communication. It is important to stress that these sources of literature, which are often original and of recent origin, cannot always be found easily through conventional channels. Any critical systematic review of the literature must consider including a review of pertinent grey literature.

What does grey literature include?

There are many sources of grey literature and may include among others:
- doctoral theses and other dissertations;
- academic cconference proceedings;
- government documents such as healthcare policies;
- research reports;
- clinical protocols or clinical guidelines;
- reports from esteemed bodies such as the Royal College of Nursing or the Nursing and Midwifery Council.

Where can I find grey literature?

Perhaps the easiest starting point for locating new and relevant grey literature is to go online to the many specialist sites. Good sources include the following bodies.
- The Healthcare Management Information Consortium (HMIC) database contains records from the Library and Information Services Department of the Department of Health (DH) in England.
- The King's Fund Information and Library Service. This site includes all DH publications including circulars and press releases. These combined databases are a good source of grey literature on topics such as health and community care management, organisational development, inequalities in health, user involvement, and race and health.

Reference and further reading

Alberani, V., Pietrangeli, P. & Mazza, M.R. (1990) The use of grey literature in health sciences: a preliminary survey. *Bulletin of the Medical Library Association* **78**, 358–362.

Gelfand, J. and Tsang, D. (2014) Data: is it grey, maligned or malignant? *The Grey Journal* **11**(1). Available at http://escholarship.org/uc/item/80w006rz#page-1

Glasper, A. & Rees, C. (2013) *How to Write Your Nursing Dissertation*. Chichester: Wiley-Blackwell.

Why does research need evaluating?

Figure 10.1 Why research needs evaluating.

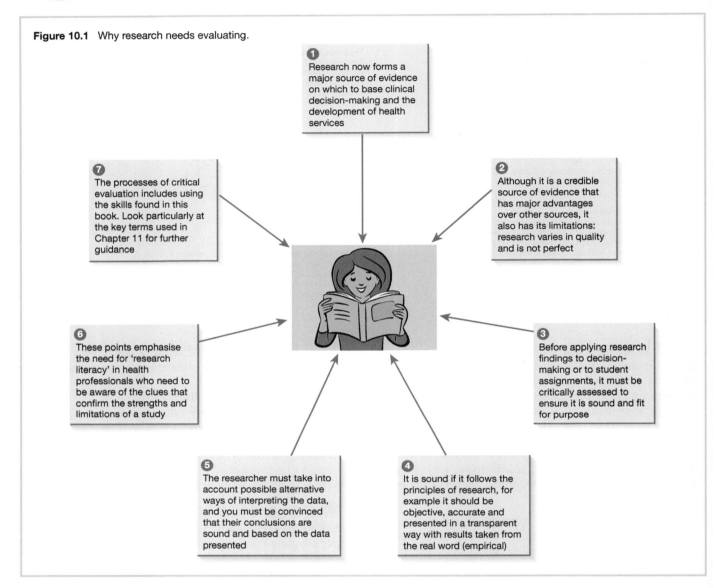

1 Research now forms a major source of evidence on which to base clinical decision-making and the development of health services

2 Although it is a credible source of evidence that has major advantages over other sources, it also has its limitations: research varies in quality and is not perfect

3 Before applying research findings to decision-making or to student assignments, it must be critically assessed to ensure it is sound and fit for purpose

4 It is sound if it follows the principles of research, for example it should be objective, accurate and presented in a transparent way with results taken from the real word (empirical)

5 The researcher must take into account possible alternative ways of interpreting the data, and you must be convinced that their conclusions are sound and based on the data presented

6 These points emphasise the need for 'research literacy' in health professionals who need to be aware of the clues that confirm the strengths and limitations of a study

7 The processes of critical evaluation includes using the skills found in this book. Look particularly at the key terms used in Chapter 11 for further guidance

Since its introduction, evidence-based practice has become accepted throughout the world and in all healthcare professional groups as a sensible and logical basis for clinical decisions. Fundamental to that success is the principle that clinical decisions should be based on sound knowledge supported by evidence of its likely effectiveness. The major source of this evidence comes from research studies, as their accuracy stands up to the greatest level of scrutiny compared to other sources of knowledge such as custom and practice and expert opinion. Does this mean we can accept all research without question as a guide to best practice? The answer is no; all research should be evaluated before it is used (Figure 10.1).

This raises a question: Why, if research is carried out by experts whose work is published, should it need evaluating? The answer is that research is never perfect, and most research studies will have their limitations. Therefore, all research needs to be assessed to establish how much weight can be put on the results.

The quality of studies varies in many ways, for example the results are influenced by the accuracy of the tool of data collection. The use of *self-report* methods of collecting data that relies on the honesty and accuracy of what people say they do, rather than their observed behaviour, is an example of why we need to consider the limitations built into studies. The sample size can also influence whether a study is strong enough to allow us to generalise the results without considering the possibility of bias due to unrepresentative members in the sample. All these factors reinforce the need to scrutinise research before we apply it to clinical practice.

The evaluation of research depends to a large extent on the critical skills and research knowledge of the reader. Research articles are written following what for some is an unfamiliar and 'scientific' process, and can also be difficult to read because of the specialised language and statistical processes used. This makes some articles impenetrable in places and difficult to understand for those not used to reading research. Many clinical staff find it easier to follow the guidance or example of others by adopting custom and practice or prefer to follow expert opinion. Where individuals do read the research themselves, they may be tempted to only read key points, conclusions and recommendations.

However, this kind of selective reading has its limitations; for example, concentrating only on the results without examining the methods section leads to an inadequate assessment of whether the study is safe to use. We must evaluate the research design of studies to ensure that the way results are produced conforms to essential principles in research. These include carefully following the research process appropriate to the form of research used, ensuring that potential pitfalls have been considered and reduced as far as possible, and basing conclusions only on the results gathered and not on the researcher's own views or prejudices (maintaining objectivity).

The first stage in evaluating research is to consider its source: does it come from a peer-reviewed journal or website where it has already been considered by experts to offer insights into the topic based on appropriate methods? This does not mean it is without fault, only that it could be useful and has some authority compared to other sources of evidence. The reader still has to use his or her own judgement.

It does not require very high levels of research knowledge to assess most studies, but it does require enough to understand the clues provided that will give you confidence in its quality. These can be found by applying the knowledge you have gained reading this book. You might start by developing your skills in evaluating studies using the concepts of reliability, validity, bias and rigour outlined in Chapter 11. These evaluative concepts of assessing research should be incorporated into a structured method of critiquing studies, as outlined in Chapter 12.

As well as individual studies, evidence can be found in reviews of the literature, particularly systematic reviews where the critical evaluation of high-quality research has already been carried out by a small team of experts and synthesised into a guide for practice. These, too, need some knowledge of how they are produced and should also be critically assessed to ensure that their advice is sound and applicable to the local clinical area, or to the student assignment you are writing.

In conclusion, most studies have their weaknesses; there is no such thing as the perfect research study as there is always the chance of errors that affects the accuracy of results. Researchers also vary in their experience and expertise, particularly in drawing accurate conclusions from research data. While it is wise to gather evidence from peer-reviewed sources, you will still need to use your own judgement and knowledge to ensure that a study is sound and fit for purpose.

Further reading

Holland, K. & Rees, C. (2010) *Nursing: Evidence-based Practice Skills*. Oxford: Oxford University Press.

Polit, D. & Beck, C. (2012) *Nursing Research: Generating and Assessing Evidence for Nursing Practice*, 9th edn. Philadelphia: Walters Kluwer/Lippincott Williams & Wilkins.

11 Key issues in evaluating research

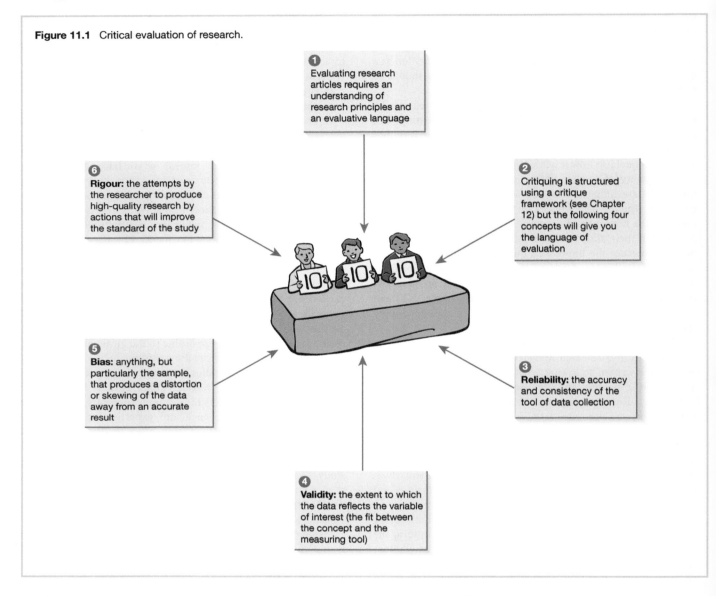

Figure 11.1 Critical evaluation of research.

1 Evaluating research articles requires an understanding of research principles and an evaluative language

6 **Rigour:** the attempts by the researcher to produce high-quality research by actions that will improve the standard of the study

2 Critiquing is structured using a critique framework (see Chapter 12) but the following four concepts will give you the language of evaluation

5 **Bias:** anything, but particularly the sample, that produces a distortion or skewing of the data away from an accurate result

3 **Reliability:** the accuracy and consistency of the tool of data collection

4 **Validity:** the extent to which the data reflects the variable of interest (the fit between the concept and the measuring tool)

In the previous chapter the case was made for why we need to evaluate all research studies and not simply take them on face value; no research is perfect and all research should be carefully examined prior to use. This chapter will offer a number of key concepts used in the process of critical evaluation and will enable you to develop your skills in this essential aspect of research literacy. They will allow you to demonstrate your knowledge of key aspects of research and increase your skill in critically evaluating studies. Critical evaluation is not just a matter of finding faults or being negative about a study; it is the careful evaluation of factors that influence its quality and highlight the difference between a strong study and one with limitations.

Chapter 12 discusses the different critiquing frameworks; this chapter lays the foundation for that work by highlighting just four key methodological concepts related to the research process that play a large part in critical analysis. Understanding these

concepts will enable you to shape and structure your thoughts and comments fundamental to the critical evaluation of studies. For quantitative research, the key concepts are reliability, validity, bias and rigour (Figure 11.1).

Reliability

Reliability relates to the accuracy and consistency of the measurements produced by a research tool for data collection. In evaluating studies, identify how data were collected and the extent to which the researcher persuades you that the tool was carefully selected for its accuracy. This will usually take the form of a named tool (e.g. Faces Pain Scale-Revised) and perhaps confirm that it is frequently used to measure this variable, or has been successfully used in previous studies. If it is designed specially for a study, it should be piloted and tested

Nursing and Healthcare Research at a Glance, First Edition. Alan Glasper and Colin Rees. © 2017 by John Wiley & Sons, Ltd. Published 2017 by John Wiley & Sons, Ltd.

for accuracy. Some specialist tools may also require those using it to have training in its use and this should be mentioned where appropriate. These points illustrate the kinds of clues to look for when reading a research report and may be useful for mention in your written analysis. They are usually found in the methodology section of a study.

It should also be remembered that the degree of accuracy in measuring variables can vary, for example tools exist to measure blood pressure, temperature, pain and anxiety but the possibility of accurate measurements for each one differ. Consequently, measurements of blood pressure and temperature are likely to be more accurate (but not perfect) compared to those for pain and anxiety, which are more subjective.

Validity

Validity is often discussed at the same time as reliability and this can lead to confusion as to what the difference is between these two concepts. Whereas reliability relates to the accuracy of the data collection tool, validity relates to the data and how closely they match the concept being measured: have the researchers been able to capture data relating to the exact concept they set out to measure? The more abstract the variable being measured, the more difficult it is to be certain that what is being measured is in reality an example of that variable. For example, we are reasonably satisfied with pain and anxiety scales now, despite them being abstract, but other concepts such as *resilience* or *emotional competence* present a challenge to researchers to demonstrate that their data reflect these concepts.

Reliability and validity are often mentioned together as they are both important issues related to data. With reliability, the data must be gathered by a tool (questionnaire, scale, physical measuring instrument such as weighing scales) that has been tested and confirmed as accurate. However, although an instrument can be accurate (e.g. calibrated weighing scales), it may not be relevant in the measurement of the variable the researcher is examining; for instance, suggesting that personal weight is an indicator of self-confidence and that the more a person weighs the greater their level of self-confidence. In other words, the tool can be reliable, but the data it produces may not be a measurement of the concept examined, as with weight and self-confidence.

Bias

Bias is the result of any factor that distorts or skews the data collected and so produces inaccurate results. The term is frequently used in relation to the sample in a study, but can apply to any part of the research process, such as the review of the literature, that is skewed or distorted.

In quantitative research, a major concern is to produce results that can be applied broadly and not just to the particular location where the study was conducted; this is the concept of *generalisability*. For this to happen, those involved in a study (individuals, objects or events) must be typical of those likely to be encountered in other places or settings. Examples might include using a sample to represent people over the age of 85, those with a chronic illness, or women who have given birth to twins.

The researcher's problem is to select those who can be identified as typical of that group. Where there is an under- or over-representation of a particular subgroup within a sample, there is a risk that the results will be influenced or skewed by an unrepresentative total group. Bias in the sample may lead to distortion in the results and lead to an error in the conclusions.

In randomised controlled trials, bias can occur when a number of people leave or drop out of one group and so upset the original balance between the experimental and control groups. This bias might affect the outcome as the researchers would no longer be comparing like with like. Similarly, in studies that depend on people volunteering to take part: such people may be different from those who choose not to volunteer. The results could be biased as they may not represent the total group but only those who are likely to 'opt in' to studies. The hesitant wording of the last sentence ('could be') is important as it is not certain that this would be the case, but it must be considered. Care must be taken in expressing concerns that are based on such assessments and judgements and a more cautious or tentative language should be used (e.g. writing 'may', 'could' or 'might') as it is by no means certain but may be a reasonable risk factor where present in a study. Bias in a study is a major concern, as measurements are not really useful where they are taken from a biased group or where a study has been biased by some other factor that makes the results unrepresentative.

Rigour

Therefore, in evaluating the quality of studies, a number of indicators can be identified that are components of different types of quantitative research design. The tool of data collection raises issues of *reliability*, the extent to which the data represent or measure what they are supposed to measure indicates *validity*, and anything that may negatively influence the outcome is *bias*. Putting all these together, if researchers demonstrate that they have thought about these areas and tried to implement systems and processes that will result in high-quality data, then they are illustrating *rigour*.

Rigour is an attribute of researchers, and describes how they can be said to be 'striving for excellence' (Burns & Grove, 2009) by the way in which they have carried out the study. It is demonstrated by the researchers trying to conduct the study following scientific principles of research as far as possible in order to safeguard the quality of the results.

This is illustrated in various ways depending on the type of study. For example, in a randomised controlled trial, one example relates to the 'blinding' or 'masking' of participants and those collecting the data to ensure that it is not known who was in which group in order to ensure that the results are as accurate as possible and not biased by the knowledge of group membership. Similarly, for surveys using questionnaires, or randomised controlled trials using tools such as pain scales, it ensures that either the tool has been demonstrated to work well in a previous study or, if it is a new tool, that it is constructed following a close examination of the literature to inform what should be included, and then assessed by experts and piloted. Descriptions of all such activities are indicators of the rigour of the researcher.

You now have a command of some of the most important technical words that will clearly demonstrate your fluency in evaluating research studies.

Reference and further reading

Burns, N. & Grove, S. (2009) *The Practice of Nursing Research: Appraisal, Synthesis and Generation of Evidence*, 6th edn. St Louis: Saunders.

Gerrish, K. & Lacey, A. (2010) *The Research Process in Nursing*, 6th edn. Chichester: Wiley-Blackwell.

Polit, D. & Beck, C. (2012) *Nursing Research: Generating and Assessing Evidence for Nursing Practice*, 9th edn. Philadelphia: Walters Kluwer/Lippincott Williams & Wilkins.

12 Critically reviewing a research paper

Figure 12.1 Critiquing a research paper.

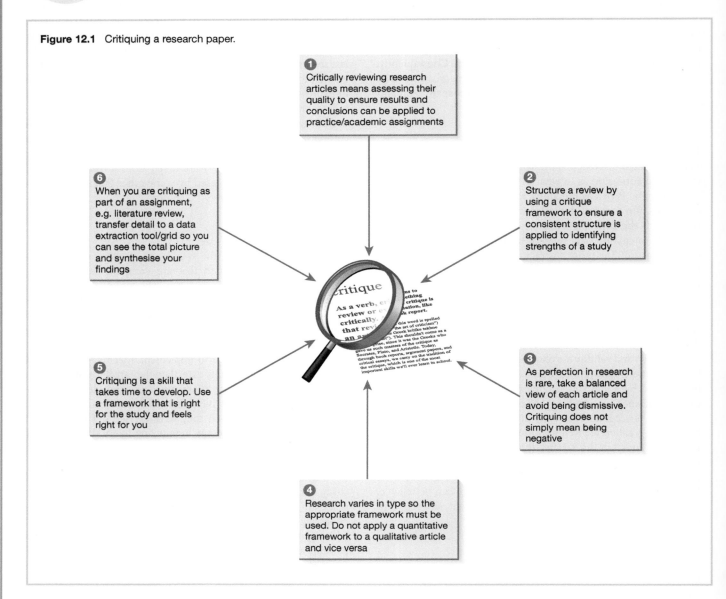

1. Critically reviewing research articles means assessing their quality to ensure results and conclusions can be applied to practice/academic assignments

2. Structure a review by using a critique framework to ensure a consistent structure is applied to identifying strengths of a study

3. As perfection in research is rare, take a balanced view of each article and avoid being dismissive. Critiquing does not simply mean being negative

4. Research varies in type so the appropriate framework must be used. Do not apply a quantitative framework to a qualitative article and vice versa

5. Critiquing is a skill that takes time to develop. Use a framework that is right for the study and feels right for you

6. When you are critiquing as part of an assignment, e.g. literature review, transfer detail to a data extraction tool/grid so you can see the total picture and synthesise your findings

Research should not be taken at face value and believed to 'prove' something on the basis of its finding. This is because research is not perfect and can only support or suggest a conclusion or statement. Combining a number of studies into a review of the literature provides better evidence to support a view or intervention. However, when reading research articles we must avoid becoming dismissive or cynical about what we read. Instead, we should take a balanced approach to carefully evaluating the strengths and limitations of research articles (Figure 12.1).

A critique framework provides a structured approach for assessing the quality of a study by examining the processes used by the researcher when carrying out a study. This should reveal the researcher's rigour in ensuring the accuracy of the results. For example, the researcher should consider the most appropriate type of research to answer the research question and anticipate likely problems or issues related to the methods to be used in data collection. Attempts should be made to reduce problems as much as possible.

Each study will contain a methods or methodology section containing clues that will allow you to assess the level of rigour. Similarly, the results section may detail some of the problems that arose in collecting information and how these were solved. All these allow an assessment of the quality of the results of the study.

Key areas to consider in critiquing include the following.
- Is there an appropriate choice between a quantitative or qualitative approach linked to the research aim?
- Are the key variables in the aim clearly defined?
- Has an appropriate tool to collect the right information been chosen and is it appropriate to the sample?
- In quantitative research, has the tool of data collection (research method) been used in a previous study or piloted to test reliability? (Remember that in qualitative studies, information is collected in a more flexible way and does not 'measure' something.)
- Are the samples clearly defined by inclusion and exclusion criteria and the numbers involved in the data collection stated?
- Are the samples representative of the group they represent and details of their key characteristics for the study included to allow such a judgement?
- Are the ethical implications of the study considered and the study approved by an ethics committee, for example a local research ethics committee (LREC) in the UK or institutional review board (IRB) in other countries such as the USA? Many articles now only provide brief details on the ethical issues, so providing there is mention of an ethics committee, you can be assured that the study is ethically rigorous.
- Have the results been processed and presented in a clear and appropriate way, with helpful description and interpretation of the results?
- Are the conclusions supported by the results and any recommendations clear and concrete, giving an indication of who should do what now?

Each critiquing model works in a similar way by proving questions or pointers to explore the decision-making path followed by the researcher. As different forms of research have a slightly different path, some elements included in a model will vary depending on the type of research. There are some major differences in the nature of quantitative and qualitative research so it is important that you choose the corresponding critiquing model for the approach.

A range of critiquing models have been reviewed by Glasper and Rees (2013) and include options such as Crombie, CASP, Parahoo and Rees, but you will find that most research or evidence-based practice books will offer a similar framework to follow. If you are currently undertaking a programme of study, you may also have one suggested to you. Learn how to use these well, as critiquing is perhaps one of the most valuable skills to learn to enable you to critically evaluate research.

Reference and further reading
Coughlan, M., Cronin, P. & Ryan, F. (2007) Step-by-step guide to critiquing research. Part 1: quantitative research. *British Journal of Nursing* **16**, 658–663.

Glasper, A. & Rees, C. (2013) *How to Write Your Nursing Dissertation*. Chichester: Wiley-Blackwell.

Polit, D. & Beck, C. (2012) *Nursing Research: Generating and Assessing Evidence for Nursing Practice*, 9th edn. Philadelphia: Walters Kluwer/Lippincott Williams & Wilkins.

Ryan, F., Coughlan, M. & Cronin, P. (2007) Step-by-step guide to critiquing research. Part 2: qualitative research. *British Journal of Nursing* **16**, 738–744.

13 The hierarchy of evidence

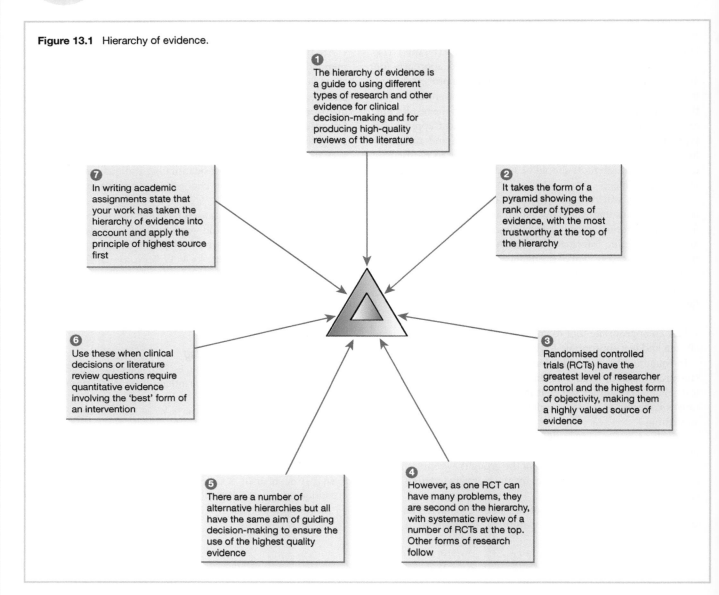

Figure 13.1 Hierarchy of evidence.

❶ The hierarchy of evidence is a guide to using different types of research and other evidence for clinical decision-making and for producing high-quality reviews of the literature

❷ It takes the form of a pyramid showing the rank order of types of evidence, with the most trustworthy at the top of the hierarchy

❸ Randomised controlled trials (RCTs) have the greatest level of researcher control and the highest form of objectivity, making them a highly valued source of evidence

❹ However, as one RCT can have many problems, they are second on the hierarchy, with systematic review of a number of RCTs at the top. Other forms of research follow

❺ There are a number of alternative hierarchies but all have the same aim of guiding decision-making to ensure the use of the highest quality evidence

❻ Use these when clinical decisions or literature review questions require quantitative evidence involving the 'best' form of an intervention

❼ In writing academic assignments state that your work has taken the hierarchy of evidence into account and apply the principle of highest source first

Evidence-based practice involves the search for 'best evidence' to make effective clinical decisions. In academic work, too, the quality of the evidence will influence your final mark. So, how do you select best evidence?

The guide to best evidence is found in the hierarchy of evidence (Figure 13.1). This usually takes the form of a triangular figure that ranks from top to bottom the highly regarded forms of evidence based on the confidence we can have in the accuracy of the information it contains. Such evidence should allow the results of one study to be generalised outside the context in which it was created. So, small local audits may be very accurate but have limited ability to apply to situations in other clinical areas. This is why audit is not usually seen as relevant to evidence-based practice.

However, one of the long-standing respected sources of evidence is the randomised controlled trial (RCT), as it has maximum control and objectivity. When published in peer-reviewed journals, RCTs are carefully scrutinised before publication. They can usually be safely generalised to other locations because those taking part are picked to represent those typical of the broader group.

However, single studies can still be open to limitations and it is unwise to change practice on the basis of one study alone. For this reason, systematic reviews of the literature are taken as one of the most valuable sources of accurate evidence.

One of the earliest and still most widely quoted hierarchies was that developed by Sackett *et al.* (1996). This placed the various types of evidence in the following order, where 1 is the most highly valued.

1 Systematic reviews of the literature and meta-analyses of RCTs.
2 At least one RCT.
3 Cohort studies and case–control studies.
4 Surveys.
5 Case reports.
6 Qualitative research studies.
7 The opinion of experts.
8 Anecdotal evidence.

This is not a perfect guide to choosing evidence and neither does it guarantee the results. More recent hierarchies have sensibly added evidence from well-designed controlled trials without randomisation, in the form of quasi-experimental studies between numbers 2 and 3.

Hierarchies can be used to guide clinical decision-making, or academic work such as reviews of the literature. They encourage the use of the higher levels of evidence before those at a lower level. However, not all questions can be answered numerically and not all can be answered through an RCT, particularly in nursing, so use hierarchies with care.

Reference and further reading

Aveyard, H. & Sharp, P. (2013) *A Beginner's Guide To Evidence-based Practice*, 2nd edn. Maidenhead: Open University Press.

Holland, K. & Rees, C. (2010) *Nursing: Evidence-based Practice Skills*. Oxford: Oxford University Press.

Sackett, D., Rosenberg, W., Muir Gray, J., Haynes, R. & Richardson, W. (1996) Evidence based medicine: what it is and what it isn't. *British Medical Journal* 312: 71–72.

14 Factors influencing research design

Figure 14.1 Factors influencing designs.

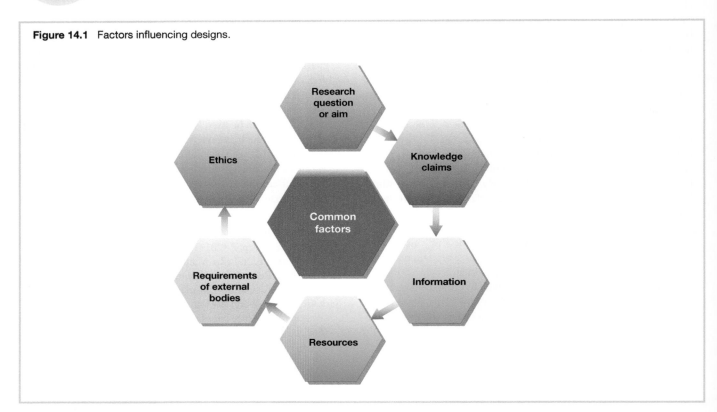

The research design of a study refers to the overall approach taken to investigate a research topic. The term is often used interchangeably with phrases such as 'research strategy' but is generally understood as directing the methods relating to a project. For example, in social research the researcher may adopt a qualitative research design, a quantitative design, or combine both to produce a mixed methods approach. Within a chosen design, a corresponding methodology reflects the main principles of the selected design or approach. In this way, a grounded theory analysis would be compatible with a qualitative research design and, similarly, descriptive univariate statistics would be consistent with a quantitative design. Research designs may vary but common to all is the collection of data, albeit in different ways and for different purposes. Identifying the factors that will influence the research design is important because they inform the scope of the study (Figure 14.1).

Nursing and Healthcare Research at a Glance, First Edition. Alan Glasper and Colin Rees. © 2017 by John Wiley & Sons, Ltd. Published 2017 by John Wiley & Sons, Ltd.

Key question for researchers: what factors should I consider when designing my research project?

Question or aim

The research question or aim is the driving force behind the choice of a research design. This involves a consideration of the characteristics of qualitative and quantitative research designs and which would best meet the aim of the research project. For example, qualitative research lends itself well to research where a deeper understanding of the phenomenon is required rather than facts as in quantitative research. Questions such as 'how', 'what', 'who' and 'why' are appropriate for qualitative research designs and may explore unexamined assumptions (Coyle, 2006). In contrast, quantitative research designs propose questions such as 'how many', 'how often' and 'what are the differences'.

Knowledge claims

According to Cresswell (2003), any inquiry should include:

> consideration of what knowledge claims are being made by the researcher, that is, the ontological position of the researcher (the fundamental nature of knowledge or being) and epistemological approach (what constitutes valid knowledge). The ontological position informs the procedure, sampling strategy, data collection methods, and analysis.

For example, a positivist or quantitative design aiming to establish facts would reflect a realist ontology supporting notions of a single independent reality. In comparison, qualitative research aligns itself with idealism, subjective realities and the construction of meaning by individuals.

Prior research

A thorough search of the literature will reveal the leading researchers in the field, the main methodologies used, and helps limit the scope of an inquiry and informs the design and focus of the proposed research (Hart, 2001). Central to any search for information will be the availability of scientific information through the internet, research groups, conferences, library facilities, search engines, government and organisational sources.

Resources

Data

Resources include accessibility to sufficient data to meet the research aim. This may be dependent on 'gatekeepers' who have the power to deny or grant access to participants. For example, in research involving children, gatekeepers would include those with a duty of care for the child, such as parents and/or teachers or guardians.

Finance

The degree of financial support will influence the design. For example, online or postal questionnaires are a relatively economic means of data collection compared with interviews, which incur costs of travel and participant expenses. A longitudinal design will incur extra costs as researchers and participants have to be reimbursed over a longer period. Translation costs may have to be considered in cross-cultural research.

The researcher

The researcher's availability, knowledge and skills (technical understanding and technical background) will influence the research design. In participatory research designs, participants may be co-researchers and any design should accommodate financial resources for lay research training.

Requirements of external bodies

Researchers may be required to adopt an approach specified by funders, journals, and research exercises and therefore make it less likely that they would be rejected. This may advantage the researcher as it is more likely to be accepted but may limit what is studied and how it is studied. However, following frequently used designs for the topic may inhibit advancement in a particular research field.

Ethical considerations

The research design should encompass ethical principles, such as respect for autonomy, non-maleficence (doing no harm), beneficence (doing well) and justice (Beauchamp & Childress, 2001). These may be embedded in research projects by ensuring the following.

- Are safety considerations built into the design for both participants and researchers? Have relevant professional research associations been consulted for guidance?
- Has a risk–benefit ratio calculation been conducted by using all available information to make an appropriate assessment of people and places. Do the benefits outweigh the risks? Risk assessment may involve considering short- or long-term physical and/or psychological risks. Take into account means by which to manage adverse events.
- Is there participant deception incorporated into the design? Some studies may involve a degree of deception and this would require justification. This may be necessary where revealing the researcher would alter natural occurrences. For example, if you want to learn about decision-making practices of nurses without influencing their practice style, you may consider telling them you are studying communication behaviours more broadly.
- Last but not least, privacy and confidentiality concerns have to be considered.

References and further reading

Beauchamp, T.L. & Childress, J.F. (2001) *Principles of Biomedical Ethics*, 5th edn. Oxford: Oxford University Press.

Coyle, A. (2006) Discourse analysis. In: G.M. Breakwell, C. Fife-Shaw, S. Hammond & J.A. Smith (eds) *Research Methods in Psychology*, 3rd edn, pp. 366–387. London: Sage.

Cresswell, J.W. (2003) *Research Design: Qualitative, Quantitative and Mixed Methods Approaches*, 2nd edn. London: Sage.

Denscombe, M. (2010) *The Good Research Guide*, 4th edn. Maidenhead: Open University Press.

Hart, C. (2001) *Doing a Literature Review*. London: Sage.

15 Patient and public involvement in research

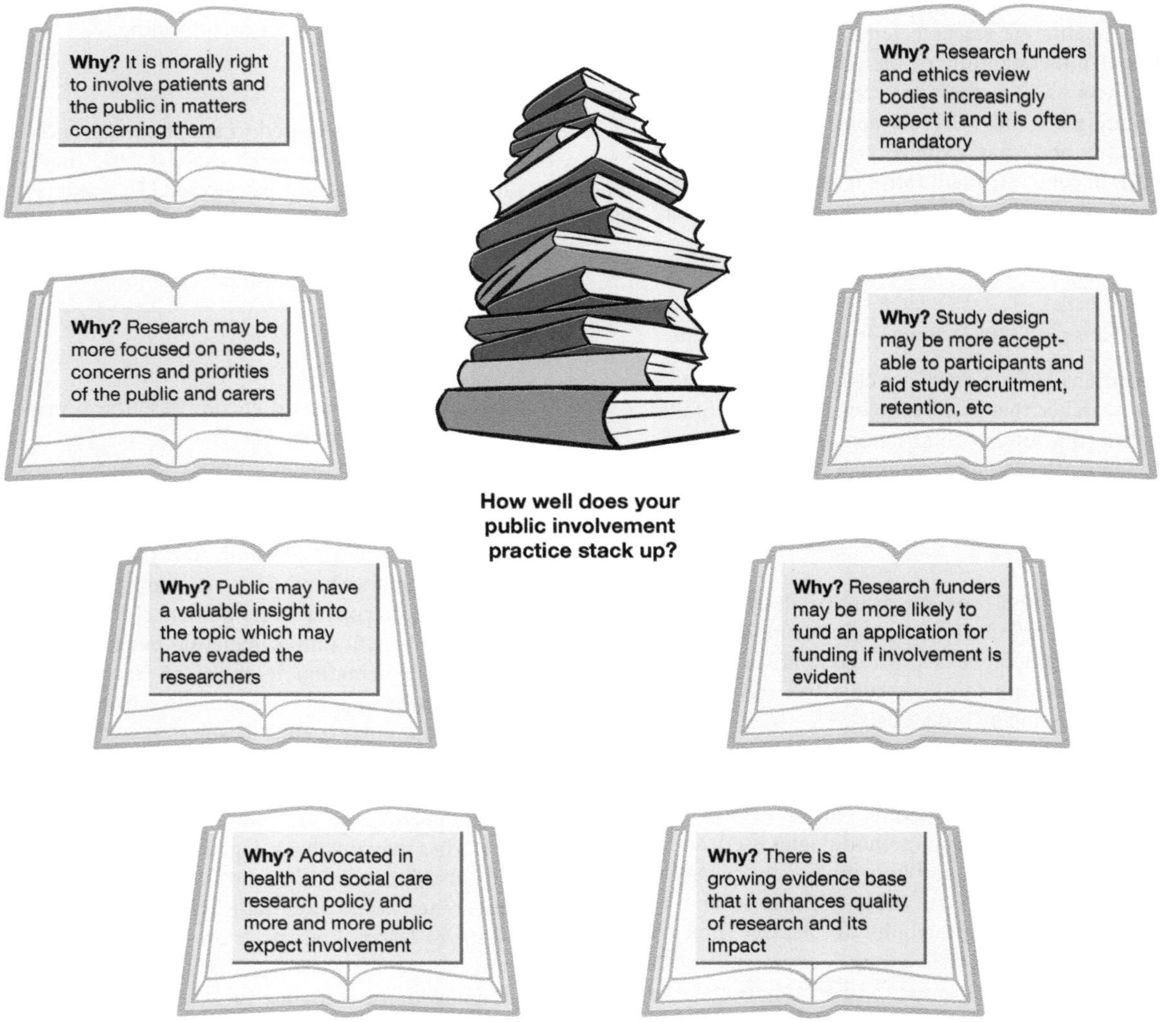

Figure 15.1 Public involvement in research concerns the public contribution to research design and implementation and not involvement as a research subject or participant.

Why? It is morally right to involve patients and the public in matters concerning them

Why? Research funders and ethics review bodies increasingly expect it and it is often mandatory

Why? Research may be more focused on needs, concerns and priorities of the public and carers

Why? Study design may be more acceptable to participants and aid study recruitment, retention, etc

How well does your public involvement practice stack up?

Why? Public may have a valuable insight into the topic which may have evaded the researchers

Why? Research funders may be more likely to fund an application for funding if involvement is evident

Why? Advocated in health and social care research policy and more and more public expect involvement

Why? There is a growing evidence base that it enhances quality of research and its impact

Why involve

Patients and the public have perspectives about their conditions or health and social care experiences that can be invaluable in informing research ideas. Public money often funds involvement in research and it is morally correct to ensure such funds are spent on topics of concern to the public themselves. The public can help with identifying research topics and prioritising among them, creating study designs that are fit for purpose and workable in the everyday lives of intended participants and suggest means of conducting, analysing and disseminating research. Research may have greater impact if the 'voice' of the public is strong in its developing, undertaking and reporting (Figure 15.1).

When to involve

Involvement should begin as early as possible and ideally at the ideas generation stage. It is better to engage later than not at all, so at the least present a draft research proposal to appropriate patients and public. It is acceptable to involve people in bid development only, but consider the benefits of an ongoing input from the public throughout a study. Naturally, there may be constraints on this depending on the amount of funding available to research teams, but the degree of involvement should reflect the overall budget. Include costs for dissemination involvement (e.g. conference attendance for the public), as well as considering payment as a 'thank you' or some other means of recognition for their time and contribution.

Nursing and Healthcare Research at a Glance, First Edition. Alan Glasper and Colin Rees. © 2017 by John Wiley & Sons, Ltd. Published 2017 by John Wiley & Sons, Ltd.

Who to involve

Members of the public may have personal experience of a condition or have characteristics of interest to researchers. Who to involve will be influenced by the role they are to undertake or what characteristics researchers see as helpful. Individual informal contacts can be consulted about an initial research idea or a group opinion can be sought at a patient forum or community group or similar. A first-hand perspective may be preferred or the view of someone who knows about the population of interest such as a patient representative organisation (e.g. Diabetes UK). Informal carers (family, friends) can often speak on behalf of their relatives but also have their own unique perspectives that researchers may wish to explore. Researchers should make an effort to seek people who may ordinarily miss out on research involvement because of being perceived as hard to reach (e.g. people with experience of dementia or young people). Others may require help to attend, for example parents of young children may need help with meeting the costs of childcare.

Involvement is not about seeking a representative sample of the public, but about seeking a range of views and characteristics of relevance to the proposed research. This may include people new to research involvement or those more experienced. Sometimes it is helpful to work with some members of the public already skilled at research involvement, especially when undertaking roles such as study steering group member, which can be challenging.

How to involve

Ethical approval is not required in England for most public involvement in research. It is only needed when the public are accessing raw data, for example as co-researchers or as advisers reading non-anonymised interview transcripts prior to commenting. During public involvement the public are not research participants and research is not being undertaken on or by them. Researchers should check the need for ethical and research governance approvals prior to involvement as this can differ between organisations and countries. Research teams should explore their need for public involvement and discuss this with potential members of the public to be involved. Provision of written information about the involvement role is helpful and should include details of the study, proposed involvement type, involvement duration, payment or reward mechanisms, and reassurance that training and support will be given. Importantly, it should be written and reinforced verbally that payments may affect the financial position of some participants and that it is up to them to check if payments affect them in terms of welfare benefits, taxation, etc. It is customary to involve people using mechanisms such as social media or face-to-face meetings that suit their needs and not just those of the research. Meetings in person should be at accessible venues and reimbursement of travel would normally be paid in full as a minimum. Often the public may prefer meetings in community venues or at existing community group meetings.

Consult organisational (e.g. university, NHS) policies on payments or read guidance from organisations such as INVOLVE. Ideally have someone skilled at facilitation or with experience of public involvement to lead the participation of the public.

One-off informal contacts with the public are acceptable, as are consultation events and discussion groups. If researchers want to build a more enduring relationship with one or more members of the public, they can discuss roles such as lay study adviser with them. Alternatives include participation as critical friends, reference group members or indeed study steering group members. Choice of role depends on whether researchers simply want the public's views or want them to have a more active role in study processes and management. Members of the public themselves will have views about how much they can contribute to a study and at what frequency and duration. Whatever role members of the public undertake, they need adequate preparation and support to do it and somebody on the research team needs to be able to take responsibility for this and meet individual's needs (e.g. research training, group-working skills).

Authentic involvement

The authenticity of involvement will be indicated by a number of factors.
- Adequate time frames for involvement.
- Suitable mechanisms employed.
- Appropriate numbers and relevant characteristics of those involved.
- Payment and rewards considered/made.
- Language used, e.g. 'work with the public' not 'use the public'.
- Clear intention to identify and act on support and training needs of the public.
- An identified team member responsible for managing involvement.
- Training and preparation of research team members for public involvement.
- Evidence of the difference that involvement made, e.g. changes to a study participant information sheet or trial design.
- Appropriate amount of study budget apportioned to public involvement.

Future involvement

Learning from public involvement in a study can be evaluated even informally to identify what the team can do to reinforce good practice or improve next time. As capacity for involvement will have been increased among the public, it is good practice to offer a continuing relationship after the end of a study and seek further opportunities for involvement. Opportunities may exist for the public to disseminate findings after a study ends. Alternatively, they may be encouraged to use the experience gained to do other things, for example community engagement or employment.

Further reading
National Institute for Health Research. INVOLVE advisory group. Available at www.invo.org.uk

16 Descriptive studies

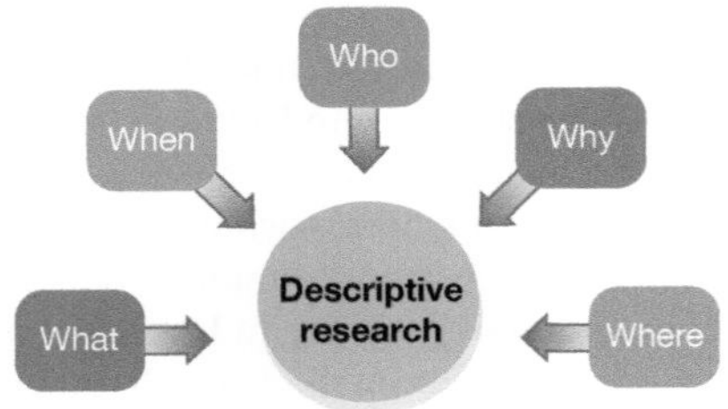

Figure 16.1 Focus of descriptive research: five Ws.

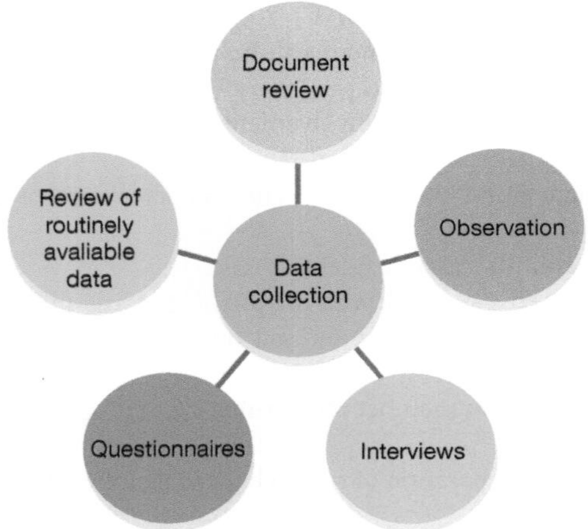

Figure 16.3 Data collection in descriptive research.

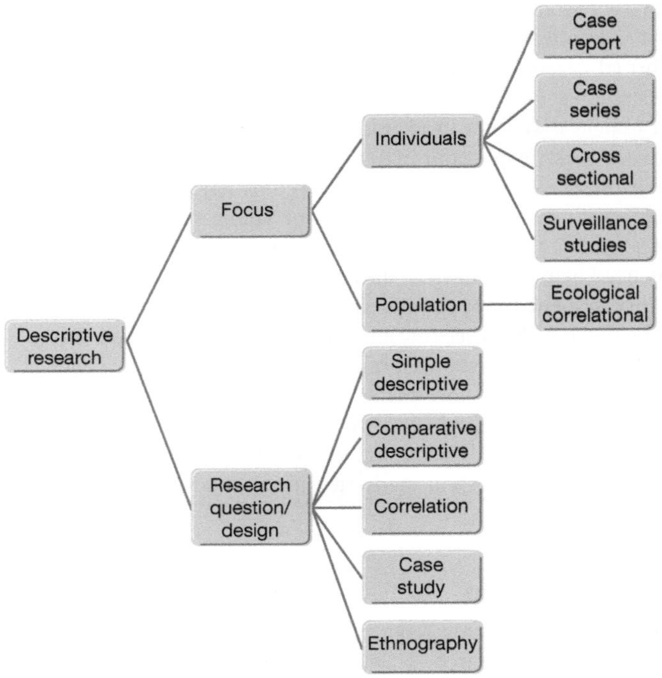

Figure 16.2 Types of descriptive studies.

Descriptive studies aim to provide a clear description of the naturally occurring phenomenon of interest or variables such as health status, attitudes and demography. The researcher does not intervene or manipulate conditions surrounding research participants but observes and describes what is happening. Descriptive studies may help in understanding associations between variables; however, these studies cannot explain or 'prove' a causal relationship between variables. Descriptive studies can be conducted using quantitative, qualitative or mixed methods.

Descriptive research on a given topic is often the initial research that helps in understanding the current situation and may provide some cues to causal relationships between variables that can then be tested through other research designs. Good descriptive research, like a good newspaper report, should answer five W questions: who, what, why, when and where (Figure 16.1).

Types of descriptive studies: by focus

Descriptive studies can be classified in various ways (Figure 16.2). Such studies may involve a one-time interaction with a group of people (cross-sectional) or a study may follow participants over a longer period (longitudinal). Descriptive studies can be divided into two major groups: those that deal with individuals and those that focus on populations. Case report, case series, cross-sectional and surveillance studies are examples of studies focusing on individuals, whereas ecological correlational studies are concerned with populations.

Case report

A case report is usually an anecdote of the case, where a clinician describes the clinical presentation of the case and details of treatment and prognosis. Case reports do not provide

Nursing and Healthcare Research at a Glance, First Edition. Alan Glasper and Colin Rees. © 2017 by John Wiley & Sons, Ltd. Published 2017 by John Wiley & Sons, Ltd.

rigorous evidence to prove something but may prompt further investigation using more rigorous designs.

Case series

A case series is concerned with aggregating more than one similar case with similar presentation. Case series may trigger further investigation of a particular condition or disease and may help in understanding epidemics. For instance, the AIDS epidemic in North America was explored after a case series of homosexual men with a similar clinical syndrome was presented.

Cross-sectional studies

Cross-sectional studies, also known as prevalence studies or cross-sectional analyses, aim to provide a snapshot of the situation at one specific point in time. Health surveys and censuses are examples of cross-sectional studies. Cross-sectional studies are conducted to describe the prevalence of diseases or conditions, or causes of disease but are not suitable for investigating rare conditions.

Surveillance studies

Surveillance studies aim to systematically collect, analyse and interpret data about a specific variable or phenomenon on a continuing and regular basis. The Global Influenza Programme run by the World Health Organisation is an example of such a study that helps in the planning, implementation and evaluation of public health practices. Surveillance can be active (data are collected by active searching) or passive (using routinely available data to answer questions). Mandatory reporting of bloodstream infection caused by meticillin-resistant *Staphylococcus aureus* (MRSA) to the Health Protection Agency in the United Kingdom is an example of active surveillance. Data collected from health records about causes of death is an example of passive surveillance.

Ecological correlational studies

Ecological correlational studies are attempts to describe an association between two or more variables in a population. An example could be the association between media violence and violence among school-age children. Such studies only help in identifying the association between exposure and outcome variables but may not prove if the association is causal.

Types of descriptive studies: by research question/design

Descriptive studies can also be classified according to their research question or design.

Simple descriptive studies

Simple descriptive studies aim to answer descriptive questions such as: What is happening here? How is this happening? Why is this happening? Who is involved?

Comparative descriptive studies

Comparative descriptive studies aim to describe and compare two groups with regard to a certain characteristic or variable, for instance comparing the rates of nosocomial infection in ward A compared to ward B.

Correlational studies

Correlational studies aim to explore and describe the association between two variables. An example could be the association between age and academic performance of undergraduate nursing students.

Case study

A case study aims to explore and understand the meaning of complex social activities and the context surrounding such activities. The focus of case study research may be an individual (one event in an individual's life or the whole life), a group (family, cultural group, class) or an institution. Case study research can be conducted using qualitative, quantitative or mixed method approaches.

Ethnography

Ethnography aims to understand social and cultural practices in their natural context. An example of ethnographic research is an exploration of end-of-shift handover practices of nurses in an emergency department.

Data collection and analysis in descriptive studies

As shown in Figure 16.3, depending on the research question, data in descriptive studies can be collected in various ways, including observation, survey questionnaires and interviews. Routinely available data, such as that from census, birth or death registers, can also be used. Data are analysed to provide descriptions of the phenomenon of interest; therefore, in quantitative research descriptive (measures of central tendencies) and inferential statistics (*t*-tests, regression analysis, comparison of groups) that describe the variable are used. For qualitative research, analysis aims to provide a description of the phenomenon of interest and surrounding context in as much detail as possible.

Advantages and disadvantages

Descriptive research can help to answer the W questions mentioned above and often help in developing and refining research questions. The research method is flexible, as the researcher can use quantitative, qualitative or mixed methods approaches to answer the question. There is no manipulation or intervention of a variable by the researcher. There are several disadvantages of descriptive research. For instance, such research can be time-consuming and expensive. The findings may be affected by recall bias or response bias. Descriptive research does not help in explaining or establishing a causal relationship between the variables.

Further reading

Watson, R., Atkinson, I. & Egerton, P. (2006) *Successful Statistics for Nursing and Healthcare*. Basingstoke: Palgrave Macmillan.

Watson, R., McKenna, H., Cowman, S. & Keady, J. (2008) *Nursing Research: Designs and Methods*. London: Churchill Livingstone Elsevier.

17 Action research

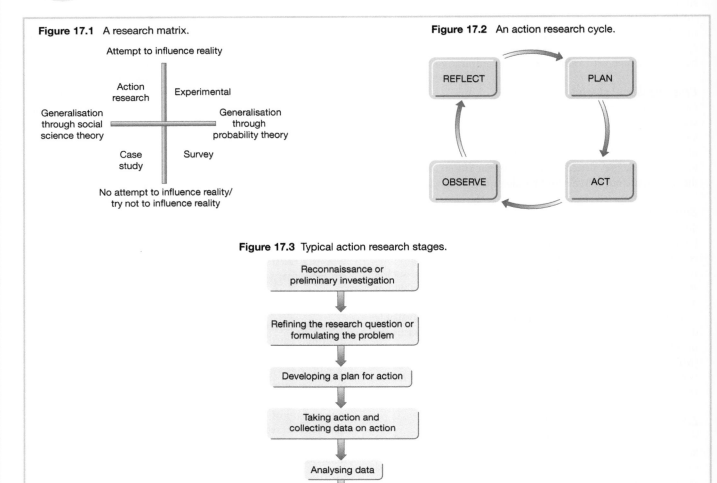

Figure 17.1 A research matrix.

Attempt to influence reality

Action research | Experimental

Generalisation through social science theory —|— Generalisation through probability theory

Case study | Survey

No attempt to influence reality/ try not to influence reality

Figure 17.2 An action research cycle.

REFLECT → PLAN → ACT → OBSERVE → REFLECT

Figure 17.3 Typical action research stages.

Reconnaissance or preliminary investigation
↓
Refining the research question or formulating the problem
↓
Developing a plan for action
↓
Taking action and collecting data on action
↓
Analysing data
↓
Reflection

A ction research (AR) is a kind of approach that involves participants in the research process. It can use both qualitative and quantitative methods of data collection. Action researchers act as agents of change and need skills not only in research but also in managing change and being reflexive. It is often used to improve practice so can have very practical outcomes as well as being a rigorous way of evaluating how things work and how best to create change.

How does AR compare with other research designs?

AR can be compared and contrasted with other types of research design, such as experimental, survey and case study. These have different ways of generalising or learning lessons to be applied elsewhere, and they vary as to whether there is an intervention or change process in play. Figure 17.1 demonstrates this on a matrix. If we choose an experimental design, there would be manipulation of variables and comparison of one group against another in terms of treatment given. Generalisation would be by applying statistical tests, i.e. using probability theory. Surveys, too, use similar analysis but unlike experiments the researcher does not seek to intervene but to 'measure' attributes as they are. Case study employs a largely in-depth qualitative examination of a relatively small number of settings or individuals and tries to describe and understand the settings and the views and experiences of participants without changing them; it has a different type of generalisation that is often called 'theoretical'. AR is like case study in its ability to learn lessons from the setting but does aim to achieve change and examine the effect of this change.

What are the principles of AR?

In AR the aim is to work *with* and *for* people rather than to do research *on* them. Typically in healthcare settings the action researcher begins by finding out from people – whether patients, staff or members of the public – what their experiences are and sometimes what problems in that setting they wish to solve. This early stage is often called a reconnaissance phase, where data are collected and consideration is given to the next stage of the research process. Consultation with participants (who may be called co-researchers) and negotiation is key throughout. The main researcher works with them to identify the data to be collected, the reflection that takes place on these data and the action that will be attempted.

Stages or phases of AR

AR is often a longitudinal process with a number of cycles of observation, reflection, planning and action. A typical model of one cycle is illustrated in Figure 17.2. Not all AR projects are cyclical though; some follow a more linear pattern. Figure 17.3 illustrates the stages of such an AR project.

Types of AR

There is no one way of going about AR and there are a number of different variants which have names such as participatory action research (PAR), cooperative enquiry, or one which uses a community of practice (CoP) approach. These all share the principles outlined above but often emphasise one aspect of AR over others, such as ensuring a high level of participation among those engaged in the research (as in PAR), or the idea of developing a group or community of people working together to create change for the common good of the group (as in a CoP).

Examples of AR projects

To illustrate the different types, consider first a PAR project which was led by a researcher who was undertaking her doctoral studies (Spears & Lathlean, 2015). Together with mentors, service users and a lecturer they worked to design, evaluate and refine a system enabling students to seek feedback from service users. The feedback concerned mental health students' interpersonal skills and occurred while on practice placement. This research aimed to explore the experiences of those concerned when nine students attempted to learn *from* rather than *about* service users. This was a 2-year study with five cycles of PAR. The findings showed that service users who volunteered to give feedback had unanimously positive experiences and the students who had a stronger sense of self were more willing and able to ask for feedback than less confident students.

Two further studies with AR designs sought to achieve organisational change. One was in a relatively deprived community setting where the aim was to encourage members of the community and professionals to work together to participate and to influence community health services mainly for families. The other tried to develop a similar group of people, a mixture of 'citizens' or members of the public and professionals (akin to a CoP) who were interested in impacting upon health services for older people. Both used group meetings and a combination of research methods such as observation and interviews to evaluate the processes that were occurring (Elsey & Lathlean, 2006).

A form of AR known as a cooperative enquiry was the choice for a project where mental health students and service users were brought into a series of group meetings to share ideas about how students feel when they are looking after patients and how the patients or service users see the contribution of students. This led to the considerable enlightenment of both parties and helped also to inform the curriculum for the students (Tee *et al.*, 2007). Again a range of research methods was chosen to evaluate the project.

Conclusion

AR is very useful where the aim is to combine rigorous methods of data collection, to involve participants firmly in the project and to create positive change in practice, policy or education.

References

Elsey, H. & Lathlean, J. (2006) Using action research to stimulate organisational change within health services: experiences from two community-based studies. *International Journal of Educational Action Research* **14**, 171–186.

Spears, J. & Lathlean, J. (2015) Service user involvement in giving mental health students feedback on placement: a participatory action research study. *Nurse Education Today* **35**, 84–89.

Tee, S., Lathlean, S., Herbert, L., Coldham, T., East, B. & Johnston, T. (2007) User participation in mental health decision-making: a co-operative enquiry. *Journal of Advanced Nursing* **60**, 135–145.

18 Participatory health research

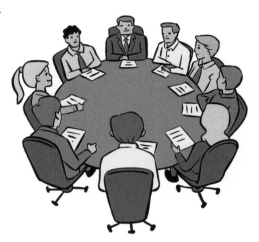

Figure 18.1 Tasks for the PHR researcher.

Planning your research

- Identifying a health-related problem amenable to PHR. Identifying possible co-researchers.
- Initial meetings to introduce each other; establish shared understanding of ways of communicating, the project vision and the proposed outcomes. To discuss any concerns, who will be involved and degree of involvement.
- Maintain regular communication and firm up ideas on how to work together, aims and objectives, ethics. If necessary, discuss how to achieve an equitable sharing of power.
- Research training for lay researchers may be required.
- Plan the action cycles; the processes for reflection, evaluation, learning, action. What constitutes data? Example: reflective diaries, meeting notes, interviews.
- Deciding how to analyse data, formulating a strategy for action and dissemination of research data and findings.
- Winding down: decisions about how to end the project are important to consider and should be negotiated according to the needs and wishes of all participants.

Participatory health research (PHR) is a collaborative research paradigm that departs from the traditional researcher/researched relationship. It draws on principles of participatory action research (PAR) to embrace the idea of researching 'with' rather than 'on' people. The purpose of PHR is to understand the experiences and self-defined priorities of those being studied and encourage people to find practical solutions to their problems. Rather than a single method, PHR encompasses a range of strategies of inquiry and analytical methods according to the project aim and collaborators' skills and interests. It is embedded in democratic principles of valuing the individual and emphasises the co-production of knowledge and action. Ultimately, PHR aims to address and improve the health and well-being of those people who are the focus of the research (Figure 18.1).

Why do PHR?

A main strength of PHR is its concern with identifying and solving real-life problems identified by the participants themselves. The research directly addresses problems in locations where the change will have a direct effect. Because of its concern with local issues, PHR is usually relatively small-scale. This challenges notions of generalisability but is regarded as effective for promoting relevant change, meaningful explanations for a health problem and empowering people that may have a wider impact (Stoecker, 2013).

Participation

Participation is the defining principle of PHR and sets it apart from other approaches in the field of health research. Participation is regarded as maximising opportunities for improving the quality of the research, identifying and providing solutions to local real-life problems, and promoting positive practical change (Wadsworth, 1998). Ideally, PHR advocates equal participation between researchers and researched. In practice, the extent to which this may be achieved is determined partly by the ability of the group to negotiate power differentials and the degree of commitment of those being researched. For example, participation may mean engagement with all or some of the following: direction of the inquiry, research design, recruitment, analysis dissemination, practical application.

Change

The purpose of PHR may be related to practical changes. It also seeks to change the way people think and act through critical reflection. PHR has its roots in critical theory that argues for empowerment through improving self-awareness and acquiring new knowledge. This is transformative learning that promotes intentions to act that may have a wider impact beyond the original more localised intentions of the study.

Transformative learning and the cyclical nature of PHR

Learning is integral to PHR. In PHR both the researcher and co-researchers learn together to co-produce transformational knowledge and gain critical consciousness that includes the different perspectives of all the participants. This process is iterative and reflective. It is usually viewed as a spiral of action research cycles consisting of phases of planning, acting, observing and reflecting. Trust, negotiation and empathy are intrinsic to the communication processes of the research team that in turn generates action based on the research findings.

Ethical pointers for PHR researchers

The blurring of boundaries between researcher and those being researched raises particular ethical issues in PHR.

Informed consent

Consent may have to be gained from individuals but also collective group consent from a group of patients or a community organisation. Consent may also have to be gained from all the co-participants whether they are lay or professional researchers; in other words, those who collect data may also be providers of data. PHR projects are usually conducted over a prolonged period and this may necessitate regularly updating informed consent according to any changes in the research design or new lines of inquiry.

Handling personal information

As with all research, personal details of participants should be stored securely on password-protected computers and in locked cupboards. In PHR where the researchers may be lay members, it is important to establish from the outset the need for safeguarding personal data in the community.

Confidentiality

PHR may involve collecting data from those known to the co-researchers. It is therefore important to formulate a written agreement about the treatment of any compromising information and the basis upon which information should and should not be used in the research dissemination.

References and further reading

Masters, J. (1995) The history of action research. In: I. Hughes (ed.) *Action Research Electronic Reader*. University of Sydney, Australia. Available at http://www.behs.cchs.usyd.edu.au/arow/Reader/rmasters.htm (accessed 16 April 2014).

Stoecker, R. (2013) *Research Methods for Community Change: A Project-Based Approach*. Thousand Oaks, CA: Sage.

Wadsworth, Y. (1998) What is participatory action research? *Action Research International*, Paper 2. Available at http://www.scu.edu.au/schools/gcm/ar/ari/p-ywadsworth98.html

Further resources

International Collaboration for Participatory Health Research (ICPHR), http://www.icphr.org

19 The ethics of healthcare research

Figure 19.1 Advice for the ethical researcher.

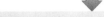

Planning your research
- Study key texts which focus on the ethical aspects of research.
- Be knowledgeable of research codes and regulations.
- Understand the three ethical principles which underpin research and consider these in relation to your own research.
- Attend research governance training seminars provided by research bodies and universities.
- Access ethical guidelines on research provided by your professional body or academic discipline.
- Discuss and be advised on the ethical aspects of your research by your supervisor

Preparing your application for submission to the ethics committee
- Ensure your study is scientifically valid: spurious research is unethical and wastes the time of research subjects/participants as well the busy researchers sitting on the ethics panel.
- Highlight what steps you have taken to ensure the following:
  - The recruitment of the subjects/participants will be done with their full consent to show that no coercion, unfairness or exploitation is involved.
  - Subjects/participants have enough information and time to make a considered decision about whether to take part in the study.
  - Subjects/participants know of their absolute right under the Helsinki Declaration to withdraw from the study at any time without this affecting them in any way (this is especially important if they are hospital patients or perhaps children in the care system).
  - Any special measures you have put in place to seek informed consent from vulnerable groups such as young children or people with learning difficulties.
  - What you will do if, for example, a subject/participant is unwell or upset during a research procedure or an interview.
  - How you will ensure the anonymity and confidentiality of the data you have collected.
  - How you will ethically disseminate your findings through publications and conference presentations

During data collection
- Take time to ensure that every research subject/participant understands the research they are taking part in; this may mean going over the information you have already given them again.
- Acknowledge that informed consent is not just about signing an informed consent form but rather about ensuring the individual research subject/participant is fully informed.
- Ensure that every research subject/participant is protected from harm and is treated respectfully.

Dissemination of findings
- Ensure anonymity of data, e.g. remove identifiable data such as names, places, details of rare condition and even place names if necessary.
- Ensure confidentiality of data, e.g. protect and destroy data to comply with local and national guidelines.

The ethical aspects of health research came under international scrutiny following the Nuremberg Trials that exposed inhumane and spurious research by the Nazi regime during World War Two. The resulting Nuremberg Code (1947) set out, for the first time, an international code for research involving human experimentation (Figure 19.1). It made absolute the need for informed consent, the right of subjects to withdraw from participation in any study and placed responsibility on the physician/researcher to protect the research subject. The 1964 Declaration of Helsinki (revised 1975, 1983, 1989 and 2000) set out further health research ethical standards, with later versions including identifiable human tissue and data. It states that the well-being of human subjects takes precedence over the interests of science and society and sets out the duties of the researcher, which include due regard to the life, health, privacy and dignity of the human subjects. It stresses that informed consent must be sought from those taking part, with special consideration given to those who because of legal incompetence, such as people with learning difficulties, are unable to give consent. Moreover, it states that every patient entered into a randomised controlled trial (RCT) must have access to the best proven prophylactic, diagnostic and therapeutic methods identified by the study.

These codes and declarations have not always been upheld. In the USA, a study of 48 major hospital studies (Beecher, 1966) found that informed consent had not been sought from patients and that their participation in studies had led to significant harm. This included the withholding of effective treatments, induced illness and new and novel procedures that caused death. The infamous Tuskegee Study (1932–1972), involving 399 black men infected with syphilis and a control group of 200 who were uninfected, was a case in point. This longitudinal study monitored both groups through to autopsy; all the recruits were poor African-American black sharecroppers. Those with syphilis were not informed of their disease or treated and many died or infected their wives/partners. When exposed, this study led to a national outcry, and public concerns about unethical research led to a National Commission and the Belmont Report (1979), which set out the following three principles to guide research.

Respect for persons

Researchers have a duty to respect the person's right to hold views, make choices and take actions based on their personal values and beliefs (Beauchamp & Childress, 2009). Informed consent must be sought from every individual involved in any research study and special consideration given to vulnerable groups, such as those with learning difficulties or bereaved people. Withholding information, as in the Tuskegee study, is unethical as it overrides the principle of respect for persons by denying their autonomy and right to make their own choices and decisions.

Beneficence

The obligation to do no harm, to maximise benefits and minimise risk means the researcher must ensure that vulnerable groups, such as children, are protected. In the UK, the General Medical Council guidelines state that the assent of children should be sought in any research study and they should not be involved if they appear to object 'in either words or actions' even if their parents' consent (General Medical Council, 2007, p. 17). For example, taking a blood sample from a child may be regarded as causing harm if the child is distressed by this and should be stopped immediately.

Justice

The Belmont Report (1979, p. 4) asked 'Who ought to receive the benefits of research and bear its burdens?' It has already been shown that the poor and disadvantaged, as in the Tuskegee study, may be targeted by unscrupulous researchers because of their vulnerability. Every study recruit must be given clear information about the research and be made aware of any risks and/or benefits to them.

Despite these principles unethical research continues. The Alder Hey Hospital Inquiry (House of Commons, 2001) found that organs (defined as human tissue under the Declaration of Helsinki) were removed from children after death without the knowledge or consent of parents. This not only caused distress to the families affected but led to a breakdown of public trust into the conduct of research and highlighted the need for robust peer review systems for research.

Peer review of research and ethical committees

Within the developed world, ethics committees now carry out the function of peer review on all health-related research (Hedgecoe et al., 2006). European countries also comply with the European Clinical Trials Directive (2001) and the European Data Protection Act (1995). Failure to seek ethical approval from the relevant body may result in severe penalties. The General Medical Council took disciplinary action against the author of The Lancet paper that linked the measles, mumps and rubella vaccine with autism, because ethical approval was not sought (McGuinness, 2008). Finally, without the participation of human subjects there would be no research; researchers owe it to them and the public to ensure all health research is conducted ethically.

References

Beauchamp, T.L. & Childress, J.F. (2009) Principles of Biomedical Ethics, 6th edn. New York: Oxford University Press.

Beecher, H. (1966) Ethics and clinical research. New England Journal of Medicine 274, 1354–1360.

European Union (1995) Data Protection Directive 95/46/EC of the European Parliament and of the Council of 24October 1995 on the protection of individual with regard to the processing of personal data and on the free movement of such data. Available at http://eur-lex.europa.eu/LexUriServ/LexUriServ.do?uri=CELEX:31995L0046:en:HTML

European Union (2001) Directive 2001/20/EC of the European Parliament and of the Council of 4 April 2001 on the approximation of the laws, regulations and administrative provisions of the Member States relating to the implementation of good clinical practice in the conduct of clinical trials on medicinal products for human use. Available at http://www.eortc.be/services/doc/clinical-eu-directive-04-april-01.pdf

General Medical Council (2007) 0–18 Years: Guidance For All Doctors. London: General Medical Council. Available at http://www.gmc-uk.org/static/documents/content/GMC_0-18_years_2007.pdf

Hedgecoe, A., Carvallo, F., Lobmayer, P. & Raka, F. (2006) Research ethics committees in Europe: implementing the directive, respecting diversity. Journal of Medical Ethics 32, 483–486.

House of Commons (2001) The Royal Liverpool Children's Inquiry: Summary and Recommendations. London: The Stationery Office.

McGuiness, S. (2008) Research ethics committees: the role of ethics in regulatory authority. Journal of Medical Ethics , 695–700.

National Commission for the Protection of Human Subjects of Biomedical and Behavioral Research Secretary (1979) The Belmont Report: Ethical Principles and Guidelines for the Protection of Human Subjects of Research. Available at http://www.hhs.gov/ohrp/humansubjects/guidance/belmont

20 Preparing a research proposal

Figure 20.1 Preparation of a research proposal.

What is a research proposal?

- It is a map or blueprint of all the stages in your research study.
- Like a map, it should include all the key stages with some detail on how you will carry out the actual study.
- It describes what you want to do and how you will do it.
- Different institutions have different rules on structure and content so check their requirements before you start.

Purpose of a proposal

- To identify why this problem needs researching.
- To provide justification for the research.
- To outline the aims of the study.
- To describe how you will achieve the aims.
- To describe the way you will conduct the research, especially in regard to ethical issues.
- To outline possible benefits of the research.
- To plan what resources you will need to carry out the research.

Key components of a proposal

- Title page
- Abstract
- Contents page
- Introduction
- Literature review
- Methods (including ethical issues)
- Conclusion
- References
- Appendices

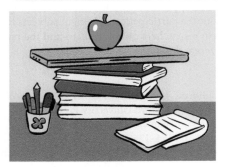

Tips: before you begin

- Before you begin, discuss your proposal ideas with your supervisor or a colleague.
- Carry out a small search of the literature to see if this problem has been researched before and what angle has been taken.
- Carefully consider what you can achieve within the time frame allowed.
- Take time to think carefully about the focus of your study as once this is clear then the rest should follow easily.

Tips: writing the proposal

- Keep the title short, about 10 words approximately.
- Abstract is a brief summary, about 300 words.
- Introduction should include key reports and define the terms.
- Literature review should include recent studies (within last 5 years). Older studies should be included if important pieces of work.
- Methods is where you describe the procedures for how you will carry out the research.
- Resources: what you will need (time, money, people, equipment) to do the research.

Tips for writing style

- Have clear headings.
- Aim to link each section by using a sentence at the end that leads to the discussion in next section.
- Avoid repetition and 'waffle'.
- Keep headings style consistent throughout.
- Number all pages.
- Perform spell check before submitting.
- Use short sentences.
- Use paragraphs rather than a solid block of text.
- Check that formatting and layout corresponds to your institution's requirements.

Nursing and Healthcare Research at a Glance, First Edition. Alan Glasper and Colin Rees. © 2017 by John Wiley & Sons, Ltd. Published 2017 by John Wiley & Sons, Ltd.

The purpose of these guidelines is to provide you with a simple framework for preparing a research proposal for live data gathering (Figure 20.1). The guidelines are presented as a guide and are not procedural steps that you must follow rigidly, as requirements can differ between courses and between universities. These guidelines should be read in conjunction with your college, school and programme guidance.

Types of proposals

In some nursing degree courses students can be required to complete a research proposal as part of their studies. In the past the research proposal was usually limited to empirical research (i.e. live data gathering), which means collecting data from participants. However, over time, the format of a proposal has changed to allow students to pursue other types of research. The types are summarised as follows:

- research with participants (patients, families healthcare staff);
- systematic review (of published studies);
- advanced concept analysis (of a concept in the literature);
- historical research (documents of events in the past).

Developing your ideas for a proposal

It can be hard at times to think what topic you would like to research. You could start with thinking about what are current issues in nursing and what is problematic. Sometimes working in the clinical area you may encounter aspects of practice that you think could be done differently. It is always helpful to discuss your ideas with your supervisor as he or she may help refine and clarify the focus of the proposal. Having a clear focus is critical before you begin, as it will ensure that the proposed study is workable and not too broad. The study must be achievable in the time allowed.

Getting support from your supervisor

Students are usually allocated a supervisor, usually a lecturer, for their research proposal. It is important that you see this person as a resource and a guide throughout the development and writing of the proposal.

Components of a proposal

Most proposals consist of a number of front pages, which are generally standard in content, and then four main chapters. The proposal should be seen as the blueprint of what you intend to do for your thesis. It is a map of how you will go about accomplishing the proposed study. It is usually couched in terms of 'this proposal will'.

Front pages

1 Front page: title of the proposal, student number, and course title.
2 Declaration: signed statement that it is all your own work.
3 Abstract: short summary of the essential components of the proposal on one page.
4 Contents page: page numbers for all the chapters and subsections.

Four main chapters

Each chapter should start with a small introductory paragraph and end with a short concluding paragraph.

Chapter 1: introduction to the proposal

This is usually a short chapter that addresses the following.
- Background to the topic: brief summary of the topic usually supported with references to key reports.
- Definition of the topic chosen.
- Brief explanation as to why this topic is important and needs to be researched.
- Brief explanation of how this proposal will add to existing knowledge in this area.
- What method you will use to address the research topic.
- The importance of your study for clinical practice and society.
- Conclusion: briefly describe what will be covered in the subsequent chapters in the proposal.

Chapter 2: review of the literature

It is important to know what kinds of studies have been already done on the topic and to provide a good critical summary and highlight any gaps. This can be used to justify the approach you will describe in the methods chapter. It can be overwhelming when faced with many studies on the topic. The best way to approach it is to select studies completed within the last 5 years, and group the studies under key themes that are clearly relevant to the topic.

Chapter 3: methods

This chapter usually begins with an overview of the philosophy underpinning the approach you have decided to use, whether qualitative or quantitative or a mix of both. It is important to explain why you have chosen the particular approach. Most students choose either descriptive quantitative (survey) or descriptive qualitative (interviews). This chapter must include details on the following.
- Sampling method: description of the participants.
- Recruitment and access: how you will obtain participants and inclusion and exclusion criteria.
- Data collection: how you will collect data.
- Data analysis: procedure for analysing the data.
- Ethical considerations: ethics approval process.
- Ensuring quality: reliability and validity in quantitative data, trustworthiness of qualitative data.

Chapter 4: conclusion

This provides a summary of the proposal and how the research will add to the existing body of knowledge. You may need to include suggested dissemination strategies (e.g. conferences, papers, summaries). This should be followed by:
- appendices (including such elements as interview schedule, questionnaire, letter to ethics committee, letter of invitation to take part, information leaflet, consent forms for participants);
- budget outlining costs of the proposal (sometimes required).

21 Developing a patient research information pack

Figure 21.1 Participant consent form: example.

Title of the Study

Name of Researcher:

Participant Identification Number

Please initial box

1. I confirm that I have read and understand the information sheet for the above research and have had the opportunity to ask questions ☐

2. I understand that my participation is voluntary and that I am free to withdraw at any time without giving any reason ☐

3. I understand that my views will be tape rcorded ☐

4. I understand that my responses will be anonymised before analysis ☐

5. I give permission for members of the research team to have access to my anonymised responses ☐

6. I agree to take part in the interview ☐

_____   _____   _____
Name of participant   Date   Signature
(or legal representative)

_____   _____   _____
Researcher   Date   Signature

Copies:
A signed and dated copy of this consent form will be given to you at the beginning of the interview for you to keep. A second copy will be filed in the research records, and stored securely at the xyz organisation

Figure 21.3 Examples of various readability formulas.

- Flesch–Kincaid Grade Level
- Gunning–Fog Score
- Coleman–Liau Index
- SMOG Index
- Automated Readability Index

Figure 21.2 Readability scores: a description.

Readability is a way to match the reading level of written material to the 'reading with understanding' level of the reader

Readability formula: helps in performing calculations on a text (mainly on sentence and word length) and provides a numerical score

Readability calculation method using Fog score
- Count the words and sentences
- Divide the number of words by the number of sentences
- Count the long words with more than two syllables
- Divide the long words by total words, and multiply by 100
- Add the two scores together and multiply by 0.4

Examples of application of Fog score of a:
- Newspaper advertisement   = 4
- Popular novel   = 8
- Report on information technology   = 20

Figure 21.4 Points to remember while developing an information sheet.

- Information packs are only one part of the process of obtaining informed consent.
- Information should be appropriate for the target audience.
- The length and complexity of the information pack should reflect the length and complexity of the research study.
- Information packs should be written in simple and jargon-free language.
- Information sheet should be written as an invitation to participants to consider participation in the study.

A participant research information pack aims to provide concise but clear information about the specific and essential aspects of the research. The information pack aims to help potential participants decide whether the study is of interest to them and if they wish to explore further details about the study in order to decide whether to participate or not. Participants are given the information pack to retain and to refer back to as and when needed. A research information pack may contain three elements that include invitation letter (optional), information sheet and a consent form (Figure 21.1).

Format of the participant research information pack

The format of a research information pack varies depending on the type of study, prevailing practices in the study setting and the complexity of the study. For example, a survey requiring responses to a questionnaire may only need brief explanation at the beginning of the questionnaire or accompanying cover letter. The research information pack can also be in the form of an invitation letter, a leaflet or a booklet. Information can be presented as bullet points, under headings and subheadings, or through question and answer points. The information should be written using simple terminology, short sentences and non-technical language. It is recommended that the readability of the information pack is checked to ensure that it is easily understandable by a lay audience (Figure 21.2), and various readability formulas are available (Figure 21.3). It is recommended that research information packs should be understandable to a child of 12–13 years of age (7th or 8th grade).

Presentation of the research information pack

The research information pack (or at least the first page of the pack and the consent form) should be printed on the headed paper of the organisation where the research is taking place and should contain relevant contact details. The information sheets and consent forms should have a version number and date in the header or footer and should be written in a font size appropriate for the needs of the potential participants. For instance, an information pack for older adults may need to be written in a larger font. Likewise, information packs for children should use appropriate pictures, graphics and colours. There are various points that researchers should remember while developing information sheets (Figure 21.4).

Content of the patient research information pack

Title of the study: This should be self-explanatory and comprehensible for a lay person. It should be written in simple language avoiding acronyms or abbreviations.

Invitation paragraph: The purpose of this paragraph is to invite the potential participant to take part in the study.

What is the purpose of the study? The purpose of the study needs to be clearly and succinctly presented. A brief background to the study can also be provided.

Why have I been invited to participate in the study? Here, why and how the participant was chosen should be explained including, for example, the reasons for choosing participants from a particular ethnic group, age group, gender or profession. The intended number of other participants for the study should also be mentioned.

Do I have to take part? Voluntary participation and the fact that the participant can withdraw from the study at any time should be included.

What will happen to me if I take part? An explanation of the participant's potential involvement in the research process should be provided, including how long the participant will be involved in the research, the duration of the research, the frequency of contact with the researcher, practical details (e.g. clinic visit, home visit) and the process of data collection (completing a questionnaire, interviews, focus group discussion, any blood test or sample collection). Diagrams and flow charts can be used to explain the research process and participants' involvement. It is also important to clearly describe if any expenses (travel, meal and childcare) or 'thank you' vouchers are available.

What will I have to do? What is expected of the participant (any lifestyle change, dietary restrictions, keeping diaries, or any other expectations) should be clearly explained.

What are the possible disadvantages and risks of taking part? Any disadvantages, discomforts, inconvenience or risks (e.g. side effects of medication, potential injury, distress caused by recall of sensitive experiences in the past) should be explained. It is also important to describe how such occurrences will be dealt with (e.g. referral to appropriate services).

What are the possible benefits of taking part? Any benefits associated with participation in the study should be explained. Where there are no benefits, it should be stated clearly.

What if there is a problem? Information about who to contact and how to contact them if the participant has a concern or wishes to complain about the research study should be provided.

Will my taking part in the study be confidential? This section should provide details of how participants' information will be kept confidential during and after the study. Explain how the data will be collected, stored (and how long for), handled (who will have access) and disposed of at the end of the study. Some studies require involvement of the participant's general practitioner and this needs to be explained.

What will happen to the results of the study? It is important to let participants know about the results of the study and how these results will be used and disseminated. It is also important to state that the report will not contain any identifiable information about participants.

Who is organising or sponsoring the research? The name of the organisation funding and/or the one organising the research should be provided.

Contacting the researcher: Contact details (phone and email address) of the research team (at least the lead researcher) should be provided.

Further reading

Medicines and Healthcare products Regulatory Agency (2012) *Best practice guidelines on patient information leaflets*. Available at https://www.gov.uk/government/publications/best-practice-guidance-on-patient-information-leaflets

National Patient Safety Agency. *Information sheets and consent forms: guidance for researchers and reviewers*. Version 3.0, December 2006. Available at www.nres.nhs.uk

Resources

Examples of various templates of research information sheet are available at http://www.hra-decisiontools.org.uk/consent/examples.html

22 Getting the most from supervision

Figure 22.1 Getting the most from supervision.

Project Plan	
Time period	Action proposed

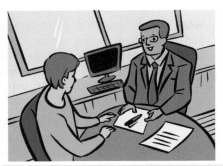

Many students find a Gantt chart or project plan helpful in structuring their supervision meetings

It is vital to maintain a professional attitude to your project as this will show your supervisor that you are taking it seriously

It is important to be realistic about access to the supervisor. They may have other students to look after, usually heavy teaching loads and if they are active researchers themselves, large research projects to manage

Suggestions for anticipating and preventing problems during supervision.

Usually a supervisor is allocated to you

- Establish an effective relationship with your supervisor
- By agreement draw up a research contract with your supervisor and agree a method of contact, including how often you will meet, what you will do when you meet either in person, email or Skype etc. Put it in your dairy.
- Try not to cancel supervision meetings and be temporally efficient!
- You can expect appropriate academic support
- You must develop a strategy of self-organisation, peer support and independent learning
- You may by arrangement record your supervision meetings
- Bring a prepared list of questions to every supervision meeting
- Prepare a short 'agenda' for meetings and after the meeting write brief notes on what has been agreed with the supervisor
- As you progress through the year, reflect and set goals with your supervisor for your supervision meetings
- The chances of being successful and gaining a good degree without regular supervision are greatly reduced.

Figure 22.2 Sample Gantt chart for an undergraduate degree.

Tasks	Month 1	Month 3–5	Month 6–8	Month 9/10	Month 12	Month 14	Month 16	Month 18
See supervisor	■							
Literature searching	■							
Critique papers	■	■						
Write chapters 1 and 2		■						
See supervisor		■						
Write chapters 3 and 4		■	■					
See supervisor/write chapter 5			■	■				
See supervisor with draft dissertation				■				

How to get started

Usually supervisors are allocated according to their knowledge of the subject. You should take the initiative to contact them once you have their details. Do this early as the sooner you can get started, the more successful you are likely to be. Early contact also shows your supervisor that you are eager to start on your project and keen to get their support. It is also the beginning of a successful relationship and one that will help you to produce the best possible thesis or dissertation (Figure 22.1).

Agreeing a working pattern

At the outset you may wish to draw up a research contract with your supervisor and agree a method of contact, including how often you will meet and what you will do when you meet, and so on. As you progress through the year, reflect and set goals with your supervisor for your supervision meetings. Above all, bear in mind that the chances of gaining a good degree are greatly reduced without regular supervision.

Anticipating and preventing problems

It is important to be realistic about access to your supervisor. He or she wants you to be successful and work with you, but equally they have other students to supervise, usually heavy teaching loads and, if they are active researchers themselves, large research projects to manage. Agree with them how often you will be in contact and put it in your diary. Before a supervision meeting, prepare a short 'agenda' to make the best use of time, and afterwards write a brief note of what you have agreed with your supervisor.

It is natural to be anxious about doing well in your project and dissertation and some students are nervous about revealing their concerns to their supervisor. However, the supervisor will be familiar with this, and is there to help you with the emotional aspects of working on what may be for you an unfamiliar activity, as well as providing subject knowledge.

Good planning is the essence

Developing a realistic plan, with manageable time scales, is the key to keeping a project on track. Your supervisor will be able to help you with this, though the project and your ability to complete it is your responsibility. Many students find a Gantt chart helpful. This lists the main activities and the time periods. A typical chart could look like the one shown in Figure 22.2.

Additional support

The supervisor is there to give you support in your project; however, it is expected that you will be able to make the most of this support by yourself by being organised and taking the responsibility for your own learning. Many resources are at your disposal, through a whole variety of means. In addition, make use of your peers and colleagues as they too may have some useful hints, tips and advice.

Further reading

Lathlean, J. (2013) Getting the most from your supervisor. In: A.Glasper and C.Rees (eds) *How to Write Your Nursing Dissertation*, pp. 108–112. Chichester: Wiley-Blackwell.

Lee, N.-J. (2010) Making research supervision work for you. *Nurse Researcher* **17**(2), 44–51. Available at http://dx.doi.org/10.7748/nr2010.01.17.2.44.c7461

23 Writing a research report

Figure 23.1 Writing a Research Report.

1. Collect and Organise Information

Don't start writing until you have all your information together. If you start writing before your research is finished, return to the initial sections and rewrite to ensure coherence.

COLLECT all relevant information together in one place - clearly labelled and signposted.

COLLECT and COLLATE all relevant references/citations.

ORGANISE information according to the requirements of the report.

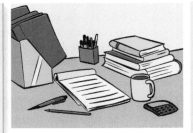

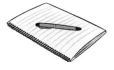

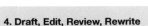

2. Write a Plan

Plan: Quantitative	Plan: Qualitative
Introduction	Introduction
Aims (including research question and/or hypothesis)	Aims
Literature Review	Literature Review
Population and Sample	Methodology/Research Framework (e.g. Phenomenology, Grounded Theory, Narratology)
Data Collection Methods	
Data Analysis	Sample and Sampling Frame
Findings	Data Collection Methods
Charts, tables and figures	Data Analysis
Discussion	Findings (including 'quotes' from the data where relevant)
Conclusion/Limitations	
Abstract	Discussion
	Conclusion/Limitations
	Abstract

4. Draft, Edit, Review, Rewrite

NEVER submit a first draft.

SEEK ADVICE from experts, colleagues, reviewers.

Edit for CONTENT, STYLE, GRAMMAR, PUNCTUATION and STRUCTURE

Keep it RELEVANT. Use KEY CONCEPTS and CURRENT DISCOURSE related to your discipline and topic. Refer to current practice guidelines and evidence.

The report should have a LOGICAL FLOW – each element should flow easily into the next.

PLOT the report. Like a good story, a research report sets the scene (introduction, literature review), gives the action (methods/what you did) and the outcomes (findings, discussion, conclusions).

3. Remember! Who, What, When, How, What Now?

WHO did what? Who collected the data? How did they collect it and record it?

WHAT data did you collect?

WHAT did you do with the data?

HOW did you analyse it – what models, methods, frameworks, tools and tests did you use?

QUANTITATIVE - include tables, p values, means and graphs or charts as appropriate.

QUALITATIVE - create a clear AUDIT TRAIL of your process of analysis.
WHEN did each stage take place?
HOW did you arrive at your conclusions?

WHAT NOW for theory, practice and future research? How will your findings impact on healthcare practice and knowledge?

The final stage of the research process is dissemination: sharing your work and findings with the wider world. The research report should be succinct, clear, understandable and clearly signposted, but most importantly it should be appropriate to its purpose and target audience. Just as the research process involves specific stages, so does the process of writing up the research (Figure 23.1).

Identify purpose and audience

The nature of the report depends on its purpose (why you are writing it) and its audience (for whom it is intended). In healthcare, research is either carried out for academic purposes or to influence or change practice (or both). The kinds of reports required will vary depending on whether the paper is to be read by academics, politicians, professionals or the public.

Nursing and Healthcare Research at a Glance, First Edition. Alan Glasper and Colin Rees. © 2017 by John Wiley & Sons, Ltd. Published 2017 by John Wiley & Sons, Ltd.

Dissemination usually requires publication in scholarly journals or in books or the production of an assignment or dissertation. It is important to establish your goals in writing the research report from the outset. Writing for publication, for example, will require writing to house styles/guidelines.

Address expectations

There are different expectations for different types of research. Quantitative research is the dominant and most widely recognised approach and the conventions of research reporting tend to be set by this approach. Qualitative research reports and systematic reviews might vary slightly in the approach to reporting, but all contain common elements.

Collect and organise information

Organisation is the key to effective writing. Gather together all the relevant information, including articles, books and other sources used in the literature review; all research data; ethical approval information; findings outputs such as charts, tables, figures or graphs; the criteria against which you are writing. Have report/writing guidelines to hand and visible.

Write a plan

Write a detailed plan for your report, utilising any guidelines, and ensuring that you include all relevant information. Keep track of all your references/citations by opening a separate document titled 'References' and put each citation into this as you go along, or use the citation manager within your word processing software. Use headings and subheadings to organise your work into logical sections, as described below.

Introduction

Set the scene as the start of the work. This should 'hook' the reader with a statement of purpose, using key words and concepts. Wider reading and an awareness of current concepts in your discipline can help. Provide the background to the research and a rationale for carrying it out.

Literature review

Healthcare research is context-dependent, · requiring an awareness of current and recent research evidence. The review should include reference to any existing major research, theories, evidence and guidelines and critique of existing research. Identify any gaps in the evidence base.

Methodology/methodological framework

Qualitative reports in particular require an exploration and explanation of the methodological framework used to guide your research process. Clarify key terms and concepts in your methodological approach here.

Population, sample and sampling frame

Define the research population and sample, justifying the choice of sample, including inclusion and exclusion criteria. Explain the sampling approach and process. Include here reference to gatekeeper approval where relevant, and to ethical issues and ethical approval.

Data collection

Describe your data collection methods clearly, and state any issues or challenges with data collection. This provides part of the 'audit' trail. Be sure to include how you recorded information and, where possible, signpost to figures or appendices which contain any data collection tools.

Data analysis

Clearly signpost every step in the process of analysis, including relevant diagrams or models. For quantitative reports, include all statistical tests. For qualitative reports, include all stages of the analysis process including any analytical frameworks used. Stick to the mantra: who, what, when, how.

Findings

Present the findings according to the convention of the discipline. This includes a prose summary of the findings (text) and any tables, figures, diagrams or charts. For quantitative research, graphical representation of findings is essential. Qualitative reports may include quotes from the data and models of the analysis process.

Discussion

This is a critical discussion of the findings of the study, making reference to the research purpose, aims or hypothesis, whether the findings were as anticipated prior to data analysis, and an evaluation of the significance of the findings. For qualitative research this will include quotes from the data.

Conclusion and recommendations for practice/future research

The conclusion provides a summary of the findings and suggests how these might be applied in practice, or how they might affect existing knowledge and understanding – the 'what now?' element. This might include a discussion of the limitations of the research, particularly for quantitative reports, and should give a final answer to the research question, giving a satisfying and strong end to the narrative journey.

Abstract

This should be written last. The format will depend on the publication/output but should include a brief summary of the research aim, methods, findings and conclusions.

Draft, edit, review, rewrite

No one submits their first draft. The key to good writing is editing. Do not fear the blank page. Write the report and then edit it, seeking feedback from a relevant person such as a tutor or expert friend (e.g. a colleague but *not* a fellow student). Focus on good-quality scholarly writing and a consistent style. Label each draft with the date you completed it and save each separately.

24 Implementation of healthcare research

Figure 24.1 Implementation of evidence-based practice (EBP).

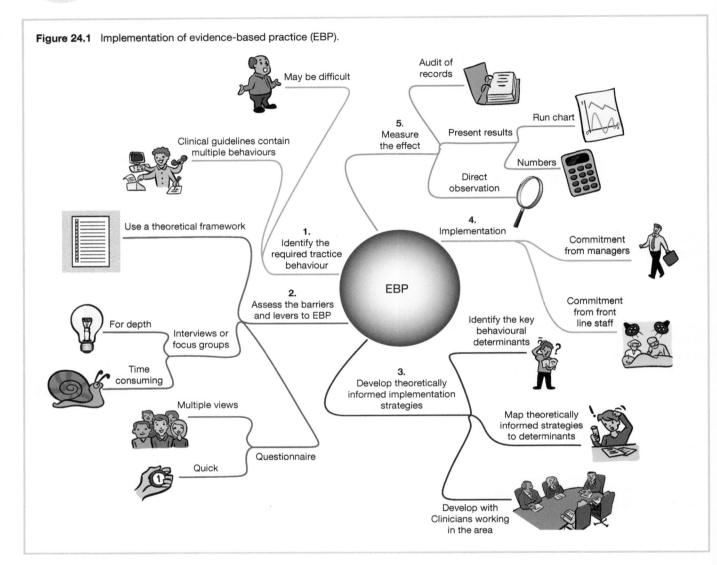

Evidence-based practice (EBP) is 'the conscientious, explicit and judicious use of current best evidence in making decisions about the care of individuals' (Sackett *et al.*, 2000). Evidence suggests that 30–40% of people do not receive care according to best practice, while 20–25% receive care that is harmful (Eccles *et al.*, 2005). The implementation of EBP practice (Figure 24.1) is important because if interventions known to be effective are offered to patients, positive health outcomes should result. Traditionally, dissemination of research findings was through peer review journals. It has been estimated that in order to be up to date a doctor would have to read 19 articles per day every day of the year (Sackett *et al.*, 2007). To make research more accessible to practitioners, best practice guidelines are commonly produced (e.g. National Institute for Health and Clinical Excellence, 2007). It was expected that guidelines would lead to a better uptake of EBP, thus improving the care patients receive. This is not the case: the impact of guidelines on care has been limited (Grimshaw *et al.*, 2004). There is a wealth of evidence to show that circulating guidelines to practitioners does not result in changed clinical practice. Furthermore, interventions to improve the implementation of EBP (e.g. audit and feedback, computerised reminder systems, opinion leaders) are not consistently effective (Grimshaw *et al.*, 2004) and the selection of interventions is often done on the basis of intuition.

In order to successfully implement EBP, it is necessary to:
1 accurately assess the barriers (things that hinder) and levers (things that help) to behaviour change in healthcare practitioners;
2 tailor implementation strategies accordingly (Baker *et al.*, 2015);
3 adopt a theoretical stance in the assessment of barriers and levers and in implementation interventions (Michie *et al.*, 2005).

Problems

Because the implementation of EBP requires the adoption of practices or behaviours by a healthcare practitioner, theories of behaviour change provide a sound theoretical platform. However, there are many theoretical models to choose from and those that exist are complex and therefore difficult to access by non-experts such as healthcare practitioners.

Solutions

To address this, the Theoretical Domains Framework (TDF) (Michie *et al.*, 2005) has been developed as an accessible, comprehensive, theoretically sound framework to support the implementation of EBP. The TDF considers the individual along with their social and environmental context. It is based on 128 constructs, which were extracted from 33 behaviour change theories and grouped to 11 key domains: knowledge, skills, social/professional role and identity, beliefs about capabilities, beliefs about consequences, motivation and goals, memory attention and decision processes, environmental context and resources, social influences, emotion and action planning. Each of these domains represent behavioural determinants that are mediators of behaviour change. Example questions to illicit barriers and levers within each domain are included for use.

To move from the assessment of barriers and levers to producing tailored implementation strategies requires a taxonomy of theory-linked defined behaviour change techniques linked to the domains of the TDF. This provides the solution most likely to influence implementation behaviour according to identified barriers (or absence of levers) and the domains within which they fit (Michie *et al.*, 2008). Examples of these techniques include graded tasks, rehearsal of skills and social pressures of encouragement, pressure and support. These can form the basis of pragmatic interventions.

Value

There are a great number of published examples of the framework being used effectively and successfully in both implementation research and to enhance the implementation of EBP. An example of both is the work of Taylor *et al.* (2013) who worked in three hospitals to support the implementation of evidence-based guidelines to reduce the risk of feeding into misplaced nasogastric tubes. The approach has also been recently adopted by organisations such as the Improvement Academy in a regional Academic Health Science Network (one of the 15 UK innovative networks set up to harness world class partnerships to transform healthcare).

References

Baker, R., Camosso-Stefinovic, J., Gillies, C. *et al.* (2015) Tailored interventions to address determinants of practice. *Cochrane Database Syst Rev*, **4**.

Eccles, M., Grimshaw, J., Walker, A., Johnston, M. and Pitts, N. (2005) Changing the behavior of healthcare professionals: the use of theory in promoting the uptake of research findings. *Journal of Clinical Epidemiology* **58**, 107–112.

Grimshaw, J.M., Thomas, R.E., Maclennan, G. *et al.* (2004) Effectiveness and efficiency of guideline dissemination and implementation strategies. *Health Technology Assessment* **8**(6), iii–iv.

Michie, S., Johnson, M., Abraham, C., Lawton, R., Parker, D. and Walker, A. (2005) Making psychological theory useful for implementing evidence based practice: a consensus approach. *Quality and Safety in Health Care* **14**, 26–33.

Michie, S., Johnston, M., Francis, J., Hardeman, W. and Eccles, M. (2008) From theory to intervention: mapping theoretically derived behavioural determinants to behaviour change techniques. *Applied Psychology* **57**, 660–680.

National Institute for Health and Clinical Excellence (2007) *How to Change Practice: Understand, Identify and Overcome Barriers to Change*. London: NICE. https://www.nice.org.uk/Media/Default/About/what-we-do/Into-practice/Support-for-service-improvement-and-audit/How-to-change-practice-barriers-to-change.pdf

Sackett, D.L., Straus, S.E., Richardson, W.S., Rosenberg, W.M. and Haynes, B. (2000) *Evidence-based Medicine: How to Practice and Teach EBM*. London: Churchill Livingstone.

Sackett, D.L., Rosenberg, W.M., Muir Gray, J.A., Haynes, R.B. and Richardson, W.S. (2007) Evidence based medicine: what it is and what it isn't. *Clinical Orthopaedics and Related Research* **455**, 3–5.

Taylor, N., Lawton, R., Slater, B. and Foy, R. (2013) The demonstration of a theory-based approach to the design of localized patient safety interventions. *Implementation Science* **8**, 123.

25 Barriers to research utilisation

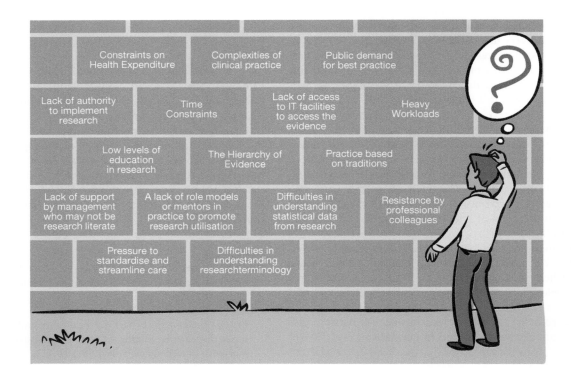

Figure 25.1 Barriers to research utilisation: 'Another brick in the wall!'

Originally, evidence-based practice (EBP) was only seen as the concern of medicine, as exemplified in Sackett *et al*.'s (1996, p. 71) definition:

> Evidence-based medicine is the conscientious, explicit and judicious use of current best evidence in making decisions about the care of individual patients.

Since then it has been recognised that all healthcare professionals need to apply EBP in order to utilise research in their own practice, to ensure clinical effectiveness and to improve patient outcomes (Fineout-Overholt *et al*., 2005). Moreover, this is seen as a means of standardising and streamlining care as well as decreasing costs (Scott and McSherry, 2008).

A useful five-step framework for research utilisation by Fineout-Overholt *et al*. (2005) identifies how EBP may be achieved.

Step 1: Asking the clinical question.

Step 2: Searching for the best evidence.

Step 3: Critically appraising the evidence.

Step 4: Addressing the sufficiency of the evidence: to implement or not to implement.

Step 5: Evaluating the outcome of evidence implementation.

However, barriers exist to achieving this in practice, as evidenced by a plethora of research studies over the last decade, much of which centred on nursing (Figure 25.1). The questionnaire Barriers and Facilitators to Using Research in Practice (Funk *et al*., 1995) has been used extensively with hospital-based nurses in countries such as Australia, Canada, China, Finland, Netherlands, Hong Kong, Ireland, Sweden, the UK and the USA to measure:

- organisation/setting in which the research will be applied;
- potential adopter of the research (i.e. their values, skills and awareness);
- communication/dissemination of the research (i.e. its presentation and accessibility);
- quality of the research itself.

Findings from these studies show that the top barriers are insufficient time to read or implement research, insufficient authority to change practice, lack of facilities, difficulty in understanding statistical analyses, and physicians not cooperating with implementation.

Other healthcare workers face barriers too, as McKenna *et al*. (2004) found in their large-scale study of primary care in the UK, including both general practitioners

(GPs) and community nurses. Using Funk's questionnaire, in conjunction with the Evidence-Based Medicine in Primary Care questionnaire, the top barrier for GPs was the uncertainty created by conflicting research results, whereas nurses ranked this in third place. Interestingly, neither group seemed aware that systematic reviews might clarify this uncertainty. GPs highlighted the limited relevance of research to practice as a significant barrier to EBP. This perhaps agrees with other discussions about the nature of evidence and what counts as evidence (Scott and McSherry, 2008). Randomised controlled trials, which are placed at the top of the hierarchy of evidence, do not necessarily translate well into the daily reality of complex practice or place the care of the individual patient or client in its actual context. Healthcare decision-making or professional judgement may rely on other forms of evidence such as qualitative findings or professional guidelines or even experiential knowledge. As Gerrish and Clayton (2004) observed, 'craft knowledge' is not usually concerned with transferability beyond the case of a particular patient or setting. Studies have shown that nurses in particular are more likely to draw on experiential knowledge, acquired through their interactions with patients and colleagues, than from textbooks and/or journals.

The practicalities of research utilisation need to be considered too. In hospital and community settings, particularly GP surgeries, decisions have to be taken fast. Practitioners cannot always access library or computer facilities for the latest findings such as Cochrane reviews, systematic reviews and meta-analyses, all of which require careful examination. Furthermore, these are not always as clear as the guidelines produced by, for example, the National Institute for Health and Care Excellence (NICE) (2012) or professional bodies. Some health professionals may have difficulties in understanding the terminology of research in academic journals, particularly statistical research. They may also have no access to EBP mentors or work in a setting with a lack of partnerships between the academic and clinical setting, all of which represent additional barriers to utilising research (Fineout-Overholt et al., 2005), even if they are keen to do so.

In nursing, there has been a discernible shift from tradition-based practice to EBP, but it faces almost insurmountable barriers. The lack of graduate-level education for many registered nurses across Europe is not conducive to creating a workforce able to critically interpret research and utilise it in practice. Aiken et al. (2014) in their recent analysis of 300 hospitals in Belgium, England, Finland, Ireland, Netherlands, Norway, Spain, Sweden and Switzerland identified that a 10% increase in the proportion of nurses with bachelor degrees in hospitals was associated with a 7% decrease in mortality, whereas an increase in a nurse's workload by just one patient increased the likelihood of a patient dying within 30 days of admission by 7%. Creating a research-literate healthcare workforce that has the time to care and utilise or translate research from 'bench to bed' is clearly in the interests of patients. However, if the many barriers to research utilisation are to be overcome, it will require a considerable investment in education, practice and research, which at a time of economic austerity may be almost impossible to attain.

References

Aiken L.H., Sloane D.M., Bruyneerl L. et al. (2014) Nurse staffing and hospital mortality in nine European countries: a retrospective observational study. *Lancet* **383**, 1824–1830.

Fineout-Overholt, E., Melnyck, B.N. and Schultz, A. (2005) Transforming health care from the inside out: affecting evidence-based practice in the 21st century. *Journal of Professional Nursing* **21**, 225–244.

Funk, S.G., Tournquist, E.M. and Champagne, M.T. (1995) Barriers and facilitators of research utilisation. *Nursing Clinics of North America* **30**, 395–407.

Gerrish, K. and Clayton, J. (2004) Promoting evidence-based practice: an organisational approach. *Journal of Nursing Management* **12**, 114–123.

McKenna, H.P., Ashton, S. and Keeney, S. (2004) Barriers to evidence-based practice in primary care. *Journal of Advanced Nursing* **45**, 178–189.

National Institute for Health and Care Excellence (NICE) (2012) Summary and implementation tools. In: *Healthcare-associated infections: prevention and control in primary and community care.* NICE Clinical Guidelines No. 139. Available at http://publications.nice.org.uk/infection-cg139/key-priorities-for-implementation

Sackett, D.L., Rosenburg, W.M.C., Muir Gray, J.A., Haynes, R.B. and Richardson, W.S. (1996) Evidence-based medicine: what it is and what it isn't. *British Medical Journal* **312**, 71–72.

Scott, K. and McSherry, R. (2008) Evidence-based nursing: clarifying concepts for nurses in practice. *Journal of Clinical Nursing* **18**, 1085–1095.

26 Designing service evaluations

Figure 26.1 Service evaluations are a way of measuring current practice with the aim of generating recommendations for improvements in service provision. This 10-step approach for conducting a service evaluation was developed by Marsh and Glendenning (2005).

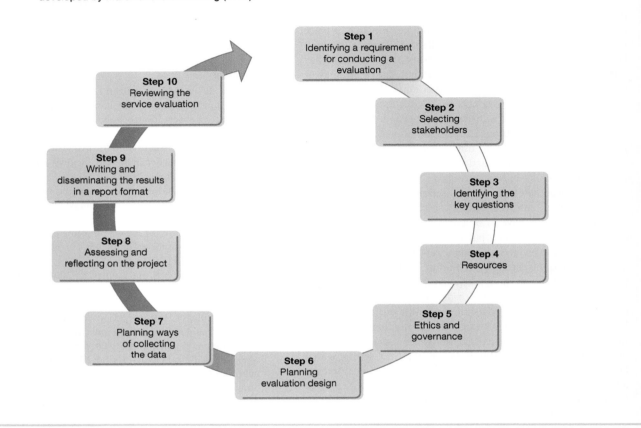

ervice evaluations are designed and conducted in order to provide a picture of the strengths and weaknesses of a service for the benefit of service users. A service evaluation provides evidence of the effectiveness of a service, resulting in changes in practice and improvements in quality of care.

Steps in a service evaluation

Marsh and Glendenning (2005) developed a service evaluation toolkit on behalf of the University of Cambridgeshire. Their model is a 10-step approach for conducting a service evaluation of any service within health and social care (Figure 26.1).

Step 1: Identify a requirement for conducting an evaluation

Often there will be something that prompts a service evaluation. For example, the service may have been in use for a long time without any evaluation; there might have been a complaint from a service user or observation from staff or peer review; an opportunity to change an aspect of the service might have arisen; there may be a greater need for using limited resources effectively; or there have been recent changes to best practice guidelines. Whatever the reasons, this first step of understanding and clarifying the drivers behind the service evaluation will enable subsequent steps, such as deciding on the stakeholders who should be involved and the development of focused and relevant key questions, to be answered. Therefore, a service evaluation is a way of providing practical information for service provision.

Step 2: Select stakeholders

When selecting stakeholders for a service evaluation it is important to consider whose voices need to be heard in order to see the complete picture of a service, or the specific part of the service, being evaluated. Getting this step right will help with the next step of identifying the appropriate questions to ask. Managers, commissioners, patients, family members, the general public and different staff members (e.g. nurses, physicians or physiotherapists) might all be stakeholders in the service under consideration. Stakeholders can be involved at every stage of service evaluation, such as planning, collecting information, interpretation and utilising the findings and dissemination of the results.

Step 3: Identify the key questions

A clear focused question helps to narrow down the service evaluation. A good question provides high-quality information and leads to an achievable and trustworthy evaluation. It can arise from the objectives of the service, the views of stakeholders or even a complaint from service users. The other criteria for selecting questions are that they should be specific, answerable, coherent, measurable and timely (Robson, 2002).

Step 4: Resources

Realistic resources in terms of availabile expertise, a firm timetable and finances need to be considered very carefully in order to maximise the output of a service evaluation.

Step 5: Ethics and governance

Conducting an evaluation requires high ethical standards, appropriate governance and an ethical manner; consent, privacy, confidentiality and risk to individuals should all be taken into consideration.

Step 6: Plan the evaluation design

The design of the service evaluation needs to be appropriate and able to answer the questions being asked. It also needs to be feasible (within the time scale and resources available) and ethical. A well-designed evaluation will provide conclusive data that result in key decisions.

Step 7: Plan ways of collecting the data

The method chosen for a service evaluation depends on the question about the service that needs to be answered. Key methods suggested are observation, focus groups, semi-structured and unstructured interviews (face-to-face or by phone), survey questionnaires, monitoring forms and searching documents. However, the chosen method also needs to be robust and provide appropriate evidence for making decisions.

Step 8: Assess and reflect on the project

A range of expertise is required when conducting the project, as well as a self-assessment for the evaluator. Therefore, there may be a requirement for training or expert support.

Step 9: Write and disseminate the results in a report format

The results of a service evaluation are usually presented in report form and shared with stakeholders, participants and interested local parties. Although the focus is often on local service issues, findings can and often do have wider resonance, so results often need to be shared nationally and internationally through publication in academic and professional journals, oral presentations and websites. However, feedback must take the audiences' culture into account. Providing an executive summary will be applicable.

Step 10: Review the service evaluation

This involves reviewing and rechecking the key points of the service evaluation's design and putting together the previous steps to ensure efficiency of evaluation (Marsh and Glendenning, 2005).

References and further reading

Marsh, P. and Glendenning, R. (2005) NHS Cambridgeshire Full Evaluation Toolkit. University of Sheffield: National Coordinating Centre for Research Capacity Development. Available at http://clahrc-cp.nihr.ac.uk/wp-content/uploads/2012/07/Full_Evaluation_Toolkit.pdf

Nolan, M. and Grant, G. (1993) Service evaluation: time to open both eyes. *Journal of Advanced Nursing* **18**, 1434–1442.

Robson, C. (2002) *Real World Research*, 2nd edn. Chichester: John Wiley & Sons Ltd.

27 Designing audit tools for measuring compliance

Figure 27.1 Designing healthcare audit tools for measuring compliance to care standards.

When auditing a service the following questions should be posed:
- Is it safe?
- Is it effective?
- Is it caring?
- Is it responsive to people's needs?
- Is it well-led?

> Audit tools can be designed to help healthcare staff make decisions and judgements pertinent to the compliance of a service to health and other policy standards.

Steps in developing an audit tool (Glasper and Farrelly, 2009)

- Investigate all policies and protocols which underpin the delivery of care to this client group.
- Selection of a topic (e.g. facilities for disabled children in hospital).
- Decide on criteria and standards for designing the tool (using for example the various policies related to childhood disability). Consider using an Excel spreadsheet with a separate worksheet for each section, with the facility to calculate percentage scores for each section.
- Pilot the audit tool to ascertain that the evidence criteria actually measure compliance.
- Determine how the data or information will be collected (e.g. how many patients' records will be surveyed).
- Collect the data following a strict time frame.
- Analyse the information and see if the results tally with the standards you have selected as the basis of your audit tool. Identify where compliance to the selected standards is suboptimal.
- Design and implement an action plan to address the areas of concern.
- Repeat the audit according to your action plan to monitor progress using the same audit tool.

Using an audit tool in practice settings

Stage 1:
Checking whether the evidence demonstrates compliance to policy standards/outcomes.

Stage 2:
If concerns are found, making a judgement about the impact on patients/families using services and the likelihood of the impact occurring.

Stage 3:
Validating the judgement.

Benchmarking

Benchmarking is simply comparing your practice against others offering similar services. Benchmarking allows both measurement (in the form of scores often using a 10-cm visual analogue, ordinal, non-parametric scale or colour coding such as Red, Amber, Green, i.e. RAG rating) and comparison and the sharing of best practice with other similar institutions of units. The metrification of audit tools is helpful for contributing to healthcare dashboard data (e.g. staffing levels).

Example of using colour ratings with percentage scores

Major concern ≤60% = Red
Moderate concern (≥60%) = Orange
Minor concern (≥70%) = Yellow
Compliant (≥85%) = Green

overnance belongs to all who work in health services not just doctors and nurses. Governance is not a top-down edict but a shared philosophy in which all can contribute as they deliver the best standard of care they can, while continually seeking improvement. Auditing services can help ensure safe high-quality care from all involved in the patient's journey and ensure that the client remains at the centre of the activities which support governance. Implementing governance to ensure that policy standards are met usually involves audit. This plays a key role in assessing how well an organisation is at meeting set standards and audit exists to improve the quality of patient care and clinical practice.

Developing a local audit topic

For example, Coles *et al.* (2007) reported measuring compliance to one of the standards of the children's national service framework in an English strategic health authority. They designed a tool that uses a five-point ordinal scale, with 1 indicating the lowest level of compliance and 5 the highest. The audit results demonstrate that there were a number of areas that required further work before all the criteria of the standard were fully met within the specified time envisaged by the Department of Health. The writers of policy and other similar documents usually couch their publications in such a way that the information embodied within can be easily converted into an audit tool. Hence, each standard in a policy document can become an individual worksheet. The Care Quality Commission, which is the healthcare regulator for England, uses key lines of enquiry in five domains to conduct audits of hospitals to ensure their compliance to national healthcare standards (Figure 27.1).

- Are they safe?
- Are they effective?
- Are they caring?
- Are they responsive to people's needs?
- Are they well-led?

Such audit tools can be used by child healthcare staff to help them make decisions and judgements about a children's hospital or a hospital ward's compliance with national child health and other policy standards pertinent to the care of children and young people in hospital.

Designing an audit tool

Many healthcare regulators prefer evidence to be metricised to facilitate percentage average scores, although some still use colour coding (RAG ratings). For example, the design of the Association of Chief Children's Nurses (ACCN) audit tool has been facilitated through the use of an Excel workbook spreadsheet, and the individual worksheets are orientated to overarching standards and benchmarks from a wide range of polices and national protocols.

The ACCN membership was supportive of metricising each of the audit sections to enable the formulation of evidence prompts (i.e. benchmarks with scores adding up to a maximum of 10) for each of the outcome subsections. In facilitating numerical scores (i.e. 0 to 10), these can subsequently be expressed as a percentage for each outcome. The Excel workbook has been designed to facilitate this function.

A discrete aspect of this audit tool has been designed to measure the compliance of individual clinical areas to those policies and standards which have been developed to illuminate best practice for the care of children with disabilities and complex illnesses. The final component of each Excel worksheet facilitates the development of an action plan for each of the measurable outcomes. This is designed to ensure that the audit tool is fit for purpose in driving up standards of care.

Some audit tools come already designed and available for use by practitioners; for example, Coles *et al.* (2013) describe how one large district general hospital was able to assess whether services for young people met English national young people friendly standards through a pan-hospital 'You're Welcome' audit tool using the *You're Welcome – Quality criteria for young people friendly health services* (Department of Health, 2011).

References

Coles, L., Glasper, E.A., Fitzgerald, C., LeFlufy, T., Turner, S. and Wilkes-Holmes, C. (2007) Measuring compliance to the NSF for children and young people in one English strategic health. *Journal of Children's and Young People's Nursing* **1**, 7–15.

Coles, L., Glasper, E.A. and Nicols, P. (2013) Are young people welcome in the English national health service? *Issues in Comprehensive Pediatric Nursing* **36**, 144–167.

Department of Health (2011) *You're Welcome: Quality criteria for young people friendly health services.* https://www.gov.uk/government/uploads/system/uploads/attachment_data/file/216350/dh_127632.pdf

Glasper, A. and Farrelly, R. (2009) Health care governance. In: A. Glasper, G. McEwing and J. Richardson (eds) *Foundation Studies for Caring*, chapter 8. Basingstoke: Palgrave Macmillan.

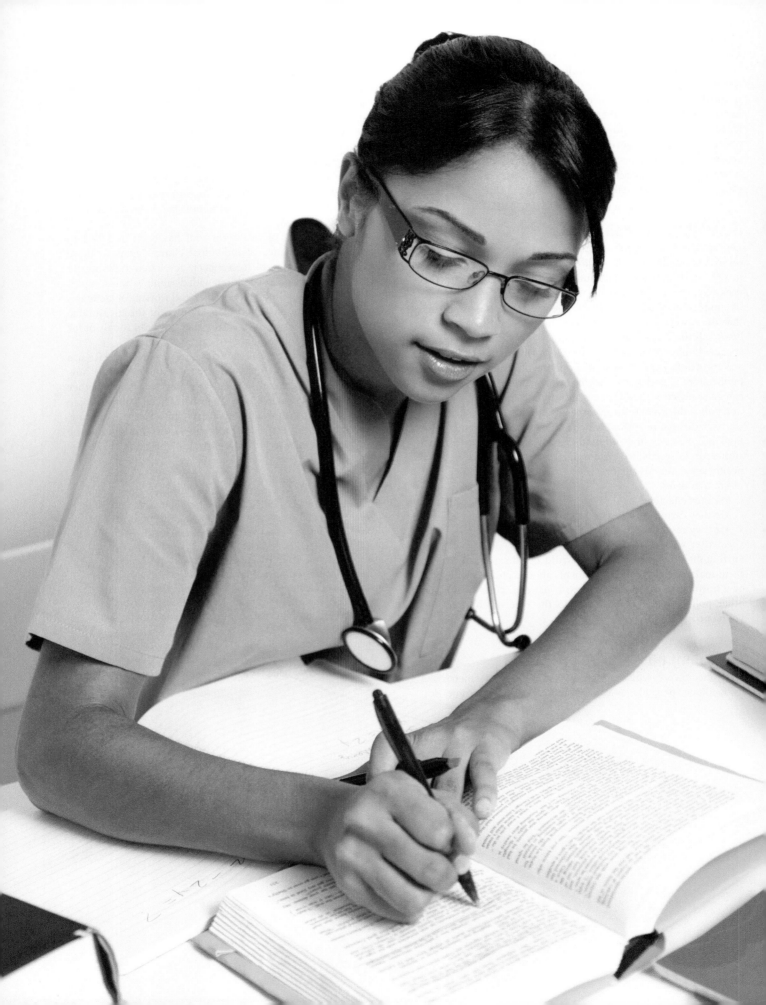

Quantitative research

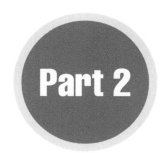

Part 2

Chapters

28 Quantitative and qualitative research approaches

Figure 28.1 Quantitative and qualitative research approaches.

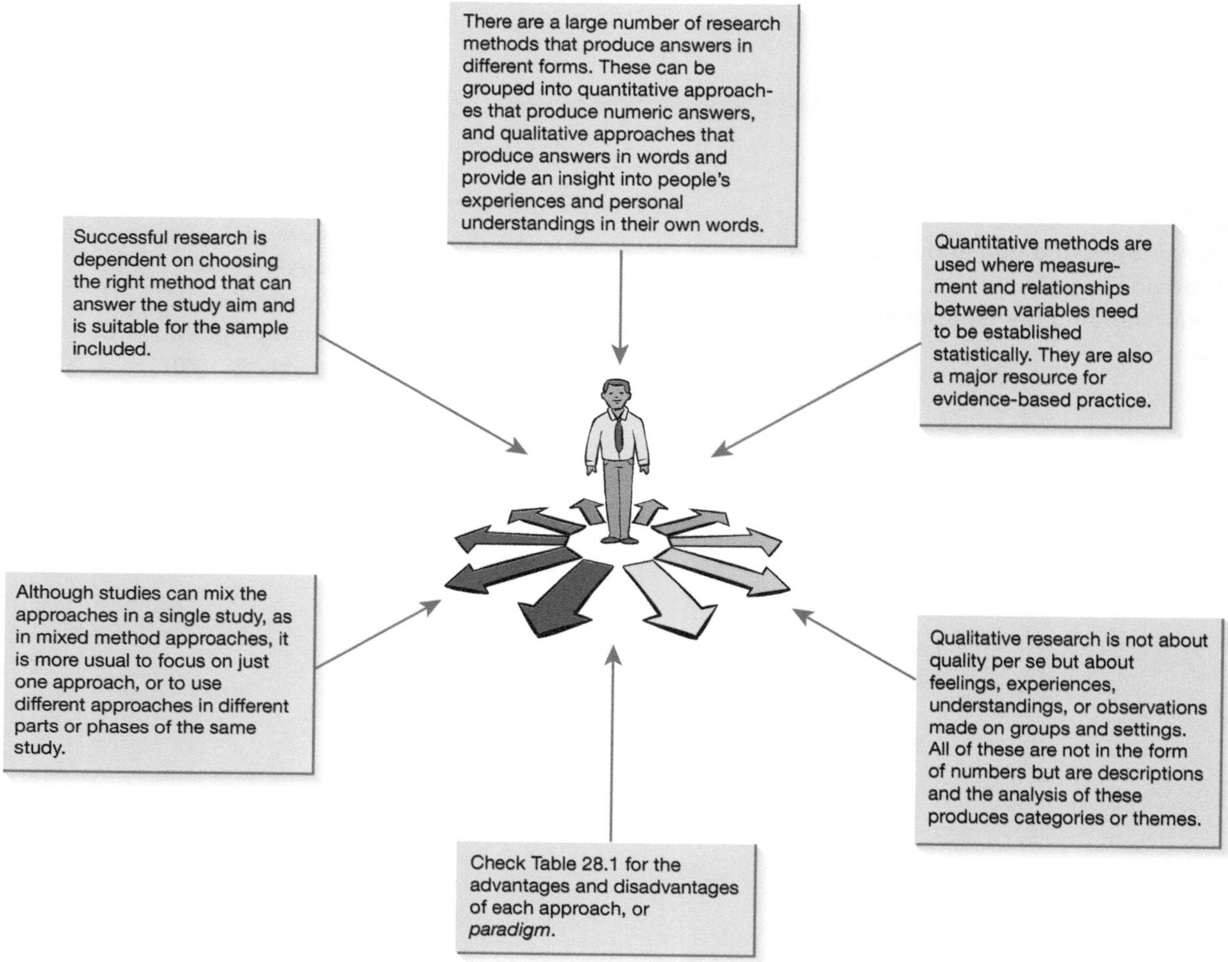

There are a large number of research methods that produce answers in different forms. These can be grouped into quantitative approaches that produce numeric answers, and qualitative approaches that produce answers in words and provide an insight into people's experiences and personal understandings in their own words.

Successful research is dependent on choosing the right method that can answer the study aim and is suitable for the sample included.

Quantitative methods are used where measurement and relationships between variables need to be established statistically. They are also a major resource for evidence-based practice.

Although studies can mix the approaches in a single study, as in mixed method approaches, it is more usual to focus on just one approach, or to use different approaches in different parts or phases of the same study.

Qualitative research is not about quality per se but about feelings, experiences, understandings, or observations made on groups and settings. All of these are not in the form of numbers but are descriptions and the analysis of these produces categories or themes.

Check Table 28.1 for the advantages and disadvantages of each approach, or *paradigm*.

Research is about getting answers to questions in an objective way using a systematic method that will provide the information required. We are familiar with many of the ways information is collected through research methods, which are the tools used to collect data, such as questionnaires, measuring scales such as pain or anxiety scales, observation and interviews. These are used in research approaches, and form the distinctive 'brand' of research such as experimental, survey and phenomenological approaches. These give the researcher the design or plan of action to follow as a template for successfully conducting the whole study. The choice of research approach is influenced by the research question and the nature of the data that will need to be collected.

Research has two major divisions that group together research approaches: quantitative and qualitative research (Figure 28.1). Each shares similarities, not only in the practical aspects of these brands, but also in the ideas and principles that underpin them. However, they differ in the way the researcher thinks about research as an activity and the role of the researcher within the whole research process. These two divisions are often referred to as research *paradigms* as they provide a total 'worldview' of the nature of the research process and how it should be conducted.

The differences between these alternative approaches can be quite stark, so it is worth identifying a number of elements they have in common. Firstly, they are both underpinned by an ethical approach that sees the safety of those taking part as a fundamental starting point. This is expressed under the principle of the avoidance of harm, whether physical, psychological, social or financial. In other words, the individual must not be put at risk as part of the research process. Similarly, a major emphasis in both paradigms is the emphasis on rigour during the study as a safeguard to producing accurate results. This takes the form of the researcher carefully following the research proposal and ensuring that each component is carried out to the highest standard. However, as can be seen from Table 28.1, there are very clear differences in the conduct of a study in each paradigm across the other stages in the research process.

Table 28.1 Major differences between quantitative and qualitative research.

Quantitative research approaches	Qualitative research approaches
Emphasis on measurement and relationships between variables	Emphasis on understanding human behaviour and presenting findings through words rather than numbers
Narrowly worded aim that requires numeric data to answer it. The emphasis is on objectivity and measurable outcomes that can be statistically processed	Broadly worded aim, often including the word 'explore', requiring a descriptive approach to answer it using the views, experiences, descriptions from individuals in their own words, or direct observational descriptions from the researcher
Early in-depth use of the literature to influence direction and content of the study	Early use of the literature avoided so ideas and analysis are not influenced by previous studies. Literature is reviewed and used once analysis has taken place to support or contrast with current findings
Use of large sample sizes to ensure results can be generalised if indicated by statistical calculations	Use of smaller samples providing in-depth data from which greater understanding can emerge from the analysis of the findings
Use of deduction as a way of analysis, starting with a theory and establishing the truth of this through the collection of the data	Use of induction as a way of analysis, starting with the findings and then constructing a theory that may explain the findings
Central focus on being able to generalise from the data and apply to other like situations	Central focus on being able to understand and gain insights from the data. Although the purpose is not to generalise from the results in detail, there is an intention that the general principles emerging from findings may have some transferability to other locations

29 Understanding the randomised controlled trial

Figure 29.1 The randomised controlled trial (RCT).

> The first recorded controlled trial is cited in the Old Testament in the book of Daniel. Verses 1–21 clearly describe this trial of diet and its effect on countenance

> The Critical Appraisal Skills Programme (CASP) offers a critiquing tool which asks 10 questions to help in understanding how RCTs function (http://www.casp-uk.net/)

> In 1747 James Lind conducts the first 'modern' trial that demonstrates the efficacy of lemon juice in preventing scurvy

Features of a randomised controlled trial

Control group
- A sample (cases)
- Random allocation to this group
- No intervention or a control standard intervention
- Measurable outcomes

Experimental group
- A sample (cases)
- Random allocation to this group
- An intervention
- Measurable outcomes

NB In an RCT crossover design, each group in turn acts as the control/experimental group

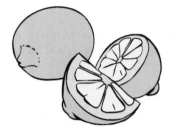

A randomised controlled trial when published in a peer-reviewed journal should answer the following questions:

1. Did the study ask a clearly focused question?
2. Was this a randomised controlled trial and was it appropriately so?
3. Were participants appropriately allocated to intervention and control groups?
4. Were participants, staff and study personnel 'blind' to participants' study group?
5. Were all the participants who entered the trial accounted for at its conclusion?
6. Were the participants in all groups followed up and data collected in the same way?
7. Did the study have enough participants to minimise the play of chance?
8. How are the results presented and what is the main result?
9. How precise are these results?
10. Were all important outcomes considered so the results can be applied?

The randomised controlled trial (RCT) (Figure 29.1) is regarded as the gold standard in research and is used primarily to measure differences in outcomes between, for example, a control group of patients who are taking standard medication for the management of hypertension and a group who are administered a new generation drug. Lattimer *et al.* (1998) will be used as an example study to explore the parameters of the RCT using the 10 Critical Appraisal Skills Programme (CASP) questions.

Did the study ask a clearly focused question?

Yes: to determine the safety and effectiveness of nurse telephone consultation in out-of-hours primary care.
- Population: 97,000 registered patients in Wiltshire.
- Intervention: a nurse telephone service.
- Outcomes: adverse events.

Was it a randomised controlled trial?

Yes: the title of the paper indicates this and this approach was deemed most appropriate given the paucity of UK data at that time.

Were the subjects appropriately allocated to an intervention and control group?

Yes. The trial year was divided into 26 blocks of 2 weeks. A random number generator on a pocket calculator was used to allocate certain out-of-hour periods, for example Tuesday evenings, to receive the intervention (the nurse-operated telephone service), the other period being allocated to the normal GP service.

Nursing and Healthcare Research at a Glance, First Edition. Alan Glasper and Colin Rees. © 2017 by John Wiley & Sons, Ltd. Published 2017 by John Wiley & Sons, Ltd.

How were participants allocated to a study group?

The setting was a 55-member general practice cooperative and the subjects were all patients contacting the out-of-hours service during specified periods over the trial year, randomly a nurse or doctor.

Were all participants, staff and study personnel blind to participants study group?

The pattern of intervention was known only to the lead investigators. Nurses and doctors were blind to the intervention until a point when they would be unable to choose or swap duty periods. Bias was therefore eliminated. The doctor versus nurse pattern was not publicised and would only have become apparent to the public on the day of calling.

Were all participants accounted for?

Yes: 7308 patient calls in the control group and 7184 in the intervention group.

Were all the participants in all groups followed up and data collected in the same way?

Yes.
• Data on workload were downloaded from the database of calls.
• Data on mortality were obtained from the Office for National Statistics.
• Data on admissions were obtained from local hospitals.
• Data on advice to attend an emergency department were obtained from cooperative records.

Did the study have enough participants to minimise the play of chance?

Yes: 'we calculated that 5,455 patients would be required in each arm of the trial using a formula described by Jones *et al*'. The study was only interested in whether the nurse service produced worse results than the normal doctor service (equivalence methodology). The trial actually used over 7000 patients in each arm.

How are the results presented and what is the main result?

• An equivalence methodology was used to assess the performance of nurses to doctors.
• Data was shown in table format and reiterated within the text.
• 49.8% of calls to nurses were managed without referral to a doctor, generating significant reductions in workload for doctors.
• No significant events in the intervention group compared to the control. For telephone management, visit to the care centre, or home visit by GP, deaths, hospital admission within 24 hours, hospital admission within 3 days, or attendance at accident and emergency department.

How precise are the results?

Confidence intervals were used to estimate the likely size of the study group behaviour, in this case deaths, admission to hospital or accident and emergency department, or GP visit. Most commonly used is the 95% interval, as in this study, in which the investigators were 95% certain that the true results would lie in the range they calculated, e.g. for deaths, 45–75 in the nurse-led group (58 actually) and 53–83 in the control group (67 actually).

Were all the important results considered so the results can be applied?

Yes, but the researchers recommended that further testing would be required of variants to the system used in this trial, 'including the selection and training of nurses and the decision support software used'.

The crossover RCT

Elbourne *et al.* (2002) discuss another type of RCT, the crossover design where all individuals receive both the intervention being tested and an alternative. In other words, by experiencing both the experimental intervention and the control intervention, they act as their own controls. Depending on the particular study this can be an alternative intervention, placebo or no treatment. The element of randomisation here is the order in which an individual experiences the two alternatives; they may have the intervention first and then the control second, or vice versa. The washout period ensures that time is given for an active intervention to pass through the body and not influence a subsequent intervention and so distort the findings.

Experimental group	Control group
Sample (cases)	Sample (cases)
Random allocation of intervention	Random allocation of intervention
Intervention	Alternative or no intervention
Outcomes	Outcomes
Washout period	Washout period
'Crossover': this is so each group in turn acts as the control/experimental group	'Crossover': this is so each group in turn acts as the control/experimental group

References

Elbourne, D.R., Altman, D.C., Higgins, J., Curtin, F., Worthington, H.V. and Vail, A. (2002) Meta-analyses involving cross-over trials: methodological issues. *International Journal of Epidemiology* **31**, 140–149.

Lattimer, V., George, S., Thompson, F. *et al.* (1998) Safety and effectiveness of nurse telephone consultation in out of hours primary care: randomised controlled trial. The South Wiltshire Out of Hours Project (SWOOP) Group. *British Medical Journal* **317**, 1054–1059.

30 Quasi-experimental study design

Figure 30.1 Quasi-experimental design: an illustration.

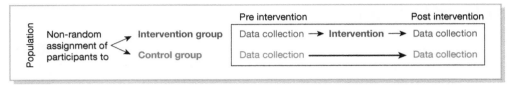

Figure 30.2 Quasi-experimental post-test/after-only design.

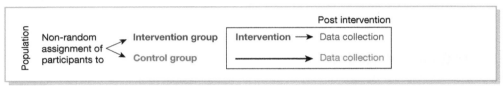

Figure 30.3 Non-equivalent control group design.

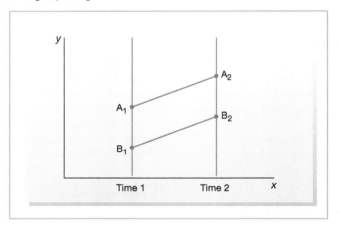

Figure 30.4 Time series design.

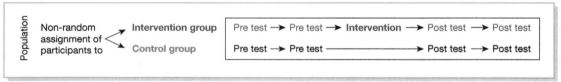

Quasi-experimental studies are those quantitative studies that aim to evaluate interventions but without the use of randomisation. Quasi-experimental designs are used when the researcher wants to explore the cause and effect relation between two variables, is able to manipulate the independent variable but is unable to use experimental design due to any issues with randomisation (e.g. ethical issues with randomisation; insufficient sample to achieve randomisation; practical or other constraints).

These designs are extensively used in the field of sociology, psychology and education. An example of a quasi-experimental study could be one where a researcher wants to explore the effectiveness of simulated teaching for a group of nursing students learning to use aseptic technique. The researcher divides the class of 50 students into two groups by using an alphabetical list of their names. The first 25 students are assigned to group A and the next 25 students are assigned to group B. Note that the researcher has not used any randomisation technique or procedure to assign these students to either group. Group A will then be taught using simulation strategies and Group B will be taught using normal teaching strategies and the results compared between the two (Figure 30.1). Data from both groups will be collected before and after the intervention. It is also possible that data are collected at one point, i.e. after the intervention (Figure 30.2).

Nursing and Healthcare Research at a Glance, First Edition. Alan Glasper and Colin Rees. © 2017 by John Wiley & Sons, Ltd. Published 2017 by John Wiley & Sons, Ltd.

Types of quasi-experimental design

There are numerous forms of quasi-experimental design and each has different strengths, limitations and applications. Some examples (but not all) are described in the following sections.

Non-equivalent control group design

This is the most commonly used design in some disciplines such as nursing and social sciences. In this design, data are collected and compared at two or more different times (Figure 30.3). Considering the example mentioned in the previous section, data will be collected from both groups (A and B) at time 1 (before using the simulation teaching method) and at time 2 (after using the simulation teaching method) and compared for the dependent variable (in this case, aseptic technique). As mentioned previously, it is also possible to collect data after the intervention only (post test) as shown in Figure 30.2.

Non-equivalent group design means the research is conducted on groups that are assumed to be similar; however, it is unlikely that the two groups are as similar as they would be if the assignment was random. In other words, groups may be different prior to assignment and that prior difference may have an impact on study outcome. This design can be further classified into other designs as follows:

- no-treatment control group design;
- non-equivalent dependent variables design;
- removed treatment group design;
- repeated treatment design;
- reversed treatment non-equivalent control group design;
- cohort design;
- post-test only design;
- regression continuity design.

Time series designs

In these designs, pre-test and post-test data are collected at different intervals (Figure 30.4). It is important to remember that the number of pre-tests and post-tests can vary. The design is used to determine the effects of the intervention over longer periods and to explore trends. Various types of time series design include:

- multiple time series design;
- interrupted time series design.

Other quasi-experimental designs

There are many other quasi-experimental designs and these may include:

- panel studies;
- proxy pre-test design;
- separate pre-post samples design;
- double pre-test design;
- non-equivalent dependent variables design;
- regression point displacement design;
- regression discontinuity analysis.

A similarity in all these methods is the lack of randomisation. Generally, a review of available evidence suggests that quasi-experimental designs can mainly be categorised into three major types: those that do not use a control group, those that use a control group but no pre-test, and those that use a control group as well as pre-test.

Advantages and disadvantages of quasi-experimental designs

Quasi-experimental designs are very effective as it is often very difficult to conduct true experiments, especially when dealing with human subjects, such as in healthcare and social research. Specifically, randomisation is not always possible in all research due to ethical, moral, legal and practical reasons. Quasi-experimental designs in such conditions can prove to be the best option and are therefore practical and feasible. In addition, the generalisability of the findings of quasi-experimental research is considered to be better compared with other non-experimental and observational designs and are time and resource efficient compared with experimental designs.

The major disadvantage of quasi-experimental design lies in the threats to internal validity (Table 30.1), which arise as a result of the absence of randomisation. Where randomisation is not used, any non-equivalence between groups will have an effect on the outcome. Similarly, in designs where people self-select to treatment or control situations, those in the groups may have different characteristics and make comparisons difficulty. In addition, where there is no control group, the effects of maturation (also known as historical effects, i.e. the changes taking place over time which may affect the outcome measures) cannot be accounted for. It is thereby difficult to control the effect of confounding factors on the findings of the study, resulting in difficulty in establishing cause and effect relationship between two variables. However, some quasi-experimental designs are more internally valid than others.

Table 30.1 Threats to internal validity.

Term	Description
Selection bias	When participants can select their own group (intervention or control) or decide themselves whether to participate or not to participate in the study
Experimental mortality	When participants discontinue/withdraw from the study
History	An event, in addition to the independent variable, that occurs during the study which has an effect on the study outcome
Maturation effect	Developmental, biological or psychological processes resulting in change in the participants' performance over time
Testing	Effect of taking a pre test on the scores post test
Instrumentation	Changes in the measurement of the variable and/or observation techniques affecting the resulting outcome

Further reading
Harris, A.D., Bradham, D.D., Baumgarten, M., Zuckerman, I.H., Fink, J.C. and Perencevich, E.N. (2004) The use and interpretation of quasi-experimental studies in infectious diseases. *Clinical Infectious Diseases* **38**, 1586–1591.
Smith, G. (2008) Experiments. In: R. Watson, H. McKenna, S. Cowman and J. Keady (eds) *Nursing Research: Design and Methods*, pp. 189–198. Edinburgh: Churchill Livingstone Elsevier.

31 Case-control studies

Figure 31.1 Case-control study design.

Sequence of events

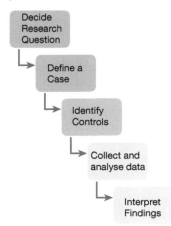

Decide Research Question

→ Define a Case

→ Identify Controls

→ Collect and analyse data

→ Interpret Findings

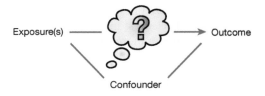

Exposure(s) ———— ? ——→ Outcome

Confounder

Measure of association: odds ratio

	Outcome present	Outcome absemt
Exposure present	a	b
Exposure absent	c	d

OR = ad/bc
If OR = 1, no association
If OR >1, positive association
If OR <1, negative association

Advantages

- Useful for generating a hypothesis
- Cheaper and quicker to conduct than cohort studies
- Useful for rare outcomes
- Can study multiple exposures/risk factors

Disadvantages

- Can only look at one outcome
- Retrospective
- Susceptible to bias
- Sampling and information bias can affect cases and controls
- Difficult to choose an appropriate control group
- Difficult to establish temporality
- Not possible to determine disease frequency

Example

Sir Richard Doll used a case–control study design in 1947 to compare the smoking history of a group of hospitalised patients with lung cancer with the smoking history of a similar group without lung cancer. A hypothesis was generated that smoking can cause lung cancer. This was further explored and confirmed in a cohort study by A.B. Hill in 1951.

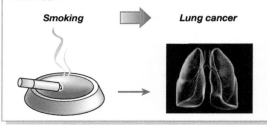

Smoking ⟹ *Lung cancer*

A case-control study is an observational study. This study design is frequently used for studying predictors of rare outcomes, such as sudden infant death syndrome (SIDS). Case-control studies are retrospective and trace backwards from an outcome to exposures (Figure 31.1). Cases are those who have developed the outcome of interest and their previous histories are compared with the histories of controls that have not developed the outcome of interest. This is a useful technique if there is a long latent period between an exposure and an outcome, for example smoking and lung cancer. Case-control studies generate hypotheses that can then be further tested in other studies of a different design, such as a cohort study or randomised controlled trial (RCT).

Conducting a case–control study

Research question
The first step when conducting a case-control study is to clearly outline the research question in terms of the study population (source of cases and controls), outcome, potential exposures/risk factors and potential confounders. A confounder is a third factor that is associated with the exposure and which affects the outcome but is not an intermediate link in the causal pathway. For example, when exploring a possible association between smoking and lung cancer, the environment could be a potential confounder.

Identify cases
Next, outline the criteria for defining a case in terms of time, place and person. In an outbreak investigation, cases from a certain time period, in a certain area and of a certain age and/or gender are included. When the outcome is a disease, the case definition should include clinical symptoms, laboratory results and diagnostic methods used. Diagnostic criteria should be sensitive and specific. Cases can be identified from disease registers or healthcare settings, such as medical records in the hospital or general practitioner's surgery.

Identify controls
The selection of controls is difficult due to the potential introduction of bias, i.e. prejudice for or against one person or group. Controls should be selected from the same source population as the cases and should be at risk of becoming new cases. The ratio of cases to controls can vary from 1:1 to 1:4; if cases are difficult to locate, the number of controls can be increased instead. Controls can be chosen from the general population in the community or from the hospital setting.

Hospital controls have several appealing features: convenience, low cost to identify and interview, comparable information quality as cases, motivation to participate, and comparable healthcare-seeking behaviour. However, hospital controls are not typical of the healthy population, for example they are more likely to smoke. If possible, bias can be reduced by using two control groups, i.e. hospital and community controls. Findings consistent across the different settings would be more robust.

Collect data
Data must conform to the principle of comparable accuracy and thus be measured in a consistent fashion for both cases and controls. Methods to measure exposures included in a study should be predetermined. Various data sources include medical records, patient interviews and surveys. Medical records are convenient as they already exist. However, only data recorded can be extracted and the accuracy of recorded data may vary between records. The use of interviews or surveys can introduce recall bias as a case may be more likely to recall exposure to a potentially toxic source. If possible, data collectors should be 'blind' (i.e. unaware) with regard to the case or control status of the participant to reduce measurement bias.

Analyse data
Cases and controls are initially compared using standard parametric and non-parametric tests to calculate means, medians and proportions. Multiple logistic regression modelling is then used to determine the association between the outcome and the exploratory variables while adjusting for confounders. Logistic regression estimates an odds ratio (OR) for the associations of key exploratory variables with the outcome of interest. The OR is a suitable measure when the disease is rare in the population and controls are selected to represent the same source population that gives rise to the cases, not just the non-cases. In this scenario, the OR usually approximates the relative risk.

An OR of 1 implies that no association exists between the exposure and the outcome. An OR >1 implies a positive association (e.g. OR = 4 for smoking and lung cancer suggests that smokers are four times more likely to develop lung cancer). An OR <1 implies a negative association (e.g. OR of 0.5 for non-smoking and stroke suggests that non-smokers are only half as likely to get a stroke compared with smokers).

Interpret findings
Extreme caution needs to be exercised when interpreting the findings of a case-control study. Consider whether bias and confounding have been adequately addressed. A careful choice of cases and controls is needed to reduce selection bias (also known as sampling bias). Consistent data collection methods for both cases and controls are needed to reduce information bias (also known as measurement, observation or classification bias).

Confounding should be controlled for in the design and/or analysis stages. One way of reducing confounding is to use a technique called matching, either on an individual basis (e.g. by pairing each case with a control of the same gender and age) or in groups (choosing a control group with an overall gender and age distribution similar to that of the cases). In the analysis stage, logistic regression further considers the effects of confounders.

Any hypothesis generated from a case-control study should be further explored using different study designs.

Example
Case–control studies that are well designed and conducted provide useful information. Various case-control studies were used to explore possible exposures associated with lung cancer. As illustrated in Figure 31.1, a link between cigarette smoking and lung cancer was observed in a case–control study and this hypothesis was subsequently further tested using a cohort study. Today, smoking is well recognised as a major risk factor in the development of lung cancer.

Further reading
Grimes, D.A. and Schulz, K.F. (2002) Bias and causal associations in observational research. *Lancet* **359**, 248–252.
Grimes, D.A. and Schulz, K.F. (2005) Compared to what? Finding controls for case–control studies. *Lancet* **365**, 1429–1433.
Schulz, K.F. and Grimes, D.A. (2002) Case–control studies: research in reverse. *Lancet* **359**, 431–434.

32 Cross-sectional design

Figure 32.1 An example of a cross-sectional design.

Cross-sectional design: Academic job stratification by years of experience

	Groups (three groups)	Method At one period of time
1	Less than 2 years experience	Interview
2	2–10 years experience	Interview
3	Greater than 10 years experience	Interview

Figure 32.2 Relationship of cross-sectional design to other studies.

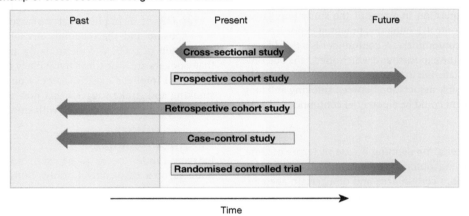

Source: Levin, K.A. (2006) Study design III: cross-sectional studies. Evidence-based Dentistry 7, 24–25. Reproduced with permission of Nature Publishing Group

Figure 32.3 Cross-sectional design: groups and time.

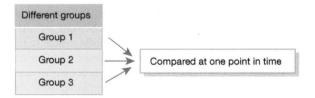

Why cross-sectional design?

Imagine you are planning to build a new home. Before you can order the materials (bricks, windows, timber, fittings, pipes, etc.) you need to have a clear idea of the building's structure or design. A suitable design is the first step and this sets the tone for all that follows. This is no different for the design of a research study and, as such, the research design ensures that the evidence collected or observed enables researchers to answer the initial question as unambiguously as possible. The research facilitated by a cross-sectional design enables researchers to avoid a random allocation of subjects to 'groups'; to collect data at one point in time; to allow for at least one independent variable with at least two categories being present; and to rely on existing variations in the independent variable(s) in the sample.

What is cross-sectional design?

In medical, health and social science research cross-sectional design is a form of observational or descriptive research that allows for the collection and analysis of data from a population or a subset of a population at one specific point in time, like a snapshot. Health surveys and censuses are examples of cross-sectional studies and they sit in the epidemiological paradigm. Cross-sectional design is also known as cross-sectional analysis, cross-sectional study, prevalence study or transversal study. Cross-sectional design research is commonly used to investigate the prevalence of medical conditions, to answer questions about the cause of disease or the results of intervention on disease. Cross-sectional design has three principal features: no time dimension, 'groups' based on existing differences rather than random allocation, and a reliance on existing differences rather than on a change following intervention.

An example of a cross-sectional design would be a one-off study that measures the levels of satisfaction academics feel at work. One approach could involve one group of academics and explore their satisfaction over time (as in a longitudinal study), but this would take many years to generate the data. Using a cross-sectional design, a study could be created with three groups: group 1, new academics with less than 2 years experience; group 2, those who have been academics for 2–10 years; and group 3, those who have been academics over 10 years (Figure 32.1). The study would then seek to explore and compare the differences in their level of academic satisfaction at one point in time. The cross-sectional design therefore allows a comparison of the three groups in terms of their difference on the dependent variable.

Time

In a standard cross-sectional design the data are collected at one point in time. As such, a cross-sectional design only measures differences between groups, rather than any change over time.

Groups based on existing differences (rather than random allocation)

Because the data in a cross-sectional design are collected at one point in time, all analysis rests on existing differences in the sample (the groups) at that point in time. This is unlike other research designs where what is sought are differences that are evident over time or with experimental designs that create variation in the independent variable with an intervention (Figures 32.2 and 32.3). A standard cross-sectional design relies on the group's pre-existing differences (in the example above, the group differences and thus allocation was based on the academics' length of service).

Reliance on existing differences rather than on a change following intervention

With experimental design, individuals are randomly allocated to groups prior to any experimental intervention so that groups are basically identical. In cross-sectional design, groups are constructed or established on the basis of existing differences in the sample. The groups are therefore established according to the category of the independent variable to which they belong. However, because there is no randomisation, the groups may well be different in other respects and this can have unforeseen impacts on the data.

Sample size

The sample size depends on funds, access to participants and time. In general, the larger the sample the better, although beyond a certain point the sample-size benefit diminishes.

Advantages

- Less expensive to undertake than some other study designs (e.g. longitudinal designs), although other designs may offer stronger evidence.
- Allows for the speedy collection of large cross-sectional data because there is no time dimension to consider in the study design.
- Although one-off cross-sectional studies lack a time dimension, this can be partly overcome with repeated one-off studies with a different sample at each point in time.
- Opportunities for external validity are greater with cross-sectional design, as gaining a representative sample of the wider population to support generalised data may be more likely.
- Offers descriptive data that can generate hypotheses.

Disadvantages

- Not suitable for the study of rare diseases.
- May not offer data about which variable is the cause, and thus the effect observed may be the result of another unsought or unknown variable. Where the data are based on issues with strong personal feelings, respondent bias may be evident.
- There may be threats to internal validity, with the main concerns relating to problems of establishing 'cause' without a time dimension and problems of establishing the level of 'meaning'. This can be addressed at the data analysis stage of the study by statistically removing differences between the groups after the data have been collected.

Further reading

de Vaus, D. (2001) *Research Design in Social Research*. London: Sage.

de Vaus, D. (2014) *Surveys in Social Research*, 6th edn. New York: Routledge.

Watson, R., McKenna, H., Cowman, S. and Keady, J. (eds) (2008) *Nursing Research: Design and Methods*. Edinburgh: Churchill Livingstone Elsevier.

33 Survey research methods

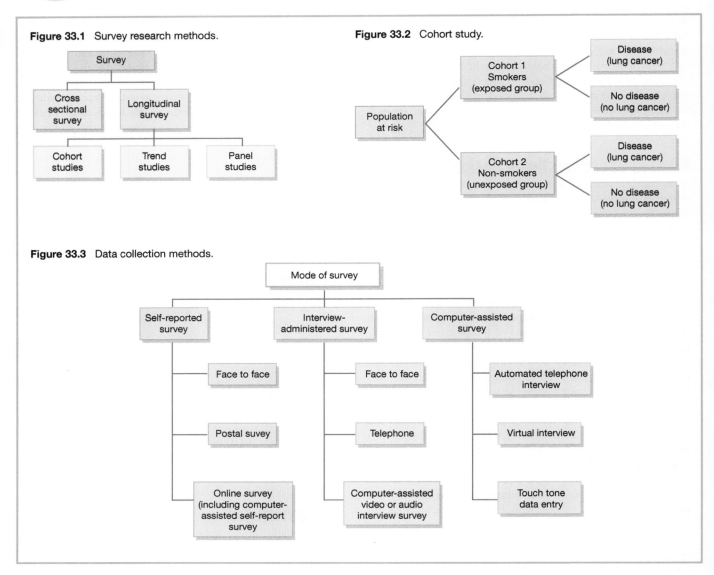

Figure 33.1 Survey research methods.

Figure 33.2 Cohort study.

Figure 33.3 Data collection methods.

A survey is a descriptive and non-experimental research method that involves the collection of information from individuals in the population through their responses to questions. It is the most popular method not only in healthcare research but in almost every field and discipline.

Types of survey

There are two main types of survey (Figure 33.1).

Cross-sectional surveys

Cross-sectional surveys provide information on a sample of a population at a single point in time, are relatively easy to conduct but may provide limited information, and can be used

for example to assess level of satisfaction of patients with triage services provided in emergency departments.

Longitudinal surveys

Longitudinal surveys are those that report on the data collected over a longer period. For instance, data are collected about the population of a city over 10 years and the researcher may use the data to study changes in demography. There are three subtypes of longitudinal study.

Cohort studies

These focus on a group of people with defined characteristics. The group is followed over time to observe the incidence of a disease of some other outcome. For instance, to explore if

Nursing and Healthcare Research at a Glance, First Edition. Alan Glasper and Colin Rees. © 2017 by John Wiley & Sons, Ltd. Published 2017 by John Wiley & Sons, Ltd.

smoking causes lung cancer, a group of smokers and a group of non-smokers will be followed over time to determine how many of them in each group develop cancer (Figure 33.2).

Trend studies

Trend studies help in exploring a pattern or trend of something in a particular population. Trend studies are used to predict future events or estimate uncertain events in the past. These studies are conducted over a longer period, but do not need to be conducted on the same population or by the same researchers. An example of a trend study would be where changes in patients' attitudes towards triage by the nurses in an emergency department are followed over time.

Panel studies

Panel studies aim to follow a specific group of people over a long period to assess changes in their attitudes towards something. Data from the same participants are collected at regular intervals using the same measures. Panel studies can be quantitative or qualitative. The British Household Panel Survey conducted by the Institute of Social and Economic Research is an example of a panel study. Panel studies can be extremely helpful for learning about a specific variable but may be difficult to conduct. Such studies are time and cost intensive and may also suffer from higher attrition rates of the participants.

Data collection methods

Data collection in survey research is mainly done through questionnaires and interviews (Figure 33.3). A questionnaire is an instrument that contains questions or statements with choices to answer for the participants. A questionnaire may be administered by the respondents themselves, or by an interviewer or researcher.

Self-administered questionnaires can be administered as paper and pencil questionnaires, postal surveys (those sent through the post) or online survey (those conducted using online tools such as SurveyMonkey®). They can be administered to individuals in private or in a group setting.

Interviewer-administered questionnaires can be administered as face-to-face interviews (where interviewer and respondents are in one place) or as telephone interviews (where an interviewer phones a respondent and ask questions and completes the questionnaire).

Computer-assisted surveys are a relatively new concept in which, as the name suggests, a computer is used to help conduct a survey. Examples include computer-assisted personal interviewing (the interviewer uses a computer to enter the data while interviewing), computer-assisted telephone interviewing (a remotely available interviewer uses a computer to enter the data while interviewing), computer-assisted self-interviewing (respondent answers the questions on a computer), and computer-assisted video interviewing (remotely present interviewer uses video calling software to interact with the respondent).

Other examples include computer-assisted automated telephone interviewing (computer with voice recognition capabilities asks questions from respondents and recognises and saves answers), touch tone data entry (respondent presses appropriate numeric key on the telephone handset to record their response) and virtual interviewer survey (questionnaire asked by a virtual interviewer over the internet).

Concerns to address when developing a survey

When considering a survey as a potential research method, a researcher needs to reflect on various issues. For instance, while contemplating the potential *population* for the survey research, the researcher needs to consider if there is a list of the survey population that can help select participants. Finding a list of all registered nurses working in Hospital A, for example, is easier than having a list of homeless people in England. The researcher also needs to think if the population to be studied is literate and therefore able to read and answer a questionnaire. Using a self-report questionnaire with young children may not be a good option. Researchers also need to consider language issues. While considering *sampling*, a researcher needs to consider if appropriate details such as addresses for postal survey or telephone numbers for telephone survey are available. When is it best to approach respondents (it may be difficult to reach respondent who work on night shifts, for instance)? What are the eligibility criteria for someone to be a respondent for the study? How many respondents need to be included in the study?

The researcher also needs to consider *questionnaire*-related issues such as the kind of questions that need to be included (sensitive questions, open or closed questions), if screening questions are needed, if more than one question is needed to explore an area, and can a sequence of questions be developed. The length of the questions needs to be considered because long questions may lead to confusion while excessively short questions may lack context or focus. Will open questions be needed or is there a need to develop a scale? Will the respondent have the required information t o answer questions? Will the respondents be comfortable answering questions? The researcher will need to consider possible *biases* such as the potential for social desirability, response bias, recall bias, interviewer distortion or interviewer subversion. The researcher also needs to consider *logistical* issues such as those related to cost or expenses, availability of required human and material resources and facilities, time scales and deadlines.

Further reading

Jackson, C.J. & Furnham, A. (2000) *Designing and Analysing Questionnaires and Surveys*. London: Whurr.

Watson, R., McKenna, H., Cowman, S. and Keady, J. (eds) (2008) *Nursing Research: Design and Methods*. Edinburgh: Churchill Livingstone Elsevier.

34 Factorial survey using vignettes

Figure 34.1 Development of vignettes.

1. Identify the independent variables (IVs)

Independent variables (IVs) for inclusion in vignettes are usually identified from literature and relevant theories. The recommended number of IVs is between five and ten (Taylor 2006).

2. Determine the levels of variables

For example, if one of the IVs is gender then the levels are male and female.

3. Identify the dependent variable (DV)

4. Write the vignette frame

- A vignette frame typically comprises a series of skeletal sentences in a fixed order to accommodate exploration of a combination of IVs that may impact on the dependent variable (DV)
- It is important to write a framework vignette in which the level of each factor could be randomly assigned to produce a variety of vignettes
- Short descriptions of a clinical scenario are ideal, in three or four sentences, to avoid overburden on the respondents.

5. Write the associated question

Questions may examine practice or attitudes and the most common response format is an analogue scale.

6. Randomly generate the vignettes

The individual vignette is the unit of analysis in a factorial survey. Therefore random assignment of levels of factors is crucial. This involves using EXCEL = RAND () function to create an $m \times n$ matrix of random numbers, where m = the number of independent variables, and n = the number of cases to be generated.

A factorial survey is a hybrid technique that incorporates the use of vignettes with multiple factors. It can provide the researcher with the opportunity to explore the interaction of various factors on the dependent variable (DV), which can produce effects that would not be predicted from exploring the relationship between the dependent variables and each independent variable (IV) individually. This acknowledges that multiple factors may be responsible for influencing any action taken. The factorial survey was initially trialed in the 1950s, then further developed into a more applicable tool for social research in the late 1970s and 1980s. The rationale for the inception of this design was acknowledgement that 'human evaluations are in part socially determined (that is, shared with others) and in part governed by individuality, the mix varying from topic to topic' (Rossi and Anderson, 1982).

A factorial survey is usually based on a factorial design and collects data in two parts, vignettes and characteristics of the respondent. The vignettes may be developed from practice, qualitative research, literature review or a combination of these sources. As noted by Polit and Beck (2008), a factorial design refers to

> An experimental design, in which two or more independent variables are simultaneously manipulated, permitting a separate analysis of the main effects of the independent variables, and their interaction.

A factorial design would typically be referred to with reference to the number of categories for each factor; for example, a '2 × 3' design refers to two factors with two levels in one category and three levels in the other. However, a factorial survey has the capacity for a larger number of factors and levels, increasing the proportion of surveys and, consequently, the proportion of observations for analysis. In the clinical area, the use of a factorial design would present ethical problems due to the difficulty of manipulating care delivery; however, a factorial survey that uses vignettes is a suitable alternative.

Vignettes

In a factorial survey vignettes are used to present the factors to be explored by the participants (Taylor, 2006). Vignettes are 'short stories about hypothetical characters in specified circumstances, to whose situation the interviewee is responding' (Finch, 1987). It is important to acknowledge that there is concern about the use of hypothetical situations to elicit opinions on clinical care; there is potential that participants' choices might not reflect the reality of the decision they may make in the clinical setting. In the past, they were predominantly used in politics and marketing; however, for a variety of reasons they have recently been used in social and healthcare research, including recognition of confusion and the need to restrain the elderly, clinical risk, patient preferences in shared decision-making, and practitioner assessments of parenting.

The development of vignettes for use in a factorial survey is presented in Figure 34.1. Multiple regression analysis is the most commonly used method of analysis for factorial survey as regression allows assessment of the relationship between the IVs, and between the IVs and the DV. However, to date there is no consensus on which type of multiple regression is most appropriate for analysing a factorial survey.

References

Finch, J. (1987) The vignette technique in survey research. *Sociology* **21**, 105–114.

Polit, D.F. and Beck, C.T. (2008) *Nursing Research: Generating and Assessing Evidence for Nursing Practice*. Philadelphia: Lippincott, Williams & Wilkins.

Rossi, P.H. and Anderson, A.B. (1982) The factorial survey approach: an introduction. In: P.H. Rossi and S.L. Nock (eds) *Measuring Social Judgements. The Factorial Survey Approach*, pp. 15–67. Beverly Hills, CA: Sage Publications.

Taylor, B.J. (2006) Factorial surveys: using vignettes to study professional judgement. *British Journal of Social Work* **36**, 1187–1207.

35 Triangulation in research

Figure 35.1 Triangulation.

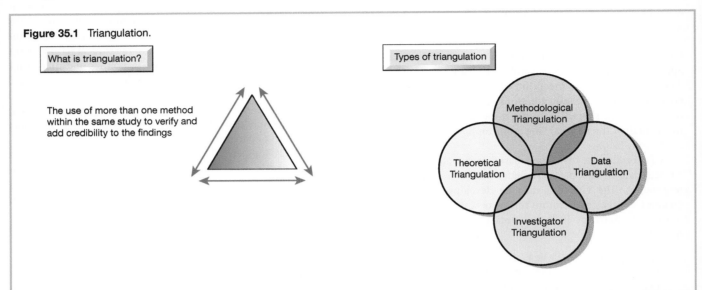

What is triangulation?

The use of more than one method within the same study to verify and add credibility to the findings

Types of triangulation

Methodological Triangulation

Theoretical Triangulation

Data Triangulation

Investigator Triangulation

Triangulation refers to the use of more than one method or data source to answer a research question with a view to one source verifying another (Figure 35.1). An example of this is when two or more blood pressure recordings are made to verify the accuracy of the reading. The term 'triangulation' was adapted from geographical surveys and navigational techniques where two known or visible points are used to find the location of a third point. The concept of triangulation was first applied to quantitative research in the 1950s where the initial idea was taking two or more measurements or calculations of something in order to check that the first measurement was correct. Triangulation was subsequently explored and applied in relation to qualitative research. It was initially used to suggest use of more than one method in a study to examine a single construct.

Why triangulate?

The purpose of triangulation is to increase confidence in the credibility and validity of research findings. It helps the researcher to develop an enriched and balanced picture of the phenomenon that is being explored by considering it from various different perspectives. It can also be used as an approach to cross-checking, or verifying, and to ensure findings are meaningful and can be trusted.

Types of triangulation

As shown in Figure 35.1, four types of triangulation were suggested by Denzin (1978).

Data triangulation

Data triangulation (or data sources triangulation) is the collection of data through different sources but using the same methods. Data are collected using the same approach but through different sampling strategies. For example, the researcher might collect data from one group at a particular time and then collect further data at a different time or from the same or a different group. This can help to identify persistent and common explanations of the phenomenon of interest but not from the same group or point in time. Data triangulation can be subdivided into three types: time, space and person. Data may be collected about different people doing the same work, at different times of the day or night, or from different places.

Data triangulation (person) can also be achieved by analysing data in various ways. For instance, *aggregate level* analysis focuses on analysing data collected from unrelated individuals; *interactive level* analysis focuses on interactions between various individuals; and *collective level* analysis focuses on a social group or community or society. All these various methods of data collection and analysis can be used to achieve data triangulation. Data triangulation is the most popular and perceived as the easiest form to implement, but carries the risk that either too much or too little data are collected or that data are not analysed in sufficient depth.

Investigator triangulation

Investigator triangulation refers to the use of more than one researcher to conduct research. More than one researcher participates in collection and/or analysis of the data using the same methods in the same study. The idea is to determine if the researcher's findings and interpretation of the findings match or correspond to each other. Investigator triangulation helps to reduce bias and increase reliability of the study findings. This might include, for example, two researchers analysing the same interview transcript to see if their interpretations merge. It requires additional resources and it may not always be easy or practical to assemble different investigators to participate in the same study.

Theoretical triangulation

Theoretical triangulation refers to the use of more than one theory in a research study in an attempt to analyse the issue under investigation from different perspectives or worldviews. The researcher may decide to use related or competing theories to develop a research question or hypothesis and develop the research methods employed. This is the most difficult form of triangulation to achieve. Use of various theories to investigate the same issue may require involvement of ideas and people from different disciplines and this can be challenging.

Methodological triangulation

Methodological triangulation uses a combination of approaches to explore one set of research questions through the careful and considered use of two or more research methods in a study design. This is the most common type of triangulation; it aims to strengthen research design and brings results together so that they substantiate and increase the credibility of the findings. Methodological triangulation is divided into two types: *within-method* analysis, which uses one method but different strategies to explore the same phenomenon; and *between- or across-method* analysis, which uses more than one method such as unstructured or semi-structured interviews along with structured questionnaires to explore the same phenomenon.

Sometimes this form of triangulation involves combining qualitative and quantitative research methods to ascertain if the findings are convergent or produce more complete findings than if the two methods were used separately. This is seen as one of the advantages of mixed or multi-method research.

Analysis triangulation

Analysis triangulation or data analysis triangulation is a further approach that involves the use of multiple methods to analyse the same set of data. For example, the researcher might use two or more statistical tests to analyse the same set of data.

In any research study more than one type of triangulation can be used. Use of more than one type of triangulation in a study is referred to as *multiple triangulation*.

Disadvantages of triangulation

Triangulation has some disadvantages. It makes research studies more complicated and it can mean that the research fails to be 'true' to any one particular method (Sim and Sharp, 1998). Of course, it is possible that two or more methods/data sources may produce inconsistent results, but this would merely serve to highlight that it would have been unwise to rely on just one method or approach to the research and that triangulation is a necessary process producing trustworthy, valid and reliable research findings.

References

Denzin, N. (1978) *The Research Act: A Theoretical Introduction to Sociological Methods*, 2nd edn. New York: McGraw Hill.

Sim, J. and Sharp, K. (1998) A critical appraisal of the role of triangulation in nursing research. *International Journal of Nursing Studies* **35**, 23–31.

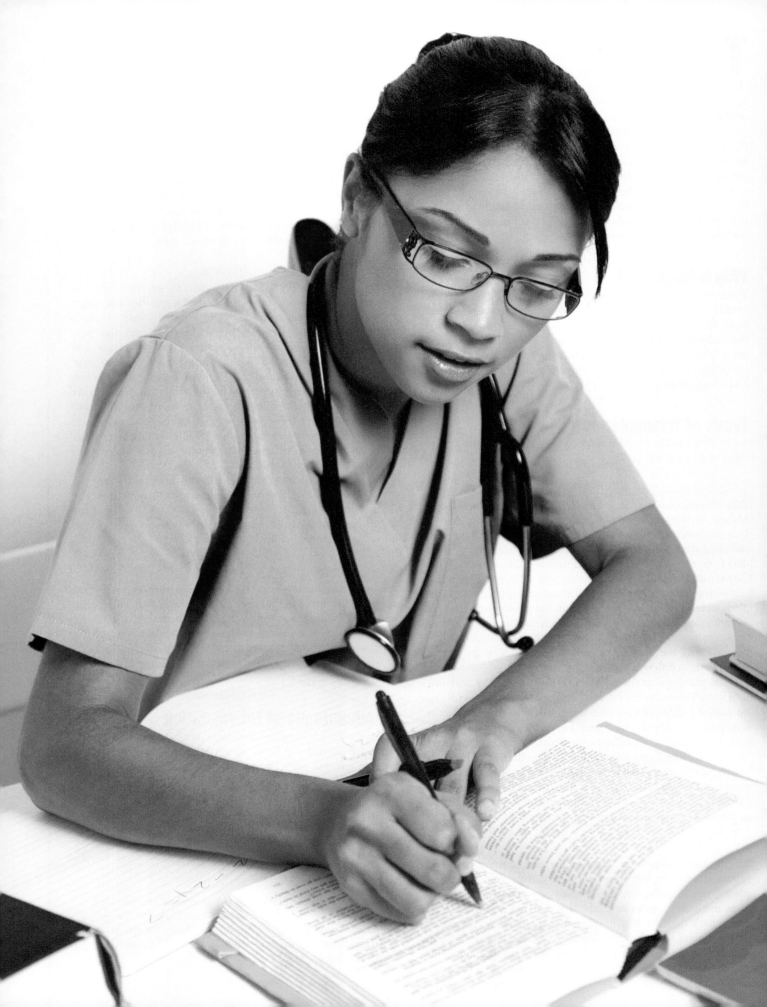

Qualitative research

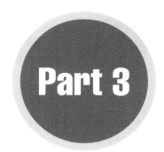

Part 3

Chapters

36 Ethnography

Figure 36.1 What is ethnography?

Understanding

Ethnographers seek to uncover the 'insider view', understanding their perspective, understanding peoples' behaviours, attitudes, beliefs and emotions; talk; space, objects, time, events, actions, relationships and interactions

What is ethnography?

Ethnography describes the research process and the research output produced from the research

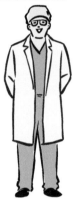

Context and culture

Ethnographers study culture or social groups in the context in which they occur. In healthcare, examples could include hospital wards, ambulances, and nursing homes

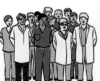

Analysing

Analysis involves organising field notes (and other data), reading, identifying and interpreting categorisations, coding data, summarising and generating conclusions to decribe what is happening and why

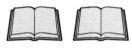

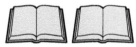

Observing

Data are collected by observing the everyday lives of a social group. This may include discussion, self-reflection and sometimes quantitative methods

Documenting

Ethnography relies on the researcher as the research instrument. Data are most commonly recorded as notes in a field diary, but audio, video, photos and diagrams can also be used

Nursing and Healthcare Research at a Glance, First Edition. Alan Glasper and Colin Rees. © 2017 by John Wiley & Sons, Ltd. Published 2017 by John Wiley & Sons, Ltd.

Ethnography is the study of a culture, subculture or a social group in order to understand the beliefs, practices and attitudes within social groups or small communities (Figure 36.1). Ethnography has its roots in social anthropology, a discipline that studies social and cultural diversity across the world. There is no single definition or interpretation of ethnography, but the term derives from the Greek *ethnos* (people or race) and *graphos* (writing). Ethnography describes both the research process (systematically observing and recording the lives of those being studied) and the research output produced from the research (the written work).

What do ethnographers 'do'?

Ethnographers seek to uncover the 'insider view', recording social groups in action, understanding their perspective, by observing – and sometimes participating – in their everyday lives. A defining feature of ethnography is that the researcher spends time in the natural setting ('in the field') over an extended period. The researcher watches what happens, listens to what is said, and asks questions about actions, interactions, experiences, beliefs, attitudes and feelings. Observation may be covert or overt, but overt is much more typical in healthcare settings. Covert observation may often be unethical. Observation is at the heart of ethnography but this is often combined with participation, discussion (interviews, informal conversations), self-reflection, analysis of documents and sometimes quantitative methods. Observational methods are described in a separate chapter.

Ethnographers write a narrative, descriptive account that conveys the social reality of the culture being studied. Ethnography is a rigorous process of scientific data collection that systematically records detailed actions, behaviour and talk, but it also involves 'telling stories' so that we are able to understand and represent a social group, culture or setting. 'Thick description' is a term often used to describe a detailed account of individuals and social groups in their cultural context. It is an attempt to capture and represent their meanings and intentions. Ethnographies may include theoretical, analytical and explanatory writing, as well as description.

Ethnography and healthcare settings

In healthcare ethnographies, the researcher spends time in settings where healthcare takes place (e.g. doctor's surgeries, hospital wards, operating theatres) so that we can understand behaviour related to health, illness or the delivery of health services. Ethnographic studies may examine healthcare at a macro level of social interaction (e.g. service provider, organisation) or at a smaller, local, micro level (e.g. single social setting such as a hospital ward). Ethnography has been applied to healthcare in many ways. Examples might include:

- examining everyday clinical work and practices of healthcare professionals in their natural setting;
- discovering the 'insider view' of patients or healthcare professionals or other staff groups to understand their beliefs and practices, and how they interact with others;
- exploring patient/professional decision-making;
- capturing patients' beliefs and experiences of healthcare (e.g. how healthcare treatment effectiveness can be influenced by patients' cultural beliefs and practices).

The sample, setting and data collection

Patients and the staff who provide healthcare are often the main participants (sometimes called informants) in healthcare ethnographies. The requirement for thick description necessitates small sample sizes. Purposive or criterion-based sampling and specific criteria to select the informants and the setting are used. Sometimes convenience sampling or *snowball techniques* are used. Whatever the method, the criteria should be explicit and systematic.

Ethnographic data collection relies on the researcher as an embodied research instrument. The researcher is an integral part of the research, the field and everyday lives of the informants. Data are most commonly collected by writing field notes in a diary, where data might be about peoples' behaviours, attitudes, beliefs and emotions; talk (informal, formal language); space, objects, time, events, actions, relationships and interactions. Researchers note their own biases, reactions and difficulties during fieldwork. Reflexivity (thinking critically about roles, ethics and responsibilities) is central to ethnography. Additional methods of recording data, such as audio, video, photos and diagrams, may also be used.

The analytical process is iterative not linear. The researcher moves backwards and forwards between data collection, forming early impressions about the data, and analysis. Analysis involves organising field notes (and other data), reading, identifying and interpreting categorisations, identifying contradictions, coding categorisations, summarising and recoding data into larger categories, and generating conclusions to describe what is happening and why.

Methodological and ethical considerations

Most healthcare settings are closed environments that require the researcher to gain permission to access them (including ethical approval to conduct research). The researcher must also negotiate acceptance by group members. Ethnographers should assess potential risks to themselves and to participants in the research. There may be health and safety considerations associated with working in a particular clinical setting. There are ethical considerations to be aware of, particularly about informed consent and data confidentiality.

Subjectivity is a limitation of ethnography. Researchers often work alone, which can make it difficult to establish the reliability of findings. Different researchers may make different interpretations, categorisations and conclusions about a social group or culture. Further, the researcher, who is a member of the group but is also an 'outsider' to the group, may affect the behaviour of the group. For example, informants may seek to present themselves (or their group) in a positive light (social desirability). The time required to conduct ethnography necessitates a small sample size. Small samples do not allow generalisation of findings to other settings. However, the aim of ethnographic research is to have a complete understanding of a particular social group in context.

Further reading

Hammersley, M. and Atkinson, P. (2007) *Ethnography: Principles in Practice*, 3rd edn. London: Routledge.

Holloway, I. and Todres, L. (2010) Ethnography. In: K. Gerrish and A. Lacey (eds) *The Research Process in Nursing*, 6th edn, pp. 165–176. Oxford: Wiley-Blackwell.

37 Qualitative observational methods

Figure 37.1 Example of the use of observation in healthcare.

Turnbull, J., Prichard, J., Halford, S., Pope, C. and Salisbury, C. (2012) Reconfiguring the emergency and urgent care workforce: mixed methods study of skills and the everyday work of non-clinical call-handlers in the NHS. *Journal of Health Services Policy* **17**, 233–240

This study examined a new type of health call-centre work in urgent and emergency care, focusing on how non-clinical call handlers' use a computer decision support system (CDSS) to support telephone triage in three healthcare settings. The main data collection method was over 500 hours of non-participant observation. Observation was chosen because:

- little was known about this group of workers and their decision-making when using a CDSS;
- it allowed observation of what people actually did in their everyday work;
- it allowed detailed study of complex social practices in real-life healthcare settings to explain how call handlers make decisions.

The researcher undertook overt non-participant observation, but data collection also included some interaction and informal conversations with participants ('observer as participant'). The researcher sat alongside call handlers taking telephone calls and observed the call handlers' actions, talk, behaviour and interactions with others. Between calls the researcher would ask call handlers about their actions and beliefs to check their understanding of what was observed. A detailed description and explanation of call handlers' skills and experience was generated from the data. The study concluded that, while these workers are often portrayed simply as 'trained users' of technology, they demonstrate high levels of experience, skills and expertise in using the CDSS.

Figure 37.2 Gold's typology of approaches to observation.

Complete participant	Participant-as-observer	Observer-as-participant	Complete observer
Fully part of the setting (often covert)	*Part of the setting and group being studied but the role is overt*	*Some participation/ engagement but the focus is on observation*	*No interaction with those being observed*

Figure 37.3 Researcher as the 'research instrument'.

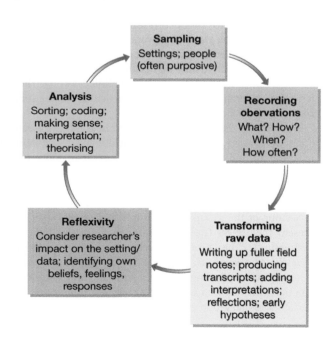

Figure 37.4 Example of initial field notes.

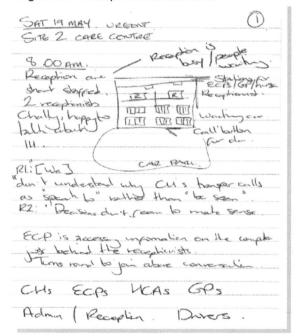

Qualitative observational methods involve direct, systematic, detailed observation and recording of people, their actions, events, behaviours, talk and interactions. Observational methods attempt to observe things 'as they are', without any intervention or manipulation of the situation itself by the researcher (*naturalistic research*). In the context of healthcare, settings could include hospitals, GP surgeries, and other healthcare organisations. The goal of this sort of research is to understand the perspective from the point of view of the participants. Observational methods can involve informal conversations and asking questions but the primary focus on observation distinguishes it from qualitative interviews.

Why is observation used?

Qualitative observational methods are often exploratory in nature. They may be used to identify, describe and explain the following.

• What people *do* rather than what people *say they do*. Biases can occur in peoples' accounts when they wish to present themselves in a positive light, or when there are difficulties with memory recall and selectivity. Actions and responses that the participants themselves may be unaware of may also be observed.
• Healthcare problems that are not clearly understood, for example patients' experiences of a new treatment, or process of care.
• Complex and multifaceted healthcare problems that require detailed data to understand 'what is going on'. Figure 37.1 shows an example of the use of observation in healthcare to examine decision making processes in telephone triage.
• Unexpected outcomes; for example, observing clinical practice or decision-making may help to uncover why there are variations in a given clinical outcome.

Types of observational research

The degree to which the researcher participates in what is being observed depends on both the nature of the research question and the study setting. Gold's (1958) typology (Figure 37.2) defines four researcher roles in undertaking observation. In practice, the degree of participation may be more a continuum, from complete participation to complete observer. To minimise the impact of the presence of the researcher on the group or the setting, the researcher may adopt a participant role (*complete participant* or *participant-as-observer*). This may be an 'insider' role where the group is unaware of the researcher's identity (covert) or a role where the identity of the researcher is made clear to those being observed (overt). Covert observation is not common in healthcare settings for ethical and practical reasons. Overt observation has fewer ethical implications, but it may have drawbacks when individuals or groups react or behave differently in response to being aware that they are being observed (sometimes called the Hawthorne effect). In non-participant roles, the researcher has less involvement or interaction with individuals or a group (*observer-as-participant*) and does not seek to be part of the setting. A *complete observer* does not take part in the setting at all (and may observe from behind glass or from a distance).

Access to settings and participants

Observation can take place in open settings (e.g. public places) or in closed settings (e.g. not open to the general public). Most healthcare settings are closed. Studying patients or healthcare staff will require permission to access settings (and require ethical approval). Gaining access can be complex, and identifying the gatekeepers (those who need to give permission and whose cooperation can facilitate access) is critical. It is important to be clear and transparent about the research aims, methods and the level of commitment the research requires. Negotiating access and building rapport with gatekeepers and participants is not a single event, but rather an ongoing process that should continue throughout.

The role of the researcher

Qualitative observational research embodies the notion of the researcher as the 'research instrument' (Figure 37.3). The researcher is required to make decisions about how and what to sample (in qualitative work sampling is often purposive, deliberately selecting particular individuals, social groups or settings). The researcher also has to decide what to focus on and record as it is impossible to record everything that is observed. There is inevitably selectivity (and subjectivity) in what is recorded, whatever the means of recording data (field notes, video, sound recording).

To ensure rigour in the data, it is crucial that observations are systematically recorded and analysed. Despite technological advances, observation is often still recorded with pen and paper. The researcher takes down notes that include details of what people do and say, as well more reflexive writing about the research process and the researchers' personal reactions or feelings. In qualitative studies, observation is usually unstructured. The researcher may have some ideas about the focus or the data 'required' but there is no checklist or coding scheme to predetermine what will be observed.

Collecting data and analysis

Where possible it is advantageous to write contemporaneous notes (i.e. while observation is taking place). It can be more difficult to recall rich detail after the event, when the researcher may also reconstruct and interpret events, rather than documenting emerging meanings, processes and early hypotheses. However, contemporaneous note taking may not always be possible. In participatory or sensitive situations for example, people may find the writing of notes disconcerting (and in turn may alter their behaviour). Initial notes or jottings are often quite personal and may only make sense to the researcher (Figure 37.4). They are used to help remember important issues, questions or solutions to problems, and they are usually written up more fully later to create a narrative account or transcript. The content of field notes may change as the researcher spends more time in the field, moving from simple observations to more complex writing that includes notes about early hypotheses, analysis and interpretation from which systems for classifying or coding data are developed. The researcher moves back and forth between data collection and analysis, to sort and make sense of the context, events and interactions observed. Data are systematically analysed by categorising and coding data, testing against hypotheses, and refining coding.

Reference and further reading
Gold, R. (1958) Roles in sociological field observation. *Social Forces* **36**, 217–213.
Green, J. and Thorogood, N. (2013) Observational methods. In: *Qualitative Methods for Health Research*, 3rd edn, pp. 131–154. London: Sage.

38 Phenomenology

Figure 38.1 Phenomenology.

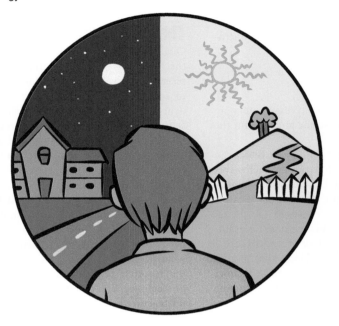

- Lifeworld
- Lived experiences
- Perspectives
- Nuance
- Person-in-world

Phenomenology is both a philosophical movement and an approach to human science research. The term is derived from the Greek word *phainomenon* meaning 'appearance'. It originates from a twentieth-century European philosophical movement founded by Edmund Husserl and has been developed by others, notably Heidegger, Gadamer and Merleau-Ponty. Essentially, phenomenology is the study of structures of how we experience the multidimensional nature of living and the meanings we attribute to these things from the subjective or first-person point of view. It is concerned with understanding the 'lifeworld' or lived experience of individuals (Figure 38.1). Central concepts include the phenomenological stance, the positioning or 'attitude' of the researcher that allows them to be open to the experience as recounted by others. Intentionality can be understood as the direction of consciousness towards understanding the world and phenomenological reduction in which the 'unessential' is removed and the essence of the phenomena is revealed.

Phenomenology can draw on phenomenological data collection through interviews and makes use of phenomenological reflection. The purpose is to study areas where little is known or which is sensitive, and to get beneath or behind the subjective experience to uncover the genuine, humanly shared nature of things. It is not a single approach but offers an opportunity to discover and reveal the 'lived experience' of research participants embedded in everyday contexts.

Application to healthcare

Phenomenology began to emerge in the healthcare literature in the 1970s. It is consistent with the values of recognising the uniqueness of individuals and the need to explore personal experiences and interrelationships. Critics argue that the approach is often poorly applied in healthcare research; for authenticity, it is essential that researchers are well versed in its philosophical roots. There is no single way of 'doing' phenomenology but a four-stage approach for empirical/phenomenological research informed by phenomenological philosophy is suggested by Todres and Holloway (2004).

1 Articulating an experiential phenomenon of interest.
2 Gathering descriptions of individuals' experiences of the phenomenon with a focus on capturing concrete examples.
3 Using intuition and 'testing' the meanings of experiences.
4 Writing a detailed, vivid, 'digested' account of the phenomenon that reflects commonalities and variations within the data. A range of procedural frameworks are offered by authors such as Colaizzi, Dahlberg, Halling, Smith, van Manen and Wertz; these developments are controversial with some debate about how they offer adaptable and accessible approaches, while there are different arguments about closeness and distance to philosophy.

A high level of skill is required to undertake all stages of the phenomenological research process; it is labour-intensive and time-consuming. Reflexivity, the art of reflecting on and critically examining the research process and considering the researcher's subjectivity and experiences brought to the study, is vital (Todres and Holloway, 2004). The investment is valuable when 'lived experiences' are faithfully illuminated and can be used to enhance clinical practice.

Data collection

After delineating the phenomenon of interest, researchers seek people who have lived the phenomenon of interest as only those who have experienced the phenomenon can communicate it to the outside world. Participants who are willing and able to describe their experiences in first-person accounts are invited to take part in unstructured, one-to-one, audio-taped interviews. Typically, interviews start with 'Tell me about your experience of…'. Subsequent questions are 'experience near', in other words they stay very close to the experience as lived and encourage sharing of concrete examples (Todres and Galvin, 2012). A strong phenomenological interview draws out descriptions and examples of the experience. Multiple interviews may be used to follow up specific issues in greater depth. The researcher adopts an open 'bridled' approach in which he or she consciously limits assumptions and presuppositions about the phenomenon, thus allowing the phenomenon to show itself in its own way and at its own pace (Dahlberg, 2007). Sample sizes are small and the data rich and insightful.

Data analysis

There are multiple approaches to data analysis and choice must be informed by the philosophical stance of the researcher, many have similar aims and analytic processes overlap. The analysis is more complex than 'content analysis' drawing on philosophical foundations. The emphasis is on revealing wholes and parts, commonalities and variance. Broadly, the process is to follow the steps described by Giorgi (2009) as a phenomenological method for psychology.

1 Collection of verbal data.
2 Reading of the data for a sense of the 'whole'.
3 Identifying meaning units within the data.
4 Organisation and expression of data.
5 Summary of the data to describe essences of the experience with universal and variable features.

Writing up

Writing up a phenomenological study involves providing an account of the research process to assure the reader of trustworthiness. An essential description of the phenomenon is provided, with extracts of data used to exemplify the phenomenon with all its nuances, commonalties and variations. The essential structure of the experience is reflected on in the context of existing literature. The aim is not to generalise but to understand shared meanings. The goal is to produce an exhaustive, vivid, essential description of the phenomenon. Findings may be used to guide practice or as a basis for further research.

References and further reading

Dahlberg, K. (2007) The enigmatic phenomenon of loneliness. *International Journal of Qualitative Studies on Health and Well-Being* **2**, 195–207.

Finlay, L. (2011) *Phenomenology for Therapists*. Oxford: Wiley-Blackwell.

Giorgi, A. (2009) *Descriptive Phenomenological Method in Psychology: A Modified Husserlian Approach*. Pittsburgh, PA: Duquesne University Press.

Moran, D. (2000) *Introduction to Phenomenology*. London: Routledge.

Todres, L. and Galvin, K. (2012) 'In the middle of everywhere': a phenomenological study of mobility and dwelling amongst rural elders. *Phenomenology and Practice* **6**, 55–68.

Todres, L. and Holloway, I. (2004) Descriptive phenomenology: life-world as evidence. In: F. Rapport (ed.) *New Qualitative Methodologies in Health and Social Care Research*, pp. 79–98. London: Routledge.

39 Grounded theory

Figure 39.1 Common features of grounded theory.

- Simultaneous data collection and analysis
- Generation of analytic codes and categories coming from data and not by pre-existing conceptualisations (theoretical sensitivity)
- Discovery of basic social processes in the data
- Inductive construction of abstract categories
- Theoretical sampling to refine categories
- Writing analytical memos as the stage between coding and writing
- The integration of categories into a theoretical framework

Figure 39.2 Type of research questions grounded theory can answer.

> **Q** What leads patients to seek healthcare assessment and treatment when they have a minor injury?

> **Q** What affects nurses' interaction with older adults with dementia in residential care settings?

> **Q** What criteria and information do patients use when they decide to trust the professionals caring for them?

Figure 39.3 Steps in developing grounded theory.

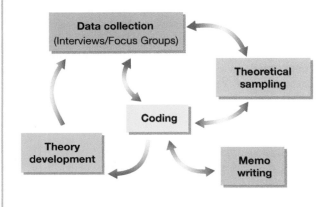

Figure 39.4 Tools of grounded theory.

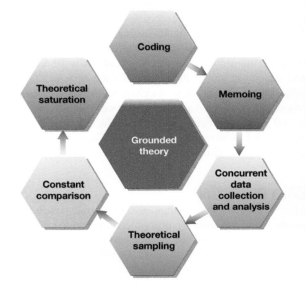

Grounded theory (GT) is a qualitative research approach that uses well-defined structured procedures to develop theory that is 'grounded' in the data (Strauss and Corbin, 1990). The approach provides a set of research tools that are used to illuminate the meaning of things (or phenomena). There is a focus on incidents and the main concerns of people in the incidents: what concerns them, what the incidents mean for them and how they think about and react to them.

GT was developed by the sociologists Glaser and Strauss, who collaboratively researched patients' and relatives' awareness of dying. Over time, both researchers followed diverging paths resulting in variations in approaches to GT that have also been developed and adapted by other researchers. One such variation is offered by social constructivists such as Annells (1996) and Charmaz (2003, 2006).

Many researchers now believe that GT can be adapted to suit the needs of research through a pragmatic flexible approach that provides the researcher with guidelines, principles and strategies for research rather than prescriptive methodological rules. However, there are certain common features of all versions of GT and these are summarised in Figure 39.1 and considered in the following sections.

The kind of research questions GT can answer

The main aim of GT in nursing and healthcare is to offer complete explanations of phenomena that are important to the people receiving healthcare and to health providers through an exploration of the social processes involved in everyday healthcare. The approach is often useful where there is no, or little, previous knowledge of the subject. The research question can be refined as the study progresses as the researcher learns more about the area of interest. Examples of appropriate GT questions are given in Figure 39.2.

Data collection and analysis in GT

There is no single method of data collection recommended for GT, although individual interviews, focus groups, document review and video recording review are commonly used. Data collection and analysis occur simultaneously alongside each other, in a cyclical process. Data analysis starts as soon as the first data have been collected and follows each point of data collection, then leading to further analysis. Various analytical tools are used in GT research (Figures 39.3 and 39.4), including coding, memoing, constant comparison, theoretical sampling and theoretical saturation.

Coding

Coding involves examining each segment of data (a word, phrase or sentence) and giving it a short name that summarises its meaning. This is a way of translating the raw data (e.g. from an interview transcript) into an interpretation of what the data says about the area of interest and developing a series of categories that summarise the data through the following processes.

1 *Open coding* (initial analysis) involves simply underlining key phrases and words. Every line of the transcript is read and each section of data is given a name that identifies the meaning in the data with the help of simple words and phrases, or descriptive labels. It is important that the words used closely relate to and reflect the data. Often the exact words used by the participants are used as a code known as 'in vivo' coding.

2 Chunks of data with similar meanings are then brought together to form 'categories'. As the data are analysed and patterns begin to emerge, further data collection decisions are made on the basis of the developing categories and concepts that emerge from the data.

3 *Axial coding* is then used to reconstruct or put the data back together in new ways by making connections between categories.

4 *Theoretical coding* involves examination of the developed categories and the connections between them. It also describes the relationships between the categories and concepts in a way that explains to others what is going on in the data. This provides a coherent, logical and comprehensive analytical story, a theory of the phenomenon under investigation.

5 Finally, a *core category* is identified that describes what has been seen in the data as clearly and succinctly as possible.

Memo writing

Theoretical memos are another important tool. The memos reflect the researcher's ideas and thoughts about what they hear and see as they collect and analyse data. Memos are usually in the form of written notes or diagrams that reflect the style of the researcher.

Constant comparison

The process of data analysis employs a constant comparison method that occurs cyclically throughout the course of the research study. As data are collected, it is constantly compared to previous data to identify similarities and differences in the emerging ideas, codes and categories developed through the coding process. This enables the researcher to understand more easily what the data are saying and to adapt the data collection and analysis accordingly.

Theoretical sampling and theoretical saturation

Participants are selected based on their ability to contribute to the theory that emerges from the analysis of the data through *theoretical sampling*: inclusion of new participants is based on the codes and categories that emerge and continue until a full explanation of the area of study is developed and can no longer be expanded. Inclusion of new participants ceases when the categories appear to be as complete as possible and no new information or data appear to further refine the categories; this is called *theoretical saturation*.

Conclusion

This chapter presents an overview of GT and the main tools and processes a researcher uses to develop theory from the cyclical data collection and analysis process. Further reading of a variety of materials relating to the conduct of GT will help you to understand these in more depth.

References

Annells, M. (1996) Grounded theory method: philosophical perspectives, paradigm of inquiry, and postmodernism. *Qualitative Health Research* 6, 379–393.

Charmaz, K. (2003) Grounded theory. Objectivst and constructivist methods. In: N.K. Denzin and Y.S. Lincoln (eds) *Stratagies of Qualitative Inquiry*, 2nd edn, pp. 249–291. Thousand Oaks, CA: Sage.

Charmaz, K. (2006) *Constructing Grounded Theory: A Practical Guide Through Qualitative Analysis*. London: Sage.

Strauss, A. and Corbin, J. (1990) *Basics of Qualitative Research*. Newbury Park, CA: Sage.

Classical grounded theory

Figure 40.1 Assessing GT studies.

- Fit: the categories developed come from the data so they fit with the data
- Work: how the theory explains the behaviour when it happened
- Relevance: the relevance of the behaviour to the theory
- Modifiability: that the theory can change with new data

Figure 40.2 Core category.

- Must be the central concept
- Re-occurs frequently
- Takes more time to saturate than other concepts
- Connections with all other concepts
- Clear and grabbing implication for theory
- Completely variable
- Is a component (dimension) of the problem
- Can be any kind of theoretical code

Figure 40.3 How is classic GT different?

- Unit of analysis is behaviour
- Conceptual framework generated from data
- Discover dominant processes in the social seen rather than describing unit under study
- Data compared to every other piece
- Data collection modified according to advancing theory: drop false leads
- Steps are concurrent not linear
- 'All is data'
- Role of the literature
- Conceptual not descriptive
- Not unit bound

Figure 40.4 Examples of core categories.

Visualising worsening progressions	How nurses detect physiological deterioration
Accommodating interruptions	Young people living with asthma
Anticipatory vigilance	Prevention of untoward incidents in the operating theatre
Emotional resilience	Coping with loved ones undergoing chemotherapy

Grounded theory (GT) was developed by Glaser and Strauss during their study of dying patients in 1965 and was subsequently written up as a methodology (Glaser and Strauss, 1967). It is an inductive approach that follows a set of procedures to systematically generate theory from data that explains behaviour in resolving or processing peoples' main concern (Glaser and Strauss, 1967). It is a process of discovery that begins with theoretical sampling and the constant comparative analysis of data as they are gathered. It taps into peoples' natural tendency to theorise and is based on the idea that we are creatures of habit. The role of the researcher is to pick up on those patterns of behaviour, what people are doing out of habit, even if these go unrecognised by the participants themselves. This is GT as originated by Glaser and Strauss and has come to be known as *classical grounded theory* (CGT) to differentiate it from other 'variations' of the method (Figure 40.1). Of importance in CGT is that the collection, coding and analysis of data proceed concurrently. In turn, this determines what data are sampled next, in a process termed theoretical sampling (Glaser and Strauss, 1967; Glaser, 1978). This is cyclical in nature, where one step leads to another until the emerging theory determines what or where next to sample. The methodology can be used with any kind of data whether generated quantitatively or qualitatively. Although commonly used with qualitative data, nonetheless it is considered a general methodology rather than just a qualitative one. Researchers are encouraged to use all forms of data (Gibson and Hartman, 2014). The criteria for judging the quality of a CGT study are outlined in Figure 40.2.

Theoretical sampling

Sampling in CGT is theoretical. This involves listening to participants and asking questions based on what is emerging rather than using an interview guide. The idea is to be led by what participants say and not by the preconceptions of the researcher. Data collection and analysis continue until saturation is reached. The idea of saturation is often misunderstood but it means collecting data until no new incidences or variations in behaviour (properties) of a concept emerge.

Constant comparison

Constant comparison is the process comparing every piece of data to every other piece. Data are then coded with previously generated concepts in mind. This involves comparing incident to incident and discovering what happened, how it happened and what caused it to happen from the perspective of participants (Glaser and Strauss, 1967). Similar incidents are coded in the same way so that researchers are not overwhelmed by generating too many concepts.

Data analysis

The emphasis in GT is on conceptualisation, which involves researchers looking for patterns of behaviour in the data and naming those patterns. This is how concepts are generated. Analysis begins by looking for incidents (an event or occurrence) of behaviour within the data, picking up on patterns. Further coding is done using constant comparison.

Memos

These are a central feature of the method, and if researchers are not writing memos then they are not doing CGT. Memos are essentially a moment capture, where the ideas and theoretical thinking of the researcher are captured. They are where the theory is developed. There is only one rule when it comes to memo writing: stop whatever you are doing and memo. It can be a word, sentence or much longer. Memos are eventually sorted into piles under the appropriate concepts and written up as the theory.

Use of the literature

A common misunderstanding attributed to this methodology is that researchers avoid reading the literature. Glaser (1978) maintains that researchers should be well read. However, what is unique to CGT is that the literature in the area under study is reviewed last, when the core category has emerged. The core category is the concept that explains how participants resolve or solve their main concern and is related to all the other concepts in explaining behaviour (Glaser, 1978) (Figures 40.3 and 40.4). The literature in the substantive area is avoided up to this point so that researchers remain open to the concerns of participants, rather than trying to preconceive what the issues are. Reasons for avoiding the literature include:
• risk of preconception (investigating what the researcher thinks are the issues for participants rather than letting them emerge);
• using concepts from the literature rather than from the analysis;
• can only know what literature to review when the researcher knows what the study is about.
Of course, researchers are very well read but can use this knowledge to make them theoretical sensitive. There is a difference between having preconceptions and using them (Gibson and Hartman, 2014). Once the theory has been generated, the literature may be used in two ways: to situate the theory in the existing literature and/or as another source of data to be analysed.

Conclusion

CGT is a general methodology for conceptualising the 'doings' of people as they engage with the problems they face in their everyday lives. It taps into a natural ability and tendency to theorise based on the idea that people are creatures of habit.

References
Gibson, B. and Hartman, J. (2014) *Rediscovering Grounded Theory*. London: Sage.
Glaser, B.G. (1978) *Theoretical Sensitivity: Advances in the Methodology of Grounded Theory*. Mill Valley, CA: Sociology Press.
Glaser, B.G. and Strauss, A.L. (1967) *The Discovery of Grounded Theory: Strategies for Qualitative Research*. Hawthorne, NY: Aldine de Gruyter.

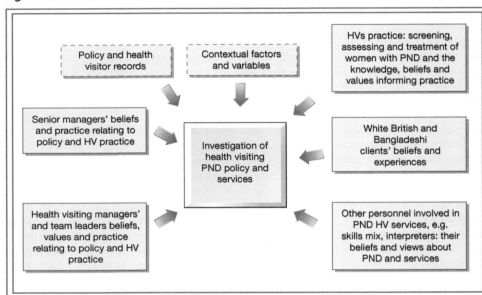

41 Case study research

Figure 41.1 The case.

The double outer line is the 'boundary' that is one health visiting service provider. Within this are further units of enquiry and these are called embedded units enquiry or analysis (single lines). Other data provided additional insights into the context or influences on health visitor (HV) practice or the service, contextual units of enquiry (broken lines).

Figure 41.2 A layered enquiry.

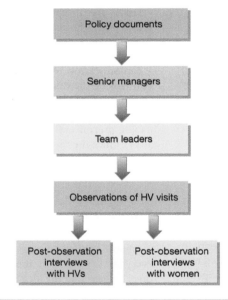

Case study research (CSR) takes a somewhat different methodological approach from studies that focus solely on variables and their influences. Instead, the concern is on collecting an extensive amount of descriptive data from one location or group, such as a clinical area, or group of health professionals or patients over a set period of time. The aim is often to understand the 'why' and 'how' of a complex situation and frequently involves collecting both quantitative and qualitative data. There is controversy over whether CSR is an approach, design, method or research strategy (Rosenberg and Yates, 2007; Anthony and Jack, 2009; Casey and Houghton, 2010; Swanborn, 2010), so this chapter will clarify its use through an example by Almond (2008).

The research question in CSR

The research question guides the study's depth and breadth, as it suggests the design and the methods be used. Almond's (2008) question was 'Are health visiting postnatal depression policies, services and practice equitable?' This question suggests who might provide data or where it might be found. Although tempting to include everything or everyone, CSR encourages the researcher to draw a boundary around which data to collect. Yin (2012) provides useful guidance on defining or classifying the case by time and place through 'bounding' or containing (Figure 41.1), for instance by identifying geographical area(s), organisation(s), incidence(s) or event(s).

Time, budget and simple pragmatics can also guide where the line is drawn, as can the need for depth or breadth. Consideration of these factors enabled Almond (2008) to select a single health visiting provider. This provider was purposively selected as it had a policy of promoting the equitable provision of services for detecting and managing postnatal depression (PND) for all women. Additionally, the provider served an ethnically diverse population, which was an important characteristic as the literature review revealed that rates of screening for PND in minority ethnic women were lower than for other women. More than one provider could have been included if the research question had sought comparisons; it would then have been called a multiple CSR design. Bounding the case by 'time' was determined by the date when the policy was launched.

Methods of data collection and analysis

In common with mixed method designs, CSR frequently includes a variety of data sources. In Almond's (2008) study, this comprised the following.
1 Observations: of screening, assessment and treatment of PND by health visitors during home visits.
2 Interviews: with senior managers, team leaders, health visitors, and health visitors' clients from high or low socioeconomic occupational class comprising white British women and Bangladeshi women (who may or may not have been British).
3 Policy documents and field notes.
4 Interviews: with personnel working with health visitors, for example nurses with a specialist or defined role in detecting and assessing PND and treating women with PND, and also interpreters and community cohesion workers.
Health visitor records were excluded as the pilot study revealed they lacked a detailed account of health visitor practice.

Since the research was interested in equity in policy, services and practice, the data were analysed using framework analysis (Spencer et al., 2003). This revealed the relationship between policy, service design and delivery, and health visiting practice and how this led to equity or inequity.

Using an assortment of methods in CSR results in a deeper, wider and complete examination of the phenomenon, which in this case study was equity. The design not only highlighted its existence but also how and why it existed. This is a further feature of CSR that illustrates its essence. Yin (2012) argues that research questions containing 'how' or 'why' lend themselves exceptionally well to CSR. However, as Almond's (2008) study has shown, CSR can also answer other types of questions.

Depth of understanding

The use of a variety of data collection and analysis methods in CSR, while challenging, adds strength to the findings and increase their trustworthiness in terms of meaning and understanding. Stake (2005) and Yin (2012) also suggest that multidimensional rather than unidimensional meanings can be generated using CSR. Almond's (2008) study adopted a single CSR design, enabling her to use a layered process of enquiry that moved from one level to another within the case and its embedded cases (Figure 41.2). It involved moving from the macro to the micro level during data collection and moving backwards and forwards through the data during the analytical phases. This iterative, fluid but methodical approach led to a greater understanding in relation to time and place of the varied influences that shaped the health visiting PND service provision and health visiting practice, and a clearer understanding of the complex phenomenon of equity.

Conclusion

CSR is a flexible research approach suited to the examination of complex situations such as healthcare. It provides the strategic framework for answering multifaceted questions, as it enables the inclusion of a range of participants, a diversity of data collection and analysis methods, and through the use of bounding the case by time and place, all of which helps the researcher to retain focus.

References

Almond, P. (2008) *A study of equity within health visiting postnatal depression policy and services*. Unpublished PhD thesis, University of Southampton.
Anthony, S. and Jack, S. (2009) Qualitative case study methodology in nursing research: an integrative review. *Journal of Advanced Nursing* **65**, 1171–1181.
Casey, D. and Houghton, C. (2010) Clarifying case study research: examples from practice. *Nurse Researcher* **17**(3), 41–51.
Rosenberg, J.P. and Yates, P.M. (2007) Schematic representation of case study research designs. *Journal of Advanced Nursing* **60**, 447–452.
Spencer, L., Ritchie, J., Lewis, J. and Dillon, L. (2003) *Quality in Qualitative Evaluation: A Framework of Assessing Research Evidence. A Quality Framework*. London: Cabinet Office Strategy Unit.
Stake, R.E. (2000) The case study method in social enquiry. In: R. Gomm, M. Hammersley and P. Foster (eds) *Case Study Method: Key Issues, Key Texts*, pp. 19–26. London: Sage.
Swanborn, P. (2010) *Case Study Research: What, Why, and How?* London: Sage.
Yin, R.K. (2012) *Applications of Case Study Research*, 3rd edn. Thousand Oaks, CA: Sage.

42 Focus group research

Figure 42.1 Focus group discussion.

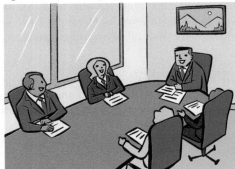

Figure 42.2 Qualities and responsibilities of a facilitator.

- Provides a conducive and supporting environment where participants feel encouraged to share their views
- Keeps participants engaged, interested and focused
- Enforces ground rules and ensures that everyone is able to share their views
- Asks open-ended questions and uses probes to stimulate discussion
- Is able to defuse arguments
- Has adequate knowledge of the topic under discussion
- Is able to control personal reactions and does not let his or her views and opinions affect the discussion
- Is sensitive to gender and cultural issues that may affect discussion
- Is able to manage challenging people and situations when needed
- Should have good listening, observation and communication skills

Figure 42.3 Qualities and responsibilities of an assistant facilitator or note taker.

- Assists facilitator in smooth running of the group
- Acts as time keeper
- Responds to unexpected interruptions during FGD
- Keeps a note of procedures and other observations during the FGD
- Takes detailed notes in situations where discussions cannot be audio recorded for any reason
- Keeps a note of participants' body language, on verbal responses, facial expressions, signs of agreement/disagreement, frustration or any other emotion displays by participants while sharing their ideas
- Handles audio recording equipment effectively
- Avoids joining in conversation and remains impartial and non-judgemental
- Should have good observation, listening and writing skills

Figure 42.4 Topic guide.

While developing and using a topic guide for FGDs, please remember that it:

- Is an outline of the points that need to be discussed in FGD
- Should be prepared in advance
- Should have minimal number of items to discuss
- Should break down major questions into small discussion points
- Should have probe questions
- May be revised after each FGD to add new issues and eliminate irrelevant questions
- Should only be used as a guide and not as a strict agenda

Figure 42.5 Example ground rules.

- One person to speak at a time
- Respect each other's opinion. It is important to listen to positive as well as negative aspects
- There are no right and wrong answers or opinions. All ideas, opinions and experiences are valuable
- Ensure confidentiality: 'Whatever is shared in the room, should stay in the room'

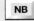 **NB** Participants may also be encouraged to suggest and agree on any other ground rules acceptable to everyone

Focus group research refers to research conducted through series of carefully planned discussions, known as focus group discussions (FGDs), with a group of individuals to explore their perceptions, perspectives and opinions about a particular phenomenon under investigation. The method was originally developed for the field of marketing research, but is now extensively used in other fields such as business management, social science, nursing and healthcare research.

The aim of such discussion is to explore diverse opinions of people about an issue in a non-threatening and supportive environment. In simple language, a focus group is a face-to-face interview method where an interviewer (moderator/facilitator) interviews a group of individuals (Figure 42.1). Usually seven to ten participants can be involved in an FGD. A group with more than 10 participants can be challenging to manage. On the other hand, a group that has fewer than seven participants may not result in meaningful and enriched discussion.

Nursing and Healthcare Research at a Glance, First Edition. Alan Glasper and Colin Rees. © 2017 by John Wiley & Sons, Ltd. Published 2017 by John Wiley & Sons, Ltd.

Why use focus group research?

A group discussion is usually more effective and generates more ideas compared with discussion between two or three people. Keeping this in mind, the use of a focus group stimulates discussion among group participants resulting in the generation of rich information about participants' perspectives about any specific research topic. Participants feel safe and comfortable in sharing their personal experiences and this acts as a trigger for other participants in the group to share their experiences. The use of FGD can also help in understanding factors that influence people's opinions or behaviours. The FGD method is effective in capturing the diverse opinions and perspectives of a group of people in a relatively short time. In addition, it is a relatively low-cost and efficient method of data collection.

Limitations of focus group research

There are some limitations in the use of the focus group research method. For instance, information generated though FGDs provides important insight about the topic under investigation, but has limited generalisability to the wider population. The discussion can be dominated by one or more vocal individuals in the group, resulting in a biased view about the topic. This may also affect other participants' ability and confidence to articulate their views. FGDs are not a suitable method when dealing with emotionally or politically charged topics or groups. Ensuring confidentiality of the information discussed in the FGD cannot be guaranteed, as it is up to the participants to not share that information outside the group. FGDs can also be affected by the moderator's bias. Finally, FGDs are often challenging to organise and manage.

Important aspects of conducting focus group research

As focus group research is based on a series of FGDs, it is important to consider various aspects in relation to the arrangement and facilitation of FGDs.

FGD team

Facilitating an FGD requires a small team consisting of at least a moderator/facilitator and a note-taker or assistant. The role of the facilitator is to guide the discussion (Figure 42.2), whereas the role of an assistant or note-taker is to help the facilitator in the smooth running of the FGD by responding to unexpected interruptions, keeping track of time and ensuring environmental conditions are appropriate (Figure 42.3).

Recruitment and initiation of participants

FGDs are conducted with a specific purpose and therefore it is important to establish inclusion and exclusion criteria to identify and recruit participants who can contribute to the discussion. Selected participants should reflect the diversity and composition of the bigger group they represent. In addition, other factors such as cultural issues that may affect participants' acceptability and ability to contribute to the focus group also need to be considered. For instance, while exploring perceptions of people about domestic violence, it may be more appropriate to conduct separate FGDs for men and women. Once identified, participants should be invited to participate 1–2 weeks in advance. It is also good practice to contact participants the day before the FGD to remind them of the time and location and to confirm their attendance.

Time and venue of FGDs

An FGD usually lasts for 1–2 hours and therefore needs to be arranged at a time of day that is most convenient for the participants. For, instance an FGD requiring the participation of mothers may be most conveniently arranged during school time when children are in school. It is also important to conduct FGDs at a convenient location for the participants. The environment of the venue where the FGD is held should have appropriate seating arrangements, lighting and ventilation, and have access to refreshments and toilets. The venue should be private and sufficiently quiet to allow uninterrupted discussion. Various public places such as a church, a community centre or a school can be good venues for an FGD.

Development of topic guide

As indicated in Figure 42.4, a topic guide is essentially an outline of the questions and issues that need to be discussed. Use of a topic guide may help effective facilitation of the FGD by providing a navigation tool for the facilitator and helps the facilitator to keep the discussion on track. Therefore, it is important to pay attention while developing a topic guide. There should be a minimal number of questions or items to be discussed to ensure availability of appropriate time for discussion.

Facilitating FGDs

In order to conduct an FGD appropriately, a facilitator requires appropriate knowledge of the topic, facilitation skills, listening abilities and patience. The FGD should start with the introduction of the facilitator and participants. It may be helpful for each member to have a name sticker to help the facilitator remember the names of the participants. The facilitator should share the aims and objectives of the research and outline the FGD at the beginning of the session. It may also be helpful to set some 'ground rules' as suggested in Figure 42.5. Obtaining consent at the start of the FGD is important. Ensure that participants understand relevant information about the study, the FGD and their rights as participants to enable them to make an informed choice. It may be more efficient to take a group-written consent than individual written consent. The facilitator should ask open-ended questions and avoid asking closed-ended question that yield 'yes' and 'no' answers only. Each participant should be given an opportunity to speak.

Further reading

Kitzinger, J. (2013) Using focus groups to understand experiences of health and illness. In: S. Ziebland, A. Coulter, J.D. Calabrese and L. Locock (eds) *Understanding and Using Health Experiences: Improving Patient Care*, pp. 49–59. Oxford: Oxford University Press.

Ritchie, J., Lewis, J., Nicholls, C.M. and Ormston, R. (eds) (2013) *Qualitative Research Practice: A Guide for Social Science Students and Researchers*, 2nd edn. London: Sage.

43 The Delphi Process

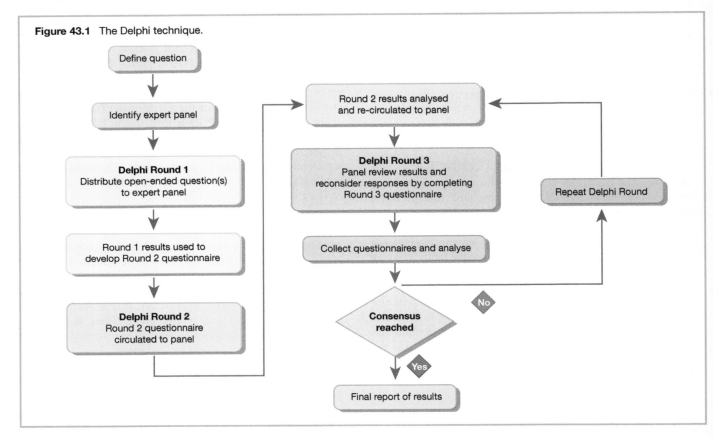

Figure 43.1 The Delphi technique.

- Define question
- Identify expert panel
- **Delphi Round 1** Distribute open-ended question(s) to expert panel
- Round 1 results used to develop Round 2 questionnaire
- **Delphi Round 2** Round 2 questionnaire circulated to panel
- Round 2 results analysed and re-circulated to panel
- **Delphi Round 3** Panel review results and reconsider responses by completing Round 3 questionnaire
- Collect questionnaires and analyse
- **Consensus reached** — No → Repeat Delphi Round; Yes → Final report of results

The Delphi technique is a systematic approach to gaining consensus among a panel of experts on an important issue. The unique structure of the Delphi technique consists of a series of sequential questionnaires, combined with controlled feedback, aimed at gaining reliable consensus from a group of experts (Linstone and Turoff, 1975).

Origins of the Delphi technique
The term 'Delphi' originates in Greek mythology, where Pythia, the resident priestess at the temple complex at Delphi, became known as the Delphic oracle for her skills of interpretation and ability to make predictions about the future (Everett, 1993). Researchers now use this technique to examine past, present and future trends. The Delphi technique was originally developed by Dalkey and colleagues at the RAND Corporation in the USA (Linstone and Turoff, 1975), where it was applied to reviewing future trends within the defence industry. Since its original development a number of Delphi techniques have evolved.

The Delphi process
The primary assumption of the Delphi process is that group opinion is more valid than individual opinion. The Delphi method therefore involves identifying experts in the area under investigation who participate and form a panel. The process is coordinated by a facilitator(s), who manages return of the questionnaires and analysis of results. The benefit of the method is that it facilitates debate between geographically separated experts who can share opinion by mail or email and reach consensus on difficult issues.

The process is initiated by sending the issue requiring consensus to members of the panel who generate solutions to statements. These are returned and collated by the facilitator. All generated solutions are then redistributed to panel members to allow them to reconsider their responses in light of the overall results. The process stops when consensus is reached, the research question is answered, saturation is achieved, or sufficient information has been exchanged (Keeney et al., 2011). This generally takes up to three rounds of questionnaires (Figure 43.1). It is recommended that a minimum of 70% return rate per round is reached to maintain rigour (Sumison, 1998).

Key features of the Delphi process
The classical Delphi process according to Rowe et al. (1991) should include the following.
- *Anonymity*: allowing free expression of opinions without social pressures from other members to conform.
- *Iteration*: refining participants' views from round to round.
- *Controlled feedback*: informing participants of the other responses, giving an opportunity to reconsider personal responses and change them.
- *Statistical aggregation of group response*: facilitating quantitative analysis and interpretation of data.

Table 43.1 Types of Delphi.

Classical Delphi	Utilises an open first round to generate ideas, elicit opinion and gain consensus. May be administered by post or email
Modified Delphi	Generally takes the form of replacing the first postal round with focus group meetings. May take the form of less than three postal or email rounds
e-Delphi	Similar process to classical Delphi, with administration by email or online web survey
Real-time Delphi	Process similar to classical Delphi, but experts may be in the same room. Consensus is reached in real time rather by post. May be referred to as a consensus conference
Online Delphi	Similar to classical Delphi but questionnaires are completed and submitted online
Technological Delphi	Similar process to real-time Delphi using technology. This may be by hand-held keypads allowing immediate responses. The technology works out the mean/median, allowing immediate feedback and opportunity to revote as a response to the group opinion
Decision Delphi	Similar process to classical Delphi, but focuses on making decisions rather than reaching consensus
Policy Delphi	Utilises the opinion of experts to reach consensus and agree policy on a specific topic
Argument Delphi	Derived from policy Delphi. Non-consensus; focused on the production of relevant factual arguments
Disaggregative Delphi	Non-consensus. Uses cluster analysis. Applies various future scenarios for discussion

The expert panel

Adler and Ziglio (1996) suggest that Delphi panellists should meet four requirements:

- knowledge and experience of the issues under investigation;
- willingness and ability to participate;
- sufficient time to participate;
- effective communication skills.

The optimum qualifications of panel members is dependent on the subject under study and the likely variance and sensitivities in the community under study. In relation to panel numbers, Delbecq et al. (1975) suggest that there should be no limit to the number of participants and that it should be representative of the population under study.

Analysis of the Delphi process

The process of analysis influences the quality of the results. Computer-mediated systems have the potential to facilitate this and expedite analysis. The electronic process can be fed into SPSS, or basic analysis can be conducted by websites such as SurveyMonkey®. Turoff and Hiltz (2008) presented specific objectives for the analysis of a Delphi study that can be easily facilitated by a computer-mediated system:

- present a clear analysis of the range of expert views and so improve the understanding of the panel members;
- highlight hidden judgemental biases and disagreements;
- detect missing information, or any ambiguity in interpretation by panel members;
- facilitate the examination of complex situations that can only be summarised by a process of analysis;
- detect patterns of data and of subgroup positions;
- highlight critical items that need greater focus.

Modifications to the Delphi process

The Delphi technique has evolved as a result of many modifications and techniques and is referred to as a 'modified' Delphi technique (Table 43.1). The most common deviation is the conduct of the first round, which may be developed by literature review, nominal group technique, idea writing or communications with stakeholders. The advantages and disadvantage of the process are highlighted in Table 43.2. Overall, the Delphi technique is increasingly applied in many areas of healthcare research to gain consensus on an issue.

References

Adler, M. and Ziglio, E. (1996) *Gazing Into the Oracle: The Delphi Method and its Application to Social Policy and Public Health*. London: Jessica Kingsley Publishers.

Table 43.2 Advantages and disadvantages of the Delphi process.

Advantages

- Method can be used to evaluate spread of opinion as well as consensus between participants
- Anonymity of Delphi participants facilitates free expression of opinions without social pressure
- The Delphi technique is adaptable and can be applied to a variety of situations and problems
- Process will generate a record of group opinions which can be reviewed at any point
- Project manager can control issues that detract from the debate
- The influence of individual personalities is removed by this process
- Improved quality of response as participants are given time to consider before responding

Disadvantages

- Requires written communication skills
- Labour-intensive and time-consuming, requires highly motivated participants
- Has not been demonstrated that results produce any better results than other judgemental techniques
- Risk of bias from the coordinating or monitor team. Debate over whether the coordinating group should be from within or outside the organisation and have experience in the subject area
- Structure of the questionnaire may lead to bias, e.g. cultural background of respondents in that they may give responses they think the panel would like to see
- In achieving consensus extreme points of view may be overlooked but may be important

Delbecq, A.L., Van de Ven, A.H. and Gustafson, D.H. (1975) *Group Techniques for Programme Planning: A Guide to Nominal and Delphi Processes*. Glenview, IL: Scott, Foresman and Co.

Everett, A. (1993) Piercing the veil of the future: a review of the Delphi method of research. *Professional Nurse* 9, 181–185.

Keeney, S., Hasson, F. and McKenna, H. (2011) *The Delphi Technique in Nursing and Health Research*. Oxford: Wiley-Blackwell.

Linstone, H. and Turoff, M. (1975) *The Delphi Method: Techniques and Applications*. Boston: Addison-Wesley.

Rowe, G., Wright, G. and Bolger, F. (1991) Delphi: a re-evaluation of research and theory. *Technical Forecasting and Social Change* 39, 235–251.

Sumison, T. (1998) The Delphi technique: an adaptive research tool. *British Journal of Occupational Therapy* 61,153–156.

Turoff, M and Hiltz, S.R. (2008) Computer-based Delphi processes. Available at http://web.njit.edu/~turoff/Papers/delphi3.html (accessed 2 September 2008).

44 The nominal group technique

Figure 44.1 The Nominal Group Technique (NGT) is an evaluative methodology which seeks consensus to a question or questions from a group of participants who wouldn't otherwise interact together. Cartoon reproduced with permission of Steven Denton.

- The process requires direct participant involvement, is non-hierarchical in nature and has the capacity to generate abundant data from only one session with participants which lasts between 1.5 and 2 hours, i.e. is time- and cost-efficient

- The technique emerged from the work of Van de Ven and Delbecq in addressing group decision-making processes

- Van de Ven and Delbecq suggest that NGT groups should be made up of no more than 5–9 participants, but larger groups can be accommodated; the technique can be used with adults and children

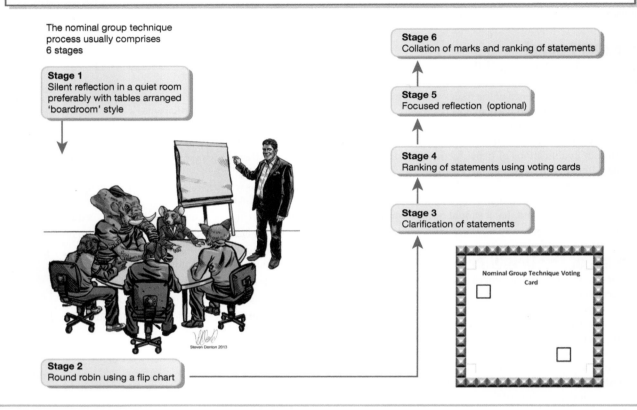

The nominal group technique process usually comprises 6 stages

Stage 1
Silent reflection in a quiet room preferably with tables arranged 'boardroom' style

Stage 2
Round robin using a flip chart

Stage 3
Clarification of statements

Stage 4
Ranking of statements using voting cards

Stage 5
Focused reflection (optional)

Stage 6
Collation of marks and ranking of statements

Nominal Group Technique Voting Card

The nominal group technique (NGT) is an evaluative focus group methodology that has both quantitative and qualitative components. These are generated from participants in response to a single posed question. Individuals are usually key informants who come together as a group nominally for the purposes of the exercise (Figure 44.1). NGT was primarily developed for use in the field of market research but has become a useful tool for researchers seeking to gain consensus answers to questions. It is a time-efficient method of collecting data, as an NGT exercise usually lasts 1.5–2 hours depending on how many questions are posed. Optimally an assistant is desirable.

Preparation

- A quiet room with tables arranged in a boardroom style.
- Flipchart with the question written on the first page in bold and different coloured flipchart pens.
- Quantity of loose A4 paper for participants to write on.
- Pens or pencils for participants.
- Adhesive Blue-Tack suitable for adhering flipchart paper sheets to walls.
- NGT voting cards ready prepared in batches of five, held together with a single paper clip in small envelopes (one envelope per participant per question).
- Preprinted question(s), one for each participant.

Stages in the NGT process

Silent reflection

After introducing yourself to the group and explaining the project and gaining written consent, sit the individuals around the boardroom table. Give each participant paper and a pen/pencil if required. Importantly, give each person a copy of the question and additionally read it verbatim from the first page of the flipchart. Ask the group if they have understood the question. This stage of the process requires the participants, without conferring, to write as many responses to the question as they can think of onto the blank piece of paper in no more than 10 minutes.

Round robin

During this phase of the process each of the participants offers the researcher one response from their list, clockwise around the group for the first question and anticlockwise for the second, and the researcher then writes that numbered response onto the flipchart starting with 1, 2, 3 and so on. There is no conferring, chatting or debate at this stage. Participants may say 'Pass' if someone else has offered a similar point but may rejoin this part of the exercise if they think of something new to add in the interim. Ask the assistant to attach each completed page to an adjacent wall. The responses are recorded from each of the participants in turn, until no responses are left to be expressed and noted, and saturation is achieved. Even small groups may generate 40 plus responses on four or more pages of flipchart per posed question.

Clarification

During this stage the researcher reads out verbatim all of the statements recorded on the flipcharts to confirm that they have accurately captured the meaning and the understanding of each of the participant's statements. Some similar statements can be amalgamated if the group agrees that this is still a true representation of their words.

Ranking of statements

Each of the participants is given five separate recording cards in a single envelope. The participants are invited to get out of their seats and examine the wall-mounted flipcharts without conferring. They are then asked to select, in no order of priority, five statements only from the lists. Using the voting cards, they are asked to write the number of the statement they have selected in the top left-hand corner box with the full written statement adjacent to it. After the participants have identified five statements by number, they are then asked to commence (again without conferring) the process of ranking each of the statements. To do this, participants are asked to hold their voting cards as if they were playing a card game. The statement that the participant feels is the most important is awarded 5 points and this is written in the bottom right-hand corner of the voting card, which is then turned face down. Then the remaining four cards are examined by the participant and the statement that is least important is awarded 1 point and again placed face down.

From the remaining three cards, the most important statement is awarded 4 points and the previous process repeated. From the final two cards, the least important statement is awarded 2 points and the remaining card is awarded 3 points. The preciseness of this stage is important to prevent participants making premature judgements. When this process is complete, the researcher then collects the paper-clipped voting cards from each participant and returns them to their envelope.

Focus reflection

This is an optional stage of the NGT process, which can be used to generate group discussion and perspectives on the statements generated and the processes involved in the NGT approach. The discussion can be recorded for later transcription and thematic analysis.

Collation of marks and ranking of statements

In this final part of the process, the researcher collates the marks awarded to the statements chosen by the participants in order to produce a hierarchy of identified statements. Although it is customary to highlight only the top five ranked statements, no data are lost and other lower scored items can be used for later inclusion in the discussion aspects of a final report. The process is repeated for subsequent questions.

Further reading

Davidson, J., Glasper, E. and Donaldson, P. (2005) Staff nurse development programme: evaluation. *Paediatric Nursing* **17**(8), 30–33.

Lennon, R., Glasper, A. and Carpenter, D. (2012) Nominal group technique: its utilisation to explore the rewards and challenges of becoming a mental health nurse, prior to the introduction of the all graduate nursing curriculum in England. *Working Papers in the Health Sciences* (Winter 2012), **1**(2).

Van de Ven, A. and Delbecq, A.L. (1971) Nominal versus interacting group processes for committee decision-making effectiveness. *Academy of Management Journal* **14**, 203–212.

45 The icon metaphor technique

Figure 45.1 The icon metaphor technique.

What is the icon metaphor technique?
Within the context of focus group work the term icon is used to refer to a small image or series of images drawn by the members of the group which embeds 'meaning' and which can be embellished with metaphors. This approach enhances the traditional focus group approach by trying to stimulate creativity and breadth and depth of discussion. It has similarities to the Zaltman metaphor elicitation technique, and the technique of using drawings as a research method both of which use images that represent the thoughts and feelings of participants to the topic of interest.

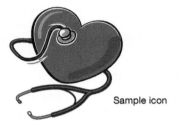

Sample icon

Method
The icon metaphor approach can be used to facilitate a focus group. The focus group facilitator also takes notes

1. Divide the main focus group into small groups of 2/3

2. Clearly delineate the topic of the focus group and the areas or questions that need addressing. Allocate a specific topic or question to each group (optional)

3. Give each group flip chart paper and felt pens

4. Ask each group to independently generate icons/drawings that symbolise their thoughts on the subject

5. On the reverse of each flip chart ask the group members to generate metaphors which elucidate the icon portrayal. Adhere each flip chart icon to an adjacent surface.

6. Each group offers its flip chart icon illustration to the remaining focus group members, who then after consideration embellish this with their own series of metaphors that help them understand the icon(s) being displayed

7. The flip chart(s) is then reversed to reveal the metaphors of the group which originated the icon drawing

8. Thus each icon in turn acts as a prompt for exploratory debate

9. This approach enhances the traditional focus group approach by trying to stimulate creativity and breadth and depth of discussion

10. The metaphor embellished icons and other notes are collected and used as data to address the topic being explored

What is the icon metaphor technique?

This interactive and fun method of conducting a focus group has similarities to the Zaltman metaphor elicitation technique and the technique of using drawings as a research method, both of which use images that represent the thoughts and feelings of participants to the topic of interest. Such techniques are often used in marketing and utilise photographs and other sensory images that consumers of products provide and which are used to explore, for example, the success of branding and customer attraction to a product.

The icon metaphor technique uses hand-drawn images, and within the context of focus group work an icon refers to a small image or series of images drawn by members of the group that embeds 'meaning' and which can be embellished with metaphors. This approach enhances the traditional focus group approach by trying to stimulate creativity and breadth and depth of discussion (Figure 45.1).

To illustrate the technique, an example published by Richardson *et al.* (2007) will be used. In this example, the researchers conducted a focus group with 18 senior members of the children's nursing community to explore the need for changes to the prevailing model of preparing pre-registration children's nurses. This came about in light of the 2007 UK Nursing and Midwifery Council (NMC) professional consultation on the future direction of pre-registration nurse training.

The 18 participants were asked to use the icon metaphor technique to explore the strengths, weaknesses, opportunities and threats of this consultation to the future preparation of children's nurses. The NMC consultation was orientated around seven discrete areas pertaining to the debate on the future direction of pre-registration nurse preparation.

Method

1 The icon metaphor approach was used within the context of a focus group. The focus group facilitator, in addition to running the event, also takes notes.
2 The main focus group was divided into seven small groups of two to three senior nurses.

3 The seven NMC topics were clearly delineated by the facilitator and each group was allocated a specific topic to discuss.
4 Each group was issued flip chart paper and felt pens.
5 Each group was asked to independently generate icons/drawings that symbolised their thoughts on the allocated subject.
6 After completion of the icon drawing, each group was asked to generate metaphors which elucidated the icon portrayal on the reverse of the flipchart. The individual group icon drawings were then adhered to adjacent walls for viewing.
7 Each group was then asked to offer their flipchart icon illustrations to the remaining focus group members for consideration. The viewers were asked to embellish the image(s) with their own series of metaphors that helped them understand the icon(s) being displayed.
8 One by one the flipchart images were then reversed to reveal the metaphors generated by the group which originated the icon drawing(s).
9 Thus each icon acted in turn as a prompt for exploratory debate.
10 This approach enhanced the traditional focus group approach by endeavouring to stimulate creativity and breadth and depth of discussion. The metaphor-embellished icons and other notes were collected and used as data to address the primary topic being explored, i.e. the future preparation of children's nurses. An analysis of these data demonstrated that senior children's nurses firmly believed in retaining a discrete children's and young people's nursing field of practice at the pre-registration level.

Reference and further reading

Guillemin, M. (2004) Understanding illness: using drawings as a research method. *Qualitative Health Research* **14**, 272–289.

Richardson, J., Glasper, E.A., McEwing, J., Ellis, J. and Horsely, A. (2007) All change in children's and young people's nurse education: the views of senior practitioners. *Journal of Children's and Young People's Nursing* **1**(8), 377–383.

Sugai, P. (2005) Mapping the mind of the mobile consumer across borders: an application of the Zaltman metaphor elicitation technique. *International Marketing Review* **22**, 641–657.

46 Interpretative phenomenological analysis

Figure 46.1 Interpretive phenomenological analysis (IPA) is a qualitative methodology that aims to understand and make sense of lived experience.

IPA was first described by Smith in 1996 and has its theoretical roots in the work of philosophers such as Husserl, Heidegger and Merleu–Ponty

Research questions aim to yield rich data about individual's lived experience

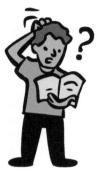

Data is collected from in-depth semi structured interviews with participants who have direct experience of the topic under investigation

Data is analysed on a case-by-case basis. Emergent themes are identified and clustered together into master themes. Finally, connections between cases are examined and a list of superordinate themes devised

Findings are presented as a narrative account and include the researcher's interpretations alongside excerpts from the transcripts. Care is taken to ensure interpretations are grounded in the data

The term 'phenomenology' is derived from the Greek words *phainómenon* ('that which appears') and *lógos* ('study'). Phenomenology is a branch of philosophy that is interested in how people understand and experience the world they live in. Interpretative phenomenological analysis (IPA) is a qualitative research methodology that is interested in how people understand and make sense of their lived experiences (Figure 46.1). IPA was introduced by Smith (1996) as a research methodology that provided researchers with an alternative way of thinking about and analysing data. IPA developed from the ideas of philosophers such as Husserl, Heidegger and Merleau-Ponty in the early twentieth century.

There are three key theoretical components of IPA: phenomenology (how we experience things), hermeneutics (the theory of interpretation, or how we make sense of) and idiography (a detailed description of how a particular person in a particular context makes sense of a particular phenomenon at a particular point in time).

IPA is a useful approach in health-related contexts as it allows practitioners an insider perspective into the 'lifeworld' of individuals, providing helpful insights into situations individuals face on a daily basis. IPA can yield helpful insights into the experiences and meanings people hold about events they have lived through (past and present) and the sense they make of them.

There is a growing body of evidence that describes IPA's theoretical basis, application and practice, particularly within healthcare settings (Smith *et al.*, 1999, 2009a, 2009b; Smith, 2004, 2007, 2009; Reid *et al.*, 2005; Eatough and Smith, 2008). Examples of studies which have used IPA in a healthcare context include: Understanding the lived experiences of people with chronic fatigue syndrome, Parkinson's disease and chronic benign lower back pain.

Given that IPA aims to give voice to the views of participants, it can be argued that it fits well with national policies promoting service user involvement in service design and development (Reid *et al.*, 2005; Department of Health, 2010).

Research questions

IPA is suited to studies where the researcher is interested in exploring and/or understanding the experience and meaning held by an individual about a particular phenomenon (Smith *et al.*, 2009c).

Sample

Because IPA is an idiographic approach, sample sizes tend to be small in order to facilitate a detailed analysis of the data generated. Participants are purposively selected to ensure a fairly homogeneous sample of participants who are able to provide rich data about their understanding and perceptions of the topic being researched.

Process

Data collection

In-depth, semi-structured, one-to-one interviews are the most commonly used methods of data collection. Interviews may take up to an hour and a half. The aim of the interview is to undertake a detailed exploration about the lived experience held by individuals about the topic area.

Data collection tool

A semi-structured interview guide allows researchers to develop open-ended questions about the topic area in order to generate rich qualitative data from participants. Interview guides can be used flexibly and usually include a maximum of 10 questions. Interviews are recorded and transcribed.

Data analysis

IPA studies require a detailed and in-depth analysis of collected data to capture the 'insider perspective' of participants (Conrad, 1987 cited in Smith *et al.*, 2009d). It is helpful for researchers to develop a framework for collating their notes and the use of a field diary is recommended. Data analysis comprises six steps. (Smith *et al.*, 2009e)

Step 1: Reading and re-reading

It is important that researchers become familiar with the data collected. It is recommended that recordings of the interviews are listened to, and transcripts read and re-read several times. This process helps the researcher get close to the participants' experience, and with repeated readings new information, ideas and areas of interest emerge.

Step 2: Initial noting

The researcher's focus at this stage is to comment on the data. This requires the researcher to 'engage' with the text, commenting on their initial thoughts and reflections and paying attention to the participants' use of language.

Step 3: Developing emergent themes

The next step is to identify emergent themes arising from the initial notes. At this stage, the researcher is moving from a descriptive to an interpretative reading of the text. Emergent themes aim to capture the participants' narrative and the researcher's interpretation.

Step 4: Searching for connections across emergent themes

Emergent themes are organised chronologically and are examined looking for connections. Themes that seem to fit together are clustered into master themes. Care is taken to make note of phrases or sentences from the transcripts which evidence the themes. This process is repeated for each participant.

Step 5: Moving to the next case

Steps 1–4 are repeated for all the interviews.

Step 6: Looking for patterns across cases

Once all the transcripts have been individually analysed, connections between cases are sought and a list of superordinate themes devised.

Findings

Findings are presented as a narrative account and include the researcher's interpretations alongside excerpts from the transcripts. Care is taken to ensure interpretations are grounded in the data. IPA acknowledges the influence that researchers have on the data collection and analysis process and the recognition of the impact of contextual factors is widely accepted.

References and further reading

Dean, S.G., Smith, J.A. and Payne, S. (2006) Low back pain: exploring the meaning of exercise management through interpretative phenomenological analysis. In: L. Finlay and C. Ballinger (eds) *Qualitative Research for Allied Health Professionals*, pp. 139–155. Chichester: Whurr Publishers.

Department of Health (2010) *Achieving Equity and Excellence for Children*. London: Department for Education and Skills.

Eatough, V. and Smith, J.A. (2008) Interpretative phenomenological analysis. In: C. Willig and W. Stainton-Rogers (eds) *The Sage Handbook of Qualitative Research in Psychology*, pp. 179–194. Los Angeles: Sage.

Reid, K., Flowers, P. and Larkin, M. (2005) Exploring lived in experience: an introduction to interpretative phenomenological analysis. *The Psychologist* **18**, 20–23.

Smith, J. (2009) Health and Illness. In: Interpretative *Phenomenological Analysis: Theory, Method and Research*, pp. 121–134. London: Sage.

Smith, J.A. (1996) Beyond the divide between cognition and discourse: using interpretative phenomenological analysis in health psychology. *Psychology and Health* **11**, 261–271.

Smith, J.A. (2004) Reflecting on the development of interpretative phenomenological analysis and its contribution to qualitative research in psychology. *Qualitative Research in Psychology* **1**, 39–54.

Smith, J.A. (2007) Hermeneutics, human sciences and health: linking theory and practice. *International Journal of Qualitative Studies on Health and Well-being* **2**, 3–11.

Smith, J.A., Jarman, M. and Osborn, M. (1999) Doing interpretative phenomenological analysis. In: M. Murray and K. Chamberlain (eds) *Qualitative Health Psychology: Theories and Methods*, pp. 218–241. London: Sage.

Smith, J.A., Flowers, P. and Larkin, M. (2009a) Collecting data. In: *Interpretative Phenomenological Analysis: Theory, Method and Research*, pp. 56–78. London: Sage.

Smith, J.A., Flowers, P. and Larkin, M. (2009b) Planning an IPA research study. In: *Interpretative Phenomenological Analysis: Theory, Method and Research*, pp. 40–55. London: Sage.

Smith, J.A., Flowers, P. and Larkin, M. (2009c) Introduction. In: *Interpretative Phenomenological Analysis: Theory, Method and Research*, pp. 1–8. London: Sage.

Smith, J.A., Flowers, P. and Larkin, M. (2009d) Introduction. In: *Interpretative Phenomenological Analysis: Theory, Method and Research*, pp. 11–39. London: Sage.

Smith, J.A., Flowers, P. and Larkin, M. (2009e) Introduction. In: *Interpretative Phenomenological Analysis: Theory, Method and Research*, pp. 79–107. London: Sage.

Todres, L. and Holloway, L. (2006) Phenomenological research In: K. Gerrish and A. Lacey (eds) *The Research Process in Nursing*, pp. 224–238. Oxford: Blackwell Publishing.

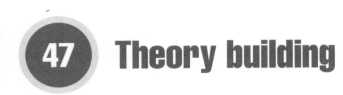

47 Theory building

Figure 47.1 What do theories do?

- A theory must specify a set of components or mechanisms that work together to produce a structure, relationship or outcome
- A theory must explain how its specified components behave and what the consequences of that behaviour are
- A theory must lead to generic explanations, propositions, or experimental hypotheses

Figure 47.2 We build a theory when we...

- Clearly identify and accurately describe a set of components or mechanisms that are at work in a context
- When we model the relationships between components and characterise the operation of mechanisms that are at work
- Develop systematic explanations that can be empirically tested through simulations, observations, or experiments

Figure 47.3 Using the NPT Toolkit to discover the normalisation potential of an innovation: www.normalizationprocess.org

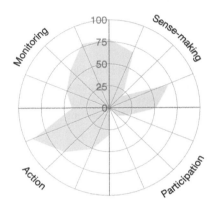

Figure 47.4 Constructs and variables of the new theory.

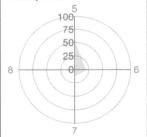
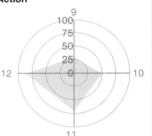
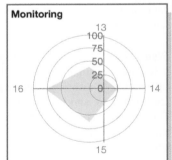

Sense-making

1. Participants distinguish the intervention from current ways of working
2. Participants collectively agree about the purpose of the intervention
3. Participants individually understand what the intervention requires of them
4. Participants construct potential value of the intervention for their work

Participation

5. Key individuals drive the intervention forward
6. Participants agree that the intervention should be part of their work
7. Participants buy in to the intervention
8. Participants continue to support the intervention

Action

9. Participants perform the tasks required by the intervention
10. Participants maintain their trust in each other's work and expertise through the intervention
11. The work of the intervention is appropriately allocated to participants
12. The intervention is adequately supported by its host organisation

Monitoring

13. Participants access information about the effects of the intervention
14. Participants collectively assess the intervention as worthwhile
15. Participants individually assess the intervention as worthwhile
16. Participants modify their work in response to their appraisal of the intervention

Nursing and Healthcare Research at a Glance, First Edition. Alan Glasper and Colin Rees. © 2017 by John Wiley & Sons, Ltd. Published 2017 by John Wiley & Sons, Ltd.

Why build a theory?

Theories are important because they provide the conceptual structure for all research. So, when we do health services research we do three things. First, we ask questions about how healthcare is organised, enacted and conceptualised. Second, we collect and analyse data that we believe will form the basis of the answer to those questions. Third, we then explain how that data analysis answers our questions, and what those answers mean. This is a basic application of the scientific method: theories form the fundamental building blocks of this work because they provide the models that inform our questions; require us to use particular research methods; and form a structure for the explanation of results.

My research team has focused on implementing telemedicine and ehealth systems: the diagnosis and management of patients using different kinds of remote management systems. From the beginning, it was clear to us that no matter how enthusiastic clinicians and patients were about these new systems, there were real problems in getting them routinely incorporated into practice. So, we had an object for our work (telemedicine systems) and a problem (difficulties in integrating them into practice) and we needed to be able to explain why that problem took the form that it did. As we started to think about this we saw that this was a generic problem: that many other complex healthcare interventions also seemed to be resistant to routine incorporation into practice. This led us to a research question: 'What factors promote or inhibit the normalisation of complex interventions in routine practice?' In turn, this would require us to answer the question: 'How can we explain the operation of these factors?'

As we looked at these problems we could see that existing theories of implementation would not help us answer these two questions. They were new, and they were interesting. We needed a new theory.

Building a theory from the ground up?

When we build a theory, we create a new explanation for an existing set of phenomena. As we looked at the implementation of complex interventions we saw that there was an implementation theory-shaped hole in implementation science. It is important to remember that the job of a theory is to do work for us, and we knew that we needed a theory to do three things: identify elements of the problem; explain the mechanisms that lead to their operationalisation; and offer hypotheses about other, similar, mechanisms so that we could transport our explanation from one problem to another (Figures 47.1 and 47.2).

We started by thinking about the data that we had available. This consisted of the results of more than 20 studies, conducted over the previous 8 years. We were able to divide this material into four groups: studies of professional–patient interaction around disease management; new technologies in clinical settings; new ways of organising care; and new ways of defining and organising evidence about practice. Against this background we conducted a set of formative analyses of these data. In each case, we started by identifying components, building a taxonomy of factors that affected the normalisation of new clinical practices. These were identified and reduced to their simplest form. Then we sorted these components, eliminating duplicates and retaining only those that had clear face validity as components of a possible theory. Components that survived this process were then written up as constructs that explained implementation processes and that could be defined as propositions or hypotheses that could be retrospectively evaluated against the known outcomes of a set of implementation processes.

We did not just do this once. Over a period of 10 years we did it three times. Each time we did it, we extended the analysis. Ultimately, we identified four major factors and 16 components that would determine whether or not a complex intervention could be normalised in practice. Then we set up an online research tool that would help researchers and health service managers think through these problems. We called the result normalisation process theory (May et al., 2007; May and Finch, 2009; May, 2013). As you can see from Figures 47.3 and 47.4, we were able to present the results of this in a simple way, showing how the variables defined by the theory related to each other when people entered data about responses to a new innovation from their staff and patients.

What did our theory look like?

At its core, our theory proposed that the normalisation of complex interventions in routine practice depended on action rather than attitudes. It was what people did, rather than how they felt, that determined whether new technologies were embedded in practice.

We stated that a complex intervention was disposed to normalisation if it conferred on its users an interactional advantage in flexibly accomplishing action, and conferred an advantage on its host organisation in flexibly executing actions. Further, it would need to fit with agreed skill-set, and improve accountability and confidence among its users. However, for this to happen, its users would have to translate their potential to enact it into actual investments in sense-making, participation, collective action and appraisal. This could happen when users translated their capacity for cooperation and coordination into work that ensured that the complex intervention could be made workable and could be integrated into their everyday practice.

Acknowledgements

Work discussed in this chapter was funded by the Economic and Social Research Council. I gratefully acknowledge this support and the contribution of Tracy Finch, Frances Mair and many others to the work described here.

References

May, C. (2013) Towards a general theory of implementation. *Implementation Science* **8**, 18.

May, C. and Finch, T. (2009) Implementation, embedding, and integration: an outline of normalization process theory. *Sociology* **43**, 535–554.

May, C., Finch, T., Mair, F. et al. (2007) Understanding the implementation of complex interventions in health care: the normalization process model. *BMC Health Services Research* **7**, 148.

48 Qualitative interviewing

Figure 48.1 Why do qualitative interviews

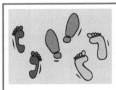
Qualitative interviews give access to how other people see the world, thus generating data on people's experiences, perceptions, concerns, and expectations

Figure 48.2 What are qualitative interviews.

In healthcare, this information is used to understand why patients or providers behave the way they do. With this understanding we can modify or change healthcare to better suit a populations' healthcare needs
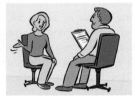

Figure 48.3 Who to interview.

What people are most likely to have the information you are looking for?

- Patient or practitioners?
- People with specific diseases?
- What other characteristics do you think may be important?

Where will you access these people?
Think about the different services they are involved with
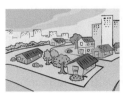

Figure 48.4 Where do you do the interview.

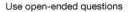
Context is important in qualitative interviewing:
- Doing an interview in your university or hospital may be convenient for you, but...
- if you interview in the participant's home or local community centre, you will learn a lot about their social environment...
- ...where is most comfortable/ accessible/quiet/safe?

Figure 48.5 Preparing for your interviews.

Checklist when going to interviews

- Accurate directions/address
- Transport/parking information
- Audio-recorder
- Spare batteries
- Topic guide
- Consent form
- Participant information leaflet
- Notepad and pen
- Mobile phone
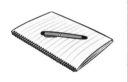

Figure 48.6 What to do in the interview.

Introduce topics into the flow of conversation

Use open-ended questions

Watch the participant's responses: Are they uncomfortable? What does this mean? Should you probe it further or leave it alone?

Allow time for silence.
If you are not talking, the patient is more likely to speak!

Active listening is essential:
give the interviewee your full attention!

Figure 48.7 Managing the data.

Write down your impressions of the interview as soon as possible or talk to another researcher about how it went (debriefing)

Keep the interview records safe and confidential
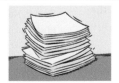

Recordings can be analysed directly or typed out and analysed from text. One hour of talking equals seven hours of typing

Computer packages are available to help you manage and store the data, but they do not do the analysis for you!

Nursing and Healthcare Research at a Glance, First Edition. Alan Glasper and Colin Rees. © 2017 by John Wiley & Sons, Ltd. Published 2017 by John Wiley & Sons, Ltd.

What are qualitative interviews?

Qualitative interviews (QIs) are a method of producing qualitative data using a flexible interview that focuses on gaining the interviewee's opinions and experiences of the issue being researched (Figure 48.1). QIs use less structure than the quantitative survey or questionnaire-based interview. The two principal forms of QI are as follows.

1 Semi-structured: a list of questions is used as a guide to ensure certain topics are discussed, but still allows room for the participant to talk in detail on particular aspects of interest to them.

2 In-depth: a few open questions are used with the aim of eliciting a rich and detailed narrative from the participant on the research issue.

QIs last from 10–15 minutes to over an hour, are generally one-on-one and are audio-recorded with the interviewee's consent.

Why use qualitative interviews?

In healthcare, QIs help us understand health behaviours, what health and disease mean to people, and what their healthcare needs, expectations and concerns are. They can also be used to explore why healthcare interventions succeed or fail (Figure 48.2). Generating good-quality data in QIs requires strong interpersonal and communication skills, many of which overlap with those used by healthcare providers in their everyday dealings with patients. However, in QI the emphasis is on the interviewee, and not the interviewer, doing the talking.

Who do you interview?

To decide who to interview, think about your research question and what you want to gain from your work (Figure 48.3). Do you need older or younger people? Is gender important? What about their jobs, level of education or home circumstances? Then consider where you will get access to these people, for example hospital clinics, advocacy groups, social support services (Figure 48.4).

Your sample may be:
• purposive (the people most likely to give you the information you are looking for);
• maximum variation (people that represent a range of characteristics within a population);
• deviant cases (people whose experiences likely represent the opposite of the norm);
• theoretical (sampling based on your increasing understanding of the research question as interviews progress);
• convenience (inviting people that you have easy access to);
• snowball (asking interviewees to recommend colleagues/contacts who may be interested in, or of interest to, your study).
The number of people interviewed is influenced by time, resources and the diversity of data in the interviews. Ideally, interviewing should continue until data saturation is reached, i.e. no new information is emerging from new interviews.

Generating the data

Good rapport between interviewer and interviewee is a key ingredient for sharing information. Be polite and non-judgemental at all times, but try not to bias the interview by explicitly agreeing with or encouraging the interviewee's opinions. You are aiming for the role of interested respectful enquirer.

The following are a range of interview techniques to consider.

1 Prepare how you will begin the interview: for example, introduce yourself and your research interests; discuss consent, confidentiality, audio-recording, and the duration and general format of the interview (if using a topic guide or not) (Figure 48.5). Opening questions should be broad and easy to answer, for example diary-type questions: 'Tell me about the first/last time you went to hospital?' or 'Can you tell me about the last time that went well/badly for you?'

2 Topic guides are lists of topics that you want to cover in the interview. Reading about other work in your field can help inform your topic guide, but be careful to keep an open mind to new ideas when in the interview.

3 Develop a deeper understanding by probing what participants say, for example 'How did you react then?' or 'How did that make you feel?'

4 Sometimes it is easier to gain access to what the participant thinks by referring to others, for example 'Some people I have interviewed have told me that they were very fearful on their last visit to hospital. What do you think about that?'

5 Clarify if your understanding of a word is the same as theirs. An example is the word 'chronic'; while healthcare providers understand this as relating to time, many lay people understand it as relating to severity. You will only know what your interviewee means if you ask them!

6 Non-verbal cues, such as active listening, maintaining eye contact and an open stance, leaving time for silence, reassure interviewees of your interest and may prompt them to continue or expand on something they have said (Figure 48.6).

7 Keep questions simple and clear, and use lay language, mirroring the interviewee's own vocabulary if appropriate. Pilot your topic guide on a non-healthcare-trained friend.

Reflexivity

Consider your professional biases, how the participant sees you (as healthcare provider or researcher) and how this will influence their responses in the interview (see also Figure 48.4).

Ethics

The impact of the interview on participants, their ability to give informed consent, and the confidentiality of interview data may require ethics committee approval.

After the interview

1 Make field notes as soon as possible, including details of the setting and surrounding environment, and your initial reactions to the interview data (Figure 48.7).

2 Listen to the interviews, the questions you asked and the participants' reaction to them: what worked and what didn't?

3 Audio-recordings are transcribed to provide an accurate account of what and how things were said, and allow repeated reviews of the data and comparisons to be made across interviews.

4 Data analysis may use one of many methodologies (e.g. phenomenology, thematic) but all begin with familiarisation with the interview data in the early stages.

Further reading

Green, J. and Thorogood, N. (2004) Qualitative Methods for Health Research. London: Sage.
Kvale, S. (1996) Interviews: An Introduction to Qualitative Interviewing. London: Sage.
Pope, C. & Mays, N. (2006) Qualitative Research in Health Care, 3rd edn. London: BMJ Books.

49 Thematic analysis

Figure 49.1 An example of the thematic analysis process.

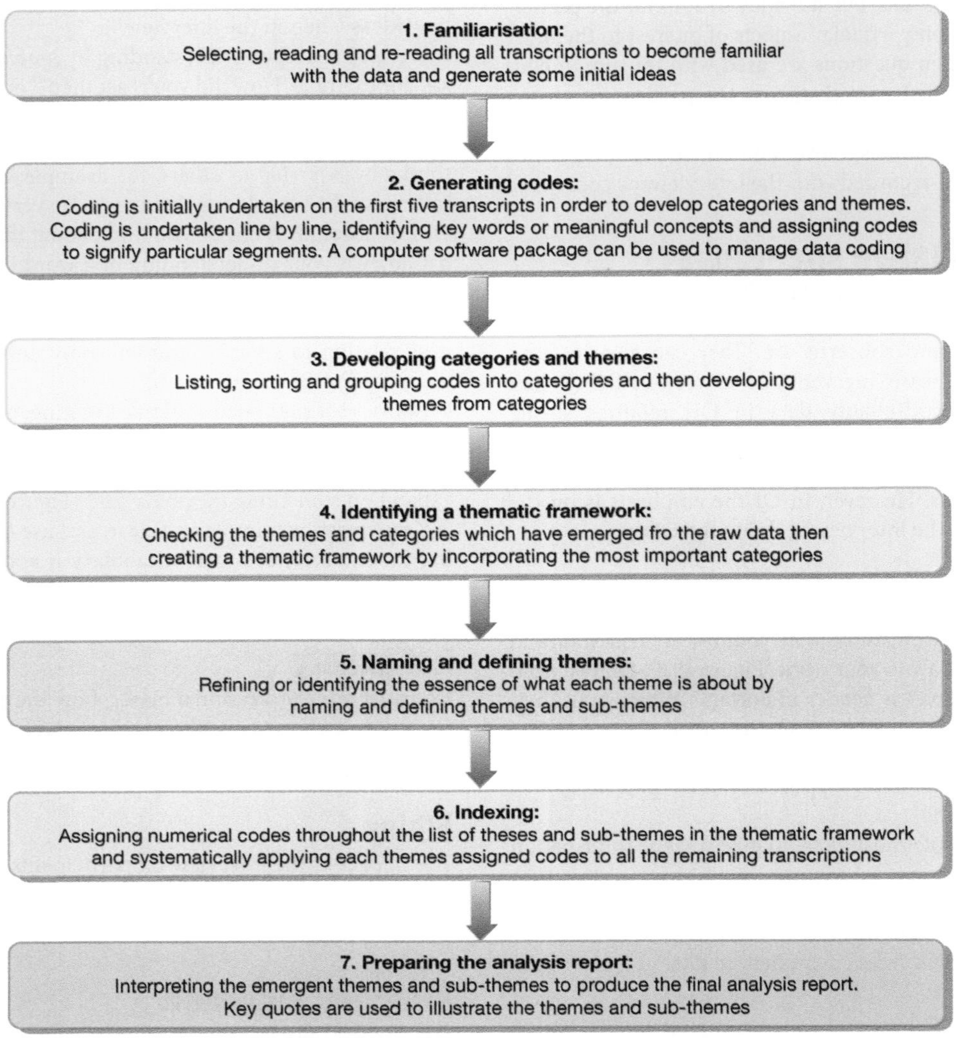

1. Familiarisation:
Selecting, reading and re-reading all transcriptions to become familiar
with the data and generate some initial ideas

2. Generating codes:
Coding is initially undertaken on the first five transcripts in order to develop categories and themes.
Coding is undertaken line by line, identifying key words or meaningful concepts and assigning codes
to signify particular segments. A computer software package can be used to manage data coding

3. Developing categories and themes:
Listing, sorting and grouping codes into categories and then developing
themes from categories

4. Identifying a thematic framework:
Checking the themes and categories which have emerged fro the raw data then
creating a thematic framework by incorporating the most important categories

5. Naming and defining themes:
Refining or identifying the essence of what each theme is about by
naming and defining themes and sub-themes

6. Indexing:
Assigning numerical codes throughout the list of theses and sub-themes in the thematic framework
and systematically applying each themes assigned codes to all the remaining transcriptions

7. Preparing the analysis report:
Interpreting the emergent themes and sub-themes to produce the final analysis report.
Key quotes are used to illustrate the themes and sub-themes

What is thematic analysis?

Thematic analysis is a common approach to analysing qualitative data, especially in healthcare research. It involves examining, identifying, developing and reporting categories and themes within data in depth. However, there is no particular way or explicit guidelines on how to perform thematic analysis, so in this chapter we share our experience of undertaking thematic analysis.

The steps of thematic analysis

The process of thematic analysis follows several steps (Figure 49.1).

Familiarisation

The initial phase consists of reading the transcripts and listening to the audio files several times in order to become familiar with data. In addition, any initial ideas that may later inform the analysis are noted.

Generating codes

Each transcript is read line by line to identify key words or meaningful concepts relating to the study's aims and research questions. Key words or concepts are then assigned codes to signify those particular segments. Commonly, computer software packages such as Nvivo are used for data management.

Developing categories and themes

All the codes from the selected transcripts are then listed and reduced, where possible, by merging codes if appropriate or deleting redundant codes. The remaining codes are then sorted by grouping similar codes into categories and categories into themes.

Identifying a thematic framework

The emergent themes from the selected transcripts are reviewed to ensure they are meaningful and clear and that they are clearly distinguishable from other themes. The themes are then incorporated into the thematic framework.

Naming and defining themes

To identify the essence of each emerged theme within the thematic framework, each theme is given an appropriate name and clearly defined. This process helps elucidate the story that each theme delivers and ensure that there is no overlap between themes.

Indexing

The list of themes and categories within the thematic framework are then assigned a numerical code. These codes are then systematically applied to all the remaining transcriptions.

Preparing the analysis report

The emerging themes and categories are interpreted. The analysis report is prepared describing the findings using key quotations to illustrate the themes and categories identified.

Further reading

Braun, V. and Clarke, V. (2006) Using thematic analysis in psychology. *Qualitative Research in Psychology* **3**, 77–101.

Pope, C., Ziebland, S. and Mays, N. (2006) Analysing qualitative data. In: C. Pope and N. Mays (eds) *Qualitative Research in Health Care*, 3rd edn, pp. 63–81. Oxford: Blackwell Publishing.

Srimuang, P. (2013) *Teachers' and students' perceptions of meditation education and its contribution to the mental well-being of young people in secondary school in Khonkaen province Thailand.* PhD thesis, University of Southampton.

50 Social network analysis

Figure 50.1 Social network analysis.

A social network is made of individuals, groups or organizations that have relations or ties between them. Social Network Analyses are techniques that analyze social networks.

1. We often associate social networks with digital services such as Facebook or Twitter, but research in social networks has a long tradition. In the 1930s, for example, Jacob Moreno studied friendship patterns, and how group relations both limited and expanded actions and, consequently, personal psychological development.

2. Social networks are often graphically depicted by network diagrams that show nodes and their connections. These can often look like complex spider webs.

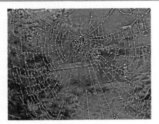

3. Nodes can represent individuals, groups, organizations, or other collective units (such as 'departments' or 'wards').

4. The ties between nodes or actors are their relational ties or social relations. These may include kinship, friendship, communication patterns, material resources...

5. The structure of the network and strength and the nature of the relationships are important elements of social network analysis because these can affect the behaviours of individuals or groups in the network.

6. Research in social network analysis is used to understand interactions in communities, the diffusion of innovations and ideas, how individuals and groups collaborate (or compete), how economic systems operate, and more.

7. Social network analysis is becoming an increasingly important research area in health and social care. It is used in health and social care to understand, for example, patient networks and patient groups, how patients manage their conditions at home, disease transmission, resource allocation, and how new knowledge is generated, shared and used.

social network is made of two elements: (i) individuals, groups, organisations or other social collectives; and (ii) the relations or ties among them. A social network does not reside only in digital networks such as Facebook or Twitter, but exist in non-digital settings. These settings can be small, such as nurses in a ward at a hospital; medium-sized, such as all nurses in a hospital itself; or large and open-ended, such as all nurses in all the hospitals in a country. The nature of social ties and their structure often affect individuals and their relations and actions. For example, groups that have a large number of weak ties (e.g. having a large number of varied acquaintances) tend to be more innovative than those with very strong bonds because they have ties with others who are *unlike themselves*. Groups that have weak ties engender more diversity than those that have close ties with others like themselves.

What are the key concepts?

The key idea in social networks is that individuals, groups and other social entities are not discrete units but instead live in a web of connections and affiliations: there are individuals and there are relations that connect those individuals. Social network analysis (Figure 50.1) is concerned with both the strength and the nature of those relations, for example a friendship, a kinship tie, a professional affiliation, a fellow community member, a fellow hobbyist, a co-worker, a member of a sports team or political party, an acquaintance who shares a mutual friend. The principle that individuals have relationships or ties suggests that actors in a social network are interdependent, the nature of the network influences the opportunities and constraints of individual action, and the flow of resources (such as information, knowledge and material) can be directed and predicted.

Why care about social networks in healthcare?

Researchers often want to know the nature of disease transmission; how patients are cared for at home; where resources are needed, how they are used, and by whom; how process knowledge and innovations are diffused; what factors influence the choices that patients make in managing their conditions. These do not happen randomly, but are influenced by the social ties that individuals and groups have. For example, networks of care groups can share practice, or social relations can

affect the transmission of disease. Conversely, understanding social relations can help to control the transmission of disease because interventions can be targeted to those who exert the most influence within a social network.

How you can study a social network

The first step is to define the population of actors or individuals. This can be a closed set of individuals, such as nurses in a ward or doctors in a unit, or a large open-ended population (such as patients who share a common disease or set of diseases). It is practical to start relatively small. Once you define your population, you then define their attributes or compositional variables. These will be influenced by the rationale of your study. Such attributes would include sex, age, occupation or role, or any set of other attributes that are relevant to your study. Then you define the relations among members of the population. This has two aspects: Who is connected to whom? What is the relation? For example, the relation can be a friendship, a co-worker, or someone who receives/gives information.

Tools that help

A simple network can be drawn with pen and paper, but large or elaborate networks require software that draws the networks as well as measures the characteristics and structure of the network. The website at http://joitskehulsebosch.blogspot.co.uk/2013/11/tools-for-social-network-analysis-from.html contains useful information for beginners.

Further reading

Giordano, R. (2007) The scientist: secretive, selfish or reticent. A social network analysis. In: *Proceedings of the 2007 eSocial Science Conference*. Ann Arbor, Michigan, USA. Available at http://citeseerx.ist.psu.edu/viewdoc/download?doi=10.1.1.125.7099&rep=rep1&type=pdf

Rogers, A., Brooks, H., Vassilev, I., Kennedy, A., Blickem, C. and Reeves, D. (2014) Why less may be more: a mixed methods study of the work and relatedness of 'weak ties' in supporting long-term condition self-management. *Implementation Science* **9**, 19. doi: 10.1186/1748-5908-9-19.

Scott, J. (2000) *Social Network Analysis: A Handbook*. London: Sage.

Wasserman, S. and Faust, K. (1994) *Social Network Analysis: Methods and Applications*. New York: Cambridge University Press.

51 Critical discourse analysis

Figure 51.1 The 3 dimensions of interactional analysis.

1. Text Analysis: focus on texts

2. Interdiscursive Analysis: focus on texts & interaction

3. Social Analysis: focus on interactions & interpretations

Figure 51.2 Fairclough's critical discourse theory on production, interaction and interpretation of text.

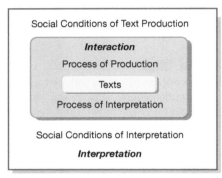

Social Conditions of Text Production

Interaction

Process of Production

Texts

Process of Interpretation

Social Conditions of Interpretation

Interpretation

Figure 51.3 Use of CDA on online text based on Fairclough's critical discourse theory.

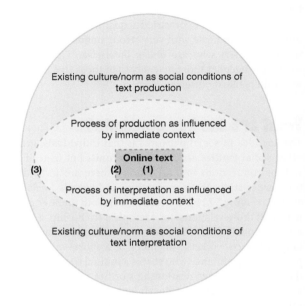

Existing culture/norm as social conditions of text production

Process of production as influenced by immediate context

Online text

(3) (2) (1)

Process of interpretation as influenced by immediate context

Existing culture/norm as social conditions of text interpretation

There are various versions of critical discourse analysis (CDA). This chapter focuses on Fairclough's (2003) textually oriented discourse analysis and its application to online discussion (Figure 51.1).

Assumptions in CDA

Texts are produced based on speech or writing in the course of social events when people act or interact. While not all social events have highly textual characteristics, all online discussions are highly linguistic; even emoticons are textual portrayals of a writer's mood or facial expressions. It is important to note that texts are shaped by social events, social practices and social structures; all in turn are shaped by text.

Conducting CDA in three stages

Consider the following analysis of text from an interprofessional text-based learning module about e-learning in healthcare by a group of healthcare professionals as Master's students:

> In other parts of England, particularly London, where my sister from Hewlett Packard has business dealings, gave me a very similar picture.
>
> *Contribution by a nursing student*

Text analysis

Whole text organisation

This involves analysing of the genre. First, note how the author is relying on the fact that Hewlett Packard (HP) is well known for computing technologies and the text refers to the author's sister who is affiliated to HP.

Clauses combination

Next, determine how dialogical the text is. In this sentence, there is no use of conjunctions or sentence adverbials ('however', 'nevertheless' or 'therefore') to connect the sentences into an argumentative thread. This sentence is therefore declarative in nature and non-dialogical.

Clauses

Now re-examine the text and see how the series of declarations made it non-dialogical; it uses 'London', which has major business districts for technologies. It also has a strong degree of commitment to truth (the sister, a sibling from HP and is therefore a reliable expert). The text is constructed to support another author based on the opinion of a reliable 'expert' who had apparently given the author a very similar picture.

Interdiscursive analysis

Examine the genres and discourse which were drawn on in the text. Continue to analyse how they work together in the text. These sequential steps allow you to establish the extent of hybridity in the text. You would then be able to determine how stable the network of practices is and how strong the boundaries between practices are.

Now return to the example: note how the text is structured as a monologue to clarify the contributor's stand, which is to support the view of another participant in the same healthcare profession (in this case, nursing). There was no sign to suggest that the text is inviting alternate views as you would see in an asynchronous discussion forum. However, the genre was established to be not only clarifying but also justifying.

Text analysis and interdiscursive analysis are conducted simultaneously and together are known as interactional analysis.

Social analysis

This final step involves the structural analysis of the order of discourse to consider how the immediate context and wider social practices have assisted with presenting this text. This means considering the author's multiple roles as student, qualified nurse and social being. This analysis is aimed at specifying the semiotic resources available to the author in the usual grammatical sense of 'paradigm'. This included the choices from the order of discourse, genres and discourse, linguistic and semiotic systems, all of which the author had selected to construct this particular text. In this case, the text is detached from nursing but associated with expertise knowledge of HP to give weight to the declarations.

Important points to note about CDA

- Uncovers any hidden power relations in text.
- Determines whose discourse is being presented (considers if alternative wording would produce the same or another discourse).
- Determines which audience group is targeted and why. Considers how events are presented and how people are characterised.
- Establishes the implicit meaning in text, the unspecified and the unsaid.
- Establishes if the use of passive voices, or strong adverbial indicates dominant discourse.

Further reading

Fairclough, N. (2003) *Analysing Discourse*. London: Routledge.

Loke, J.C.F. (2012) Researching student perspectives on interprofessional online learning via asynchronous text-based conferencing in healthcare education: a literature review. *Journal of Nursing Education and Practice* **2**, 141–150.

Loke, J.C.F., Colquhoun, D. and Lee, K.W. (2011) *Critical Discourse Analysis of Interprofessional Online Learning in Healthcare Education*. New York: Nova Science.

Loke, J.C.F., Colquhoun, D. and Lee, K.W. (2012) A reconstruction of power-relations based on caring within interprofessional online learning. In: S. Nancarrow (ed.) *Global Health Conference. First Annual International Conference, Singapore 27–28 August 2012*, Vol. 1, pp. 167–173.

Loke, J.C.F., Colquhoun, D. and Lee, K.W. (2013) A glimpse into nursing discursive behaviour in interprofessional online learning. *Journal of Nursing Education and Practice* **3**, 67–79.

52 Bricolage research methods

Figure 52.1 A different perspective.

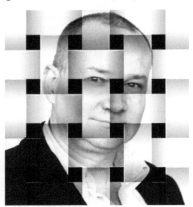

Bricolage attempts to present research findings in a way that challenges its audience to see its subject matter in an unexpected, irregular or offbeat way. A range of metaphors can be used to describe the process of producing the bricolage: including weaving

Figure 52.2 Use of existing data. Photograph by Jon Sparks.

Bricolage may include both existing (found) data – in keeping with the traditional meaning of bricolage – and new data, produced for the study itself

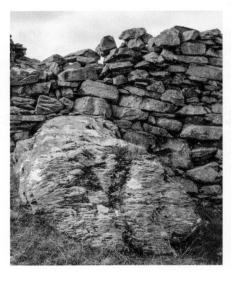

What is bricolage in research terms?

The key characteristic of bricolage as a research approach is that it presents research findings/data in a way that potentially challenges its audience to see its subject matter in an unexpected, irregular or offbeat way (Figure 52.1). It does this by careful consideration of what data should be collated or collected, and how the data should be presented or re-presented in a novel form. Data contained within a bricolage may include both existing (found) data in keeping with the traditional meaning of bricolage and new data, produced for the study itself (Figure 52.2).

Thus bricolage involves the use of more than one source of data (and usually a diverse range of data) with conscious organisation of this material within the finished research text. This sounds complicated and would seem to involve a lot more work than some other forms of research. However, perhaps a less anxiety-provoking way to think about it is to suggest that bricolage allows for bite-size chunks of research to be carried out; such 'data chunks' may well have an individual meaning, but when pieced together result in the creation of a more meaningful whole. This 'whole' should be greater than the sum of its parts in the way that it *is* pieced together. The way the different 'data chunks' are put together potentially influences the way in which meaning is constructed by the reader. Some orderings of data would suggest the way a reader should navigate the text, while other orderings may infer that such a decision should be made by the reader. Different data sources can be layered, placed on specific parts of the page, used as inter-texts (which divert from the main text) or deliberately juxtaposed to fragment or splinter reading. Alternatively, the different data sources can be reworked into a different (and 'artistic') form, such as fiction, poetry, drama and/or visual imagery.

A range of metaphors can be used to describe the process of producing the bricolage – weaving, sewing, quilting (both patchwork and embroidered), montage and collage; the fragments of data or different materials can, though, be thought of as either being drawn into an ordered whole (stained glass) or left disjointed and jarring against each other (smashed glass). If, however, we want to move beyond metaphor, what 'stages' are required to produce a bricolage. First a disclaimer: given that bricolage often employs an emergent approach to research, each of these 'stages' might be revisited at any phase of the research; such revisiting should, however, be documented in a research log/diary. Furthermore, before starting, some exemplars of bricolage should be read (Wibberley, 2012).

Possible stages in producing a bricolage

• Start a 'research log' or research diary in which you record your activities, feelings, experiences, ideas and other thoughts around an area of interest related to your intended research.

• Read the literature around your area of interest, preferably from a range of disciplinary perspectives. Keep an annotated bibliography of your reading in the research log/diary.

• Think about and explore a range of different data sources (existing or to be produced) that could be used to illuminate your knowledge and understanding of an area of interest. Subsequently, make some initial decisions as to what data will be required. Document these decisions in your research log/diary. Consider to what extent the research log/diary may be one of the data sources and whether or not the literature around your area of interest should be considered as data and/or background literature.

• Collect your required data, whether this be primary data (e.g. interviews, observations, field notes, reflective comment) or secondary data (e.g. newspaper articles, novels, autobiographies, policy documents, epidemiological reports, academic literature, perhaps from different disciplines). Add entries to your research log/diary in relation to this data collection. Undertake appropriate initial analysis of the data, drawing on relevant forms of data analysis used by other approaches to research. It is the bringing together of the different data sources subsequent to this initial analysis that is unique to bricolage. Add entries to your research log/diary in relation to this data analysis.

• Immerse yourself in this analysed data and consider the way that it provides convergent or disparate evidence. Then consider the different ways that the data could be presented or re-presented, and the implications that the placement of the data might have for the construction of meaning for a reader. Document these considerations in your research log/diary.

• Continue considering and trying out different ways of presenting or placing the data through immersion and re-immersion in the analysed data. Reordering is part and parcel of the process of bricolage.

• Use your research log/diary to articulate the steps taken in developing the bricolage, perhaps through inclusion of extracts from the log/diary. It is this articulation that ensures that the final product can be considered to be bricolage as a form of research.

Reference and further reading

Lather, P. and Smithies, C. (1997) *Troubling the Angels: Women Living with HIV/AIDS*. Boulder, CO: Westview Press.

Romano, T. (2000) *Blending Genre, Altering Style*. Portsmouth, NH: Boynton/Cook Publishers, Inc.

Wibberley, C. (2012) Getting to grips with bricolage: a personal account. *The Qualitative Report* **17**(50), 1–8.

53 Narrative inquiry

Figure 53.1 Diaries and images can be a source of stories.

A convoy to South Africa

We were in this convalescent environment and after some time many of us with strong British Military Hospital connections were granted passage home to the UK whilst the rest of us with South African Military Hospital and convalescent connections were drafted to join the South African convoy travelling south.

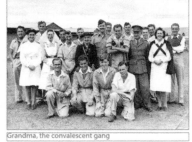

Grandma, the convalescent gang

En route to Durban via Mombasa we were able to visit many places of interest spending our nights back on board the ships. We then continued our journey southward to Dar es Salaam where we picked up a number of Italian prisoners of war to work on board our ship and also in South Africa as POWs from the Italian campaigns in East Africa.

Figure 53.2 Frank's (2010) capacities of stories. Note that a story does not have to demonstrate all capacities but should have 'sufficient' capacities.

- Trouble
- Character
- Point of view
- Suspense
- Interpretive openness
- Out of control
- Inherent morality
- Resonance
- Symbiotic
- Shape-shifting
- Performative
- Truth telling
- Imagination

Figure 53.3 Narrative interviewing creates opportunities for stories to be shared.

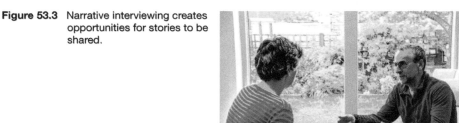

Narratives and stories

Telling stories is one of the fundamental ways in which humans relate to and communicate with each other. Stories surround us, guide us, connect us and provoke us. They are told to help shape meaning and create understanding in and about our lives. The stories people tell are often told and re-told, and are shaped depending on the audience or the reason for telling the story. Within healthcare research, researchers using narrative inquiry (NI) work with stories in order to understand the challenges and transformations that happen to people when, for example, they are ill, disabled or requiring interventions.

There are many different theoretical forms and definitions of NI, each reflecting different disciplinary perspectives. The methods of analysis are also diverse and again often reflect the researcher's disciplinary background. The terms 'narrative' and 'story' are often used interchangeably within research, although narrative is often seen as a means of describing a collection of stories with similar storylines, genres or typologies.

Within NI, stories can arise from many different spoken, written or visual source materials, including interviews, diaries (Figure 53.1), films, photographs, quilts, clinical reports, blogs and text messages. They can be told to a known audience such as the researcher or to an unknown audience (e.g. via a blog). NI can be a way for people to share difficult, sensitive stories and emerging stories and creates a safe space in which they share emotive elements of their experiences. Narrative researchers need to be conscientious, reflexive and sensitive in how they elicit and work with stories.

Elements of stories

Just as there are different approaches to NI, there are different ways of determining whether something that appears to be a story actually has the requisite elements to 'be a story'. Structural approaches examine various elements of stories; for example, *abstract*, *orientation* (e.g. time, place), *crux* (event, trouble or moral issue(s) embedded in the story), *resolution*, *evaluation* (the storyteller's attitude to what they have described) and the *return to present*. Other approaches place emphasis on the *temporality* of stories, the *changes* that occur to the actors within the story, the *actions* that occur within the story, the elements of *(un)certainty* and the *context*. Socio-narratology focuses on *how stories act* in the lives of people and the *capacities* stories have to influence our lives (Figure 53.2).

Narrative interviews

One of the primary ways of generating stories within healthcare research is through the use of interviews; most often these are undertaken face to face (Figure 53.3), although they can be undertaken remotely via the telephone or via the internet. Narrative interviews can be single or longitudinal. The basic techniques of narrative interviewing are similar to other interview methods. However, in NI the main focus is on creating opportunities for stories to be shared, with as much rich contextual detail as possible to support subsequent analysis. Rather than using a schedule or structure to guide the interview, NI researchers tend to work flexibly and start with a broad opening question such as:

• 'In your own time, tell me the story of …' or 'I'm interested in your story of … please share it with me.'

The aim is not to collect as many stories as possible within any one interview but to generate understanding and insight. While avoiding interrupting the storyteller, clarification questions can be asked to help provide more detail and depth about how and where this particular story fits into the life of the storyteller, as for example:

• In your story you mentioned you felt worried, why was this? Who were with you when […] happened? Why did you choose to tell this story and tell it in this way? Who couldn't you share this story with? Has your story changed since you first told it? What parts of your story did you find easy/difficult to tell? Why?

The researcher's engagement with the storyteller inevitably shapes or co-constructs the story and it requires skill, reflexivity and care by the researcher to be able to elicit, understand, interpret and contextualise a story.

Narrative analysis

Narrative analysis is the systematic study of narrative materials and it often draws on elements of conversation analysis and discourse analysis, although in NI the analytical lens is turned to how the stories are told, and why they are told in particular ways and the effect they have on the audience. Narrative researchers are also interested in understanding what the purpose of the story was – what lesson the storyteller hoped would be learned from the story. Some researchers focus on typologies (e.g. journey narratives, chaos narratives and recovery narratives).

The 'good' and the 'bad' of NI

NI is often proposed to be potentially therapeutic or cathartic, although there is very little substantive evidence that this is the case. Researchers sometimes worry whether they have collected 'good stories'. Good stories are often described as being those that are memorable because something interesting or troublesome happens that captures the moral imagination of the listener and which create connections between the storyteller and the listener(s). Some of this is contingent on contextual, structural and cultural factors.

There can be a tendency for storytellers to relate stories about things that have gone wrong, where there was a sense of trouble, a problem that was overcome rather than stories where everything went well. Researchers who only attend to dramatic stories can easily overlook stories that appear to be mundane. This needs to be taken into account when the researcher is re-telling the stories and generating narratives based on their research.

Stories that are exceptionally 'good' offer as many moral points and opportunities for learning as 'bad' stories.

Reference and further reading

Carter, B. (2004) Pain narratives and narrative practitioners: a way of working 'in-relation' with children experiencing pain. *Journal of Nursing Management* **12**, 210–216.

Carter, B. (2008) 'Good' and 'bad' stories: decisive moments, 'shock and awe' and being moral. *Journal of Clinical Nursing* **17**, 1063–1070.

Frank, A.W. (2010) *Letting Stories Breathe. A Socio-Narratology.* Chicago: University of Chicago Press.

54 Appreciative inquiry

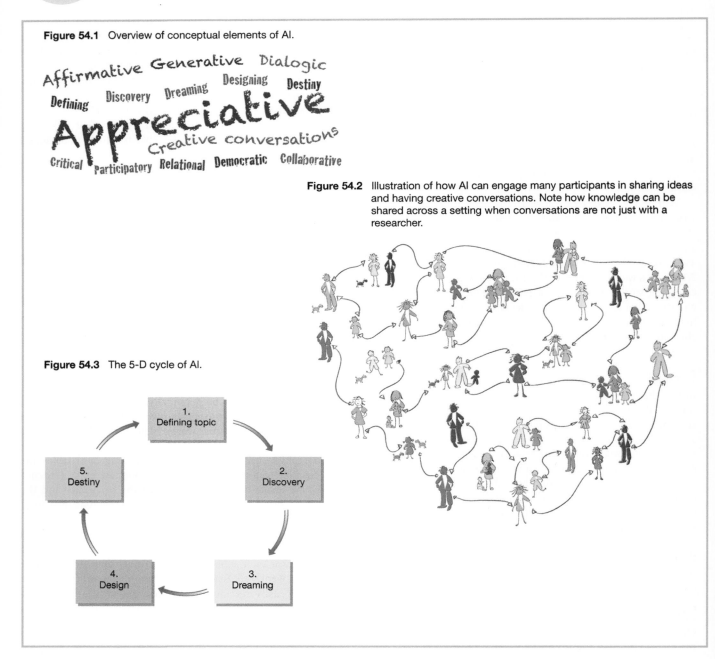

Figure 54.1 Overview of conceptual elements of AI.

Affirmative Generative Dialogic
Defining Discovery Dreaming Designing Destiny
Appreciative
Creative conversations
Critical Participatory Relational Democratic Collaborative

Figure 54.2 Illustration of how AI can engage many participants in sharing ideas and having creative conversations. Note how knowledge can be shared across a setting when conversations are not just with a researcher.

Figure 54.3 The 5-D cycle of AI.

1. Defining topic
2. Discovery
3. Dreaming
4. Design
5. Destiny

Appreciative inquiry (AI) is an affirmative, collaborative, relational and democratic approach to undertaking research (Figure 54.1). AI's roots lie in organisational change and management but more recently it has been adopted as a research approach. AI has been used in many different settings including healthcare, prisons and universities.

While it has some similarities to action research (AR) in that it is cyclical and aims to create change, it differs from traditional AR and many other problem-oriented approaches to research, as AI actively adopts an appreciative stance. AI is grounded in working with existing strengths and successes within a setting or an organisation and working collaboratively, energetically and cooperatively to build a better future. AI is underpinned by the use of generative and affirmative language.

The adoption of an appreciative mindset can lead to criticism that AI is biased. However, the skill of an AI researcher is to be both appreciative as well as critically analytical in their work. AI researchers do not disregard negative situations but encompass these within discussions.

Core resources, expertise and ethics

Core resources include the creative conversations between participants and the commitment of the participants from all levels of an organisation to drive forward change. AI researchers work in partnership with participants, drawing on participants' insights, creativity, assets, expertise and skills to generate knowledge, change and collective action. No one is seen to have overriding expertise.

Successful AI occurs when trust and good relationships (researcher–participants, participants–participants) are built over time. Conscientious preparation is essential, especially in relation to ethical matters as often the AI researcher does not have direct control over data collection. AI is based on people within a setting sharing information and insights about future directions. This means that care must be taken in gaining informed consent, ensuring effective communication and determining whether the hoped-for change is achievable.

Engagement and process

There are many different approaches to engagement, ranging from summits (e.g. many participants meeting simultaneously and intensively over several days) to small-scale work (e.g. a small team working together over several months). The process of engagement depends on the topic, hoped-for outcome and the resources available.

There is no specific method to follow to undertake a good AI study. AI researchers work flexibly, inclusively and democratically and choose tools to generate *creative conversations* (Figure 54.2) that have a good fit with the particular setting. Good AI questions are ones that create affirmative connections between people, give opportunities for creative responses and detailed contextualised insights.

Most AI studies are conversation-based; interviewing is a core method. Although preferentially interviews are face to face, remote methods (e.g. telephone or internet based) can be used successfully. Interviews can be between individuals (participant–participant or researcher–participant) or in small groups (e.g. focus groups or nominal groups).

Phases of AI

There are different iterations of the phases of an AI study but most are based on the 4-D cycle (Discovery, Dreaming, Designing, Destiny). The cycle starts with the choice of what to study and this is sometimes referred to as a fifth D (Defining) (Figure 54.3). Although the cycle looks neat on paper, the lived experience of AI often reflects a study in which there is overlap of phases. Participants are actively engaged in all phases and both participants and researcher(s) make a record of the discussions through the use of summary and action sheets throughout.

Phase 1: Defining the topic (choosing an affirmative topic)
AI topics are affirmative and are characterised by focusing on something the participants want to achieve, that they are intrigued by and which they believe will create positive change.

Phase 2: Discovery (the best of what is or has been)
Discovery focuses on what is already working well, what is already making a positive difference and what participants would like to see changed. The future-oriented change questions are often called 'miracle' or 'magic wand' questions.

Phase 3: Dreaming (what might be)
In Dreaming, a more strategic approach is adopted and the examples of best practice from Discovery are drawn together to create a collective vision of a better, shared future. This is achieved through the use of identifying themes (areas of convergence), *quotable quotes* (quotations or short stories that have value and resonance to the participants) and *provocative propositions* (statements that sum up what a better future could be and which challenge current thinking).

Phase 4: Designing (what should be)
Designing focuses on creating an ideal organisation/setting based on the grounded examples of future working developed in Dreaming. Design requires participants to prioritise what they want to change and take forward to the next phase.

Phase 5: Destiny (what will be)
Destiny focuses on creating the networks, processes, structures and new ways of working required in order to achieve the affirmative and generative desired outcome. Dissemination also needs to be participatory.

Conclusion

Using AI creates a unique and affirmative way of engaging with participants and can result in energy being created that can lead to positive strategic change and the development of knowledge. AI can also reveal stories of success that allow people to appreciate the best of what they are already doing. When the conditions are not right, AI can raise false hopes of a new and better future. However, when it works well, AI is generative and transformative.

Further reading
Carter, B. (2006) 'One expertise among many': working appreciatively to make miracles instead of finding problems. *Using appreciative inquiry as a way of reframing research. Journal of Research in Nursing* **11**, 48–63.

Carter, B. (2012) Developing and implementing an appreciative 'quality of care' approach to child neglect practice. *Child Abuse Review* **21**, 81–98.

Trajkovski, S., Schmied, V., Vickers, M. and Jackson, D. (2013) Implementing the 4D cycle of appreciative inquiry in health care: a methodological review. *Journal of Advanced Nursing* **69**, 1224–1234.

55 Qualitative data analysis software packages

Figure 55.1 Qualitative tasks supported by CAQDAS packages.

Source: Lewins A, Silver C (2007) Using Software in Qualitative Research: A Step-by-Step Guide. Reproduced with permission of SAGE Publications

Figure 55.4 The NVivo workspace.

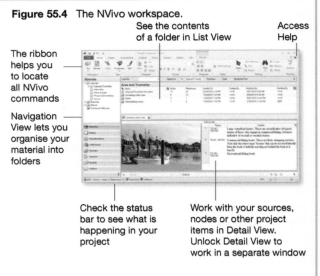

The ribbon helps you to locate all NVivo commands

Navigation View lets you organise your material into folders

See the contents of a folder in List View

Access Help

Check the status bar to see what is happening in your project

Work with your sources, nodes or other project items in Detail View. Unlock Detail View to work in a separate window

Figure 55.2 Suggested procedure.

Source: Bazeley P (2007) Qualitative data analysis with NVivo. Reproduced with permission of SAGE Publications

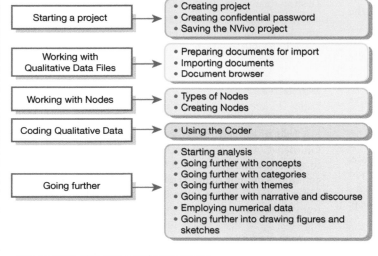

Starting a project
- Creating project
- Creating confidential password
- Saving the NVivo project

Working with Qualitative Data Files
- Preparing documents for import
- Importing documents
- Document browser

Working with Nodes
- Types of Nodes
- Creating Nodes

Coding Qualitative Data
- Using the Coder

Going further
- Starting analysis
- Going further with concepts
- Going further with categories
- Going further with themes
- Going further with narrative and discourse
- Employing numerical data
- Going further into drawing figures and sketches

Figure 55.5 Word cloud.

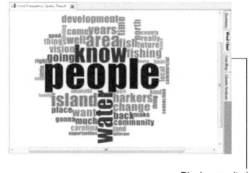

Display results in a word cloud, double-click a word to gather all occurrences in a node

Figure 55.6 The Detail View with the Coding Stripes option activated. Note the circled Coding Stripes function.

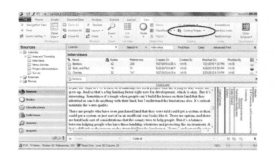

Figure 55.3 The NVivo welcome screen.

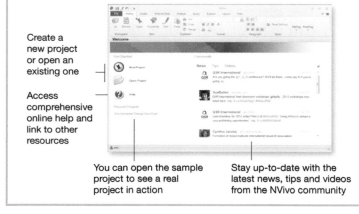

Create a new project or open an existing one

Access comprehensive online help and link to other resources

You can open the sample project to see a real project in action

Stay up-to-date with the latest news, tips and videos from the NVivo community

This chapter examines NVivo™ 10 as an example of qualitative data analysis software and considers the areas of its functionality and its use in qualitative data analysis.

Understanding qualitative data analysis

Qualitative data analysis (QDA) involves a range of processes and procedures by which qualitative data – mostly textual transcriptions obtained from interviews, ethnographies, and documents captured on audio recording or video, cameras and charts – are converted into some form of explanation, understanding or interpretation in relation to the people and situations being investigated.

Traditionally, qualitative researchers have used manual means such as folders, files, wallets, index cards, and multiple coloured pencils to gather together materials of similar themes or analytic ideas. However, with the introduction of the personal computer (PC), which has proved excellent at manipulating texts, it is clear that much of the manual processing (especially large-scale) could be done more efficiently with computer-assisted qualitative data analysis software (CAQDAS). The initial focus of CAQDAS was on text since that was easy to handle on PCs. Nevertheless, in recent times, where much audio and video is in digital form too, the software technology has been improved to support the analysis of audios, videos and text-linking capabilities.

Although the sample size in QDA may be relatively small compared with those used in quantitative approaches, datasets in QDA tend to be very large, and require intensive examination and understanding to interpret the phenomena being investigated. Therefore, selecting a CAQDAS package capable of organising, interrogating, integrating and exploring tasks, as demonstrated in Figure 55.1, could shorten the analysis time frame while providing more thorough and rigorous coding to facilitate interpretation. One such software package is NVivo 10, developed by QSR international Pty Ltd.

About NVivo for QDA

NVivo is comprehensive qualitative data analysis software that has the capability to retrieve, code and build theory, allowing users to replicate all the manual processes that would be otherwise employed. Data sources in NVivo constitute anything from video recordings to typed memos capturing thoughts and ideas. When imported into NVivo, data are categorised into internals (field notes, audio interviews, video footage, photographs or any raw data relevant to the project) and externals (including newspaper articles, web pages, books and memos).

Using the self-training elements, demo program and help files that come with the program, alongside a suggested procedure (Figure 55.2), learning to use NVivo is reasonably easy and can be done while the research is already in progress. Using the software can reduce a number of manual tasks, giving the researcher more time to discover tendencies, recognise themes and derive conclusions. Additionally, since it facilitates the combining of different aspects of a project, NVivo is considered an ideal technique for researchers who are working in a team (Wong, 2008).

Starting NVivo: importing and integrating data

The first screen encountered when opening NVivo is the welcome screen (Figure 55.3), allowing the user to start a new project, open an existing project, access the help files or join the optional community of users. Creating a new project opens the NVivo workspace (Figure 55.4) providing easy access to all project materials. Additional files can be imported from various sources using the External Data tab. Besides importing already transcribed texts into its workspace, NVivo is now able to transcribe media files directly into the project. The imported documents can then be browsed, explored, edited or coded.

Exploring data within NVivo

NVivo includes basic data mining tools such as word frequency counts (Figure 55.5), which index textual strings in tabular format, providing counts by file and across the dataset. Building on word frequency tools, text search tools allow the reader to specify which strings, words or phrases to search for. Such tools not only provide access to key words within the source file but also usually allow for a user-specified context around each 'hit' to be automatically coded. Charts, models and other visualisation techniques can be created to understand trends, test theories and make sense of what is happening in the source materials. Simple bar charts or graphs can be used to demonstrate the relationship between the conceptual and theoretical data.

Organising and managing data

Coding – a process where segments of data are identified as relating to or being an example of a more general idea, instance, theme or category – is the most important function of QDA analysis and a particular strength of NVivo. Node is used by NVivo to represent a code, theme or idea about the data, which allows the researcher to gather related materials in one place so that emerging patterns and ideas can be explored further. One way of creating nodes is by using Nodes in the Navigation View window (Figure 55.6) and the Create and Analyse tab in the ribbon of commands. In order to understand the conceptual and theoretical issues generated in the course of the study, NVivo is capable of organising a number of data documents including interview transcripts, surveys, notes of observations, and published documents which, by manual methods of analysis, may appear cluttered.

Interrogating data and reporting

Querying or searching constitutes part of an ongoing enquiry process in NVivo. Posing several questions of the data and utilising the software to answer these queries allows further interrogation and the formulating of transcript reports.

Conclusion

NVivo has the potential to facilitate different methods of qualitative analysis to significantly improve the quality of research. However, as these software packages are primarily tools to assist with qualitative research, the computer does not analyse data for the researcher, and therefore the interpretation of results still rests with the researcher.

References

Bazeley, P. (2007) *Qualitative Data Analysis with NVivo*, 2nd edn. London: Sage Publications

Lewins, A. and Silver, C. (2007) *Using Software in Qualitative Research: A Step-by-Step Guide*. London: Sage Publications.

Wong, L. (2008) Data analysis in qualitative research: a brief guide to using NVivo. *Malaysian Family Physician* **3**, 7.

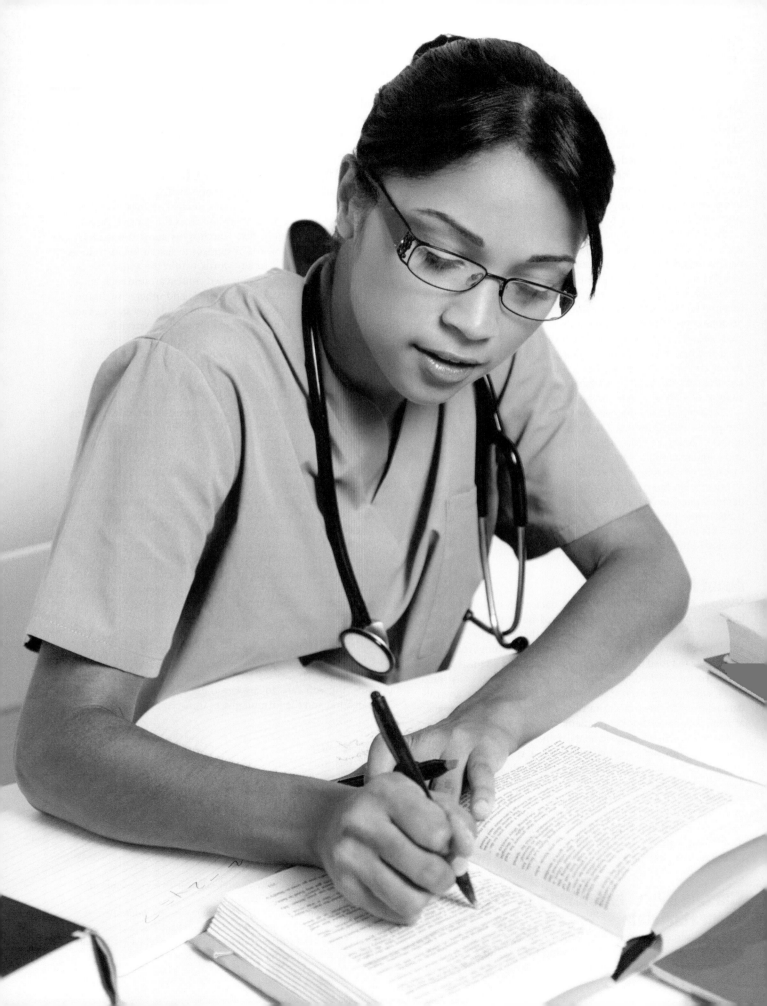

Research techniques

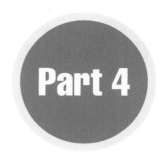
Part 4

Chapters

56 Questionnaire design

Figure 56.1 Research questionnaire design.

Important tip (for all quantitative research)

Don't do statistical tests that are (i) unnecessary – that's unethical and a waste of time and energy – and (ii) that you can't explain yourself. You may get asked about them and if your statistician isn't around, you will have to answer the question

Tips for good questions

- Never have a question that contains two questions, for example in a questionnaire about children's adherence to their medication regimen, the question said: 'Child doesn't want to take it, refuses, or is uncooperative.' Being uncooperative may be different from refusing to take it, and so this should be asked in two questions
- Make sure a question doesn't run over onto another page
- Use coloured segments to make individual questions stand out
- Make sure the questionnaire flows logically; don't jump all over the place (unless you mean to – this device can be used to ensure respondents are reading the questionnaire properly and not just ticking boxes)
- Similarly, you can put scores going in different directions to make sure people read the questions properly, but you have to be sure when entering data that the score is entered the right way round

Who makes up your panel of consumers?

You need those who represent the people you are going to study, e.g. if you are designing a questionnaire about adolescent health, you would need to have a young person on your panel. If you are studying people who are from a vulnerable group (as designated by HRECs), it is a good idea to have someone from that group. For example, in Australia, in research about Aboriginal and Torres Strait Islander people, it is imperative to include an Aboriginal or Torres Strait Islander person on the panel

Stage 1
Find themes in the existing literature

Stage 2
Small qualitative study: interviews and thematic analysis

Stage 3
Collate themes from literature and qualitative interviews

Stage 4
Work with statistician and IT person to put questionnaire together and to create and test database

Stage 5
Give the questionnaire to your family, friends and neighbours; make changes

Stage 6
Give the questionnaire to your panels of experts and consumers

Repeat Stage 6 as necessary

Stage 7
Do pilot study

Stage 8
Publish pilot study ready to begin main study

Where the statistician comes in

- Helps determine which techniques will work best for your research question
- Helps set up database in Excel or SPSS ready for data entry
- After you enter some dummy figures, your statistician will help you run statistical tests on them to see if the tests work, if flaws can be found in the way the database is set up, and if the questions are all working together

Where your IT person comes in

- Helps with formatting of questions, how they fit on the page, and presentation
- Helps you set up the database
- The database can be set up so that any wrong entry in a cell will give an error message (but this might be more trouble than it's worth – consult with your IT person and your statistician, and the person/people who will be doing the data entry)
- Will help with testing your whole system

Who makes up your panel of experts?

This depends on your topic, of course, but find people who are not just experts in the relevant field, but also those you know will be willing to help in a timely way. Don't ask someone you know is very busy and may not reply in good time. Give people the option by asking if they are willing to be part of it, and how much time they would need to reply. If they say they can't reply within a week or so each time you ask, invite someone else. A good number is four to six

Questionnaires are used a lot in nursing research, but many are designed and administered without going through the necessary rigorous and thorough processes needed to ensure a questionnaire answers the questions one is trying to ask. It is not just a matter of writing down a few questions, making them into a list, and sending them out. Many a survey or questionnaire-based study has fallen into this trap, making it unreliable and unable to be safely translated into clinical practice. Questionnaire design is very complicated but easy to get right. Two of the best resources on this topic are Oppenheim (2001) and Polit and Beck (2014). These will be used consistently throughout this chapter and so are referenced here. Both these books contain detailed explanations of how to develop a questionnaire effectively.

Preliminary work

The overarching premise of any research is that the *research question guides everything*, and this is as relevant to the design of the questionnaire as to everything else about a project. Start with a full research proposal/protocol (the words are interchangeable), planning out exactly what you are going to do. This can then be submitted to a human research ethics committee (HREC) for approval. Across countries, HRECs differ in the way they work, and some may not require approval for questionnaire design and/or a pilot study; however, journals require indication that you have at least asked your local HREC for a letter of support for this early stage of the research. Other HRECs require full-blown applications even at this early stage. It is important that you contact your local HREC and ask what they require.

Nursing and Healthcare Research at a Glance, First Edition. Alan Glasper and Colin Rees. © 2017 by John Wiley & Sons, Ltd. Published 2017 by John Wiley & Sons, Ltd.

The easiest way to develop a questionnaire is to find one that suits your purpose and adapt it. A plethora of questionnaires for a huge range of topics exists, and owners of questionnaires are usually very pleased to see their work used. It pays to ask permission, though, as it is good manners to let the authors know you are using their work, and to provide them with the results of your own study at the end of the project. Some questionnaires bear a cost; some are very expensive and are licensed to be used by one type of professional only, for example the Spielberger State-Trait Anxiety Inventory (American Psychological Association, 2014), widely used in health research, can be used only by psychologists.

So why develop one's own questionnaire? Often an existing one just will not cut the mustard, so a new one is needed. This can be quite a complicated process, but if one works through it systematically, step by step, the questionnaire you end up with will not just be fit for purpose, but once published will be used by other researchers around the world (Figure 56.1).

After writing your proposal, it is important to find the people required: a statistician, a panel of experts and a panel of consumers. Also included will be your family, neighbours and people in your community. These will be your reference point for all stages of the questionnaire design. You will also need a theoretical framework for your work to help guide you through how best to frame your study. As an example, most of my research is based on the theory of family-centred care, and so I devise questionnaires that answer questions related to that. A sound theoretical framework will keep you on track to make sure your work is relevant and answers your research question.

First stop is existing literature. What have others found out about your topic? Can you find other questions to ask from their work? This will give you a 'kick-off' point. Next, and this is where the research starts to get interesting, conduct some interviews with these questions, and some of your own, with people who are the same as your potential participants; in other words, drawn from the same population as your targeted research. You will need probably six or seven people, depending on when you reach data saturation. Accordingly, questionnaire design starts with a solid piece of qualitative research. Themes will emerge which can be combined with your themes from the existing literature, and you will see your questions for the questionnaire emerging. Put the two together, and write the questions.

Consult your statistician at this stage: look at your questions and decide the appropriate method of scoring to use, for example Likert scales, semantic differentials and various other techniques.

A very important tip: resist the temptation to put every possible question, and every connotation of a question into the questionnaire. Keep it as short as possible or people will not complete it, so *keep it simple*.

Put it all together, and get help with formatting if necessary. An IT person is invaluable here. The better a questionnaire looks, while retaining simplicity, the more likely people are to complete it. Remember, you are asking someone to give some of their time, and to give you the courtesy of the answers they feel are correct. The least you can do is make the questionnaire as easy as possible to complete.

When you think the questionnaire looks good, test it yourself a few times. Then give it to your neighbours, friends and family to do. Tell them you don't want them to give real answers, they just need to tell you if the questionnaire and the questions are easily read and easily understood, and that the techniques for answering the questions work. When you have changed and adapted it according to suggested corrections, give it to your panels of experts and consumers.

There are many tools for testing questionnaires, but often direct quotes, corrections and conversations will yield as much information. Your statistician will advise about this.

Questionnaire development is about iterations: send it to your panels, and people; they send it back with corrections and suggestions; you adapt it, send it out again, and so forth. This can be done over and over until you are sure no more changes are being suggested.

At all stages go back to your research question to ensure you are going to get the answers that will give you the information relating to the question.

Once you are confident the questionnaire is as good as you can make it, and it is serving your research question, begin the pilot study as per your initial proposal (for which you will have ethics approval).

Pilot study

Pilot studies characteristically test if a study is going to work. They use a convenience sample, the size of which is determined by the population for whom the study is designed. For example, if your target population is very large, then your pilot population might be 100; if small, 10 may do. The convenience sample can be influenced by requirements of study; for example, if you are including Aboriginal people as part of your Australian target sample, you may have to include a subset population of, say, five Aboriginal people and 20 non-Aboriginal (reflecting the smaller proportion of Aboriginal people in the wider population). Such decisions are related to the study itself and your statistician can help you devise the appropriate numbers.

Send out the questionnaires as per your protocol; as they are returned, enter the data into the database. Clean the data once they are all in, making sure there are no errors in the data entry.

Work with the statistician to run reliability statistics, for example Cronbach's alpha, test–retest reliability, split half technique, as appropriate. Once this is done, ask your panel of experts and panel of consumers to have one more look at the questionnaire, and adapt if necessary.

Your questionnaire is now ready to apply. It is a good opportunity to publish your pilot study.

At the end, and throughout the process, keep returning to your research question to check that you are really doing what you plan to do.

Notify the HREC that you have completed the pilot study, and send them a copy of any paper published from the work.

References

American Psychological Association (2014) The State-Trait Anxiety Inventory (STAI). Available at http://www.apa.org/pi/about/publications/caregivers/practice-settings/assessment/tools/trait-state.aspx

Oppenheim, A.M. (2001) *Questionnaire Design, Interviewing and Attitude Measurement*. London: Continuum.

Polit, D.F. and Beck, C.T. (2014) *Essentials of Nursing Research: Appraising Evidence for Nursing Practice*, 8th edn. Philadelphia: Wolters Kluwer Health/Lippincott Williams & Wilkins.

57 Using web-based tools to design a questionnaire

Figure 57.1 Stages in the process of creating an online questionnaire.

Researcher

Participants

Web browser

Questionnaire design

Questionnaire distributed to participants

Analysis of results

Questionnaire complete

Database

Table 57.1 Advantages and disadvantages of web-based questionnaires.

Advantages

- Questionnaire can be electronically designed to structure the content and format of questions
- Skip patterns can be incorporated to exclude non-relevant follow-up questions, order questions randomly or direct participants to other sections or versions of the questionnaire
- May cost less than paper questionnaire to administer
- Cost of paper, printing, posting avoided
- Questionnaires are returned rapidly
- Participants complete electronic questionnaires more quickly; automatic reminders can be forwarded, resulting in faster response times
- Improved data quality
- Validation check can be included, prompting respondents when they enter incomplete/implausible answers
- Data is automatically analysed
- Data entered electronically facilitating immediate analysis
- Errors in data entry and coding may be avoided
- Due to automatic electronic data collection, human errors of data entry and analysis may be avoided
- Ability to facilitate immediate participant feedback
- Facilitates methods such as Delphi process, which requires individualised participant feedback

Disadvantages

- High non-response rates compared with more traditional methods of data collection
- Potential participants may not have access to a computer or email, resulting in reduced response rates from some geographical areas or populations. Participants also require a degree of computer literacy
- Administrative problems may affect response rates
- Electronic problems such as 'bounce-back' or undelivered emails
- Concerns in relation to issues around bias
- Risk of self-selection bias: some questionnaires may result in higher response rates from certain subgroups such as the higher educated or student population
- Concerns in relation to reliability and validity
- High risk of sampling errors. May be due to bad design, more rapid reading time by participants
- Issues in relation to confidentiality and safety
- May result in a reluctance by participants to complete electronic questionnaires

Traditional modes of data collection such as paper-and-pencil questionnaires have several limitations. These include decreased response rates and high costs of time and administration, particularly with a large diverse study population. Web-based or online questionnaires are increasingly being used as an alternative tool for the design and administration of questionnaires and surveys. The rapidly increasing use of the internet provides researchers with the potential to access geographically diverse populations, utilise automated data collection and potentially reduce researcher time and cost. However, issues in relation to questionnaire design, implementation and evaluation have been reported as having an impact on reliability of data and response rates (Van Gelder *et al.*, 2010), emphasising the importance of careful design and administration. Therefore the many advantages and disadvantages of the online questionnaire should be carefully considered when selecting which method of data collection to utilise (Table 57.1).

Design of the online questionnaire

Several methods are available for the design and administration of online questionnaires.

• Utilise existing services in your organisation to create and deliver questionnaires, by applying the virtual learning environment (VLE) for your organisation (e.g. Blackboard or Moodle). However, the disadvantage would be that participants would have to have access to the VLE, which may limit sample size.
• A PC application can be added to a computer to design and administer the delivery of questionnaires. A disadvantage of this method may be that the user will require a degree of IT skills to install the required software.
• Potentially the easiest option is to use a web-based questionnaire builder. This software typically offers different levels of service, with basic services frequently being available free of charge and large questionnaires or those requiring particular functionality for composition structure or analysis usually incurring a cost. A variety of online tools are available, including:
  • SurveyMonkey® (first 10 questions are free, prompt online support);
  • Smart survey (UK-based company, has a facility for adding images to questions and answers, support via phone and email);
  • Survey methods (good analysis tools with prompt online support, US-based company).

SurveyMonkey

SurveyMonkey (www.SurveyMonkey.com) is one of the survey tools which is widely used and provides an online facility that enables the development of a survey style questionnaire. It offers a variety of formats with useful questionnaire options incorporating a user-friendly process.

   Basic question options available in SurveyMonkey include open- and closed-ended questions, Likert-style questions, semantic differential scales, checklists, textboxes (for qualitative data), drop-down menus (for categorical or nominal items) and filter questions. The author can therefore develop the content and structure of the questionnaire in order to meet the needs of the study. The results analysis option displays charts for a quick analysis as well as downloading the raw data. Qualitative data obtained from open-ended questions are easily converted to Word files, which enables analysis both manually or via computer programs. When you use SurveyMonkey data downloads directly to Excel or SPSS, data are protected by password access and are available only to the author.

Features of SurveyMonkey

• The survey tool is easy to set up and use.
• The basic version is free and allows you to create sample surveys to ensure it meets your requirements.
• The question bank gives you sample questions and answers to help you create a survey/questionnaire and potentially reduce any problems with ambiguous questions.
• Has the option to create multiple collectors, which allows you to track where people are locating your surveys.
• Results analysis has the ability to display charts, facilitating rapid analysis as well as downloading the raw data.
• Has the ability to create multiple page surveys.
• Has the ability to create customised reports.
• Data can be entered manually from other survey sources.

Structure and content of the questionnaire

The general principles involved in the design and structure of a questionnaire should also be applied to an online questionnaire (Oppenheim, 1992). However, other additional benefits linked with online questionnaires and web-based surveys relate to graphical and interactive design. The potential to utilise innovative screen design, colour, and question formatting (which are not available for paper questionnaires) may increase data collection (Titus *et al.*, 2000). A typical progression for the creation, administration and completion of an online questionnaire includes the following (Figure 57.1).

• Select method of administration, e.g. web-based questionnaire builder and register with the system.
• Complete the login process and select design.
• Create title, include organisation completing the questionnaire, information section, welcome and appreciation message.
• Create questions, selecting type of response required.
• Modify and pilot questionnaire.
• Distribute to participants, send reminders, analyse results.
• Final report/results.

Confidentiality and safety

The capture of electronic data poses specific problems which should be considered when using an online questionnaire. It is easy to duplicate and transmit, and will be collected using the internet. Therefore it is important that the usual letter of explanation is given to participants and that consent is sought. Questions around anonymity should be addressed, particularly if this is an important issue for potential participants. It is also crucial to consider security of data collected, particularly if the individual participants' records can be identified within the data.

References

Oppenheim, A.N. (1992) *Questionnaire Design, Interviewing and Attitude Measurement*. London: Pinter.
Titus, K.L., Schleyer, D.M.D. and Forrest, R.H.D. (2000) Methods for the design and administration of web-based surveys. *Journal of the American Medical Informatics Association* **7**, 416–425.
Van Gelder, M.H.J., Bretveld, R.W. and Roeleveif, N. (2010) Web-based questionnaires: the future in epidemiology? *American Journal of Epidemiology* **172**, 1292–1298.

58 Quality of life scales

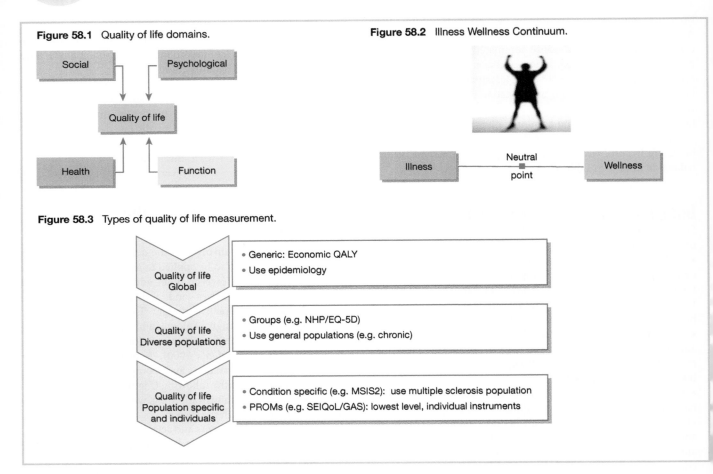

Figure 58.1 Quality of life domains.

Social → Quality of life ← Psychological

Health → Quality of life ← Function

Figure 58.2 Illness Wellness Continuum.

Illness ——— Neutral point ——— Wellness

Figure 58.3 Types of quality of life measurement.

Quality of life Global
- Generic: Economic QALY
- Use epidemiology

Quality of life Diverse populations
- Groups (e.g. NHP/EQ-5D)
- Use general populations (e.g. chronic)

Quality of life Population specific and individuals
- Condition specific (e.g. MSIS2): use multiple sclerosis population
- PROMs (e.g. SEIQoL/GAS): lowest level, individual instruments

The search for scales

Quantitative healthcare research is concerned with the measurement of variables that will lead to patient assessment or comparing the impact of interventions on outcomes between different groups. The measurement of some variables, such as temperature, weight or pulse, are reasonably easy to measure, but more abstract concepts such as pain, anxiety or resilience are more difficult and require a scaling 'instrument' in order to produce numbers that permit mathematical calculations. These can then establish the existence of correlation or cause-and-effect relationships. Quality of life (QoL) is one such abstract concept that requires a clear definition and an accurate measuring tool if it is to be included in research. This chapter considers the development of QoL scales and some of the issues surrounding them.

What is it?

In 1991 a WHO working party defined QoL as 'an individual's perception of their position in life's context of culture and value systems in which they live and in relation to their goals, expectations, standards and concerns'. It was seen as a combination of physical, functional, psychological and social aspects of health and was both a subjective and objective state existing at one moment in time. It is often broken down into constituent elements or *domains*, typically including health, function, psychological and social (Figure 58.1). In this way it echoes the WHO's 1947 definition of health as 'not merely the absence of disease, but complete physical function, social function, role function, mental health and general health perception'.

The development of QoL scales

As a result of the WHO's definition of health, indicators of QoL have expanded to encompass many aspects of life, and this has shifted the emphasis from measurements of health status to the broader elements included in QoL definitions. The focus of health activity has also changed, from simply attempting to extend life to considerations of the quality of extended life. As a result of this shifting focus from mortality to morbidity, QoL measurements have increasingly been used to assess the nature and quality of survival.

In addition, the introduction of the International Classification of Impairment, Disability and Handicap (ICIDH) also had an impact on the focus of care. The ICIDH was later revised and became the International Classification of Functioning, Disability and Health (ICF), and resulted in the integration of QoL into the biopsychosocial model of health.

The importance of these changes is that measuring instruments used before the reclassification of ICIDH in 2000 may not reflect the widening scope of health. Once QoL was introduced, there was a greater focus on individual needs. Subsequent developments included the Illness Wellness Continuum (IWC), which emerged in response to the holistic definition of health grounded in the biopsychosocial model. The IWC can be located within the salutogenic model of health (Antonovsky, 1979) which attempts to place an individual along a continuum between 'health-ease' and 'dis-ease'. Health comprises body and mind, including social factors and happiness within wellness (Figure 58.2). Illness recognises physiological state, negative emotional mood such as misery and social factors, reflecting current QoL definitions. Health is the dominant state at the wellness end, diseases at the illness end.

The application of QoL instruments

A whole range of instruments has been devised to measure QoL, each with different levels of popularity, strengths and limitations. Streiner and Norman (2008) suggest that QoL instruments can be discriminative, predictive or evaluative; for example, they can compare patient populations, predict discharge outcomes (such as the Nottingham Health Profile and Bartel Index) or evaluate the benefit of interventions.

A limitation of some QoL tools is the lack of a theoretical underpinning, which means it is unclear what such instruments measure. Clarity in the beliefs and ideas supporting a particular instrument will help to understand what they measure and their role and accuracy in assessing QoL. Some instruments do draw on a relevant theory, for example the Utility Theory that underpins Figure 58.3. This theory suggests that individuals can place different personal health outcomes along a linear scale, based on the subjective value each health outcome has for them. Quality-adjusted life-year (QALY) asks individuals to score their QoL between the worst scenario and the best, with each year being adjusted for its QoL. QALY imposes an external value system devised from aggregated grouped data taken from large-scale epidemiological studies.

Social theories linking QoL and society identify the influence of social factors on an individual's assessment of their health and desirable outcomes. The social domain is used to underpin the WHO QoL instrument (WHOQoL) and the Schedule Evaluation of Individual QoL (SEIQoL). In terms of accuracy and general use, instruments such as WHOQoL have been tested internationally across a broad range of chronic conditions and, as a result, WHOQoL is a generic tool relevant to wider populations and can be used as a discriminative instrument to compare changes in QoL between groups (Figure 58.3).

Other theories and models have further refined QoL tools. For instance, the humanist model has been used in the QoL index (QLI), Subjective QoL Profile (SQLP) and the WHOQoL. The theory of reasoned action is a goals theory explaining decision-making and is used to underpin the Goal Attainment Scale (GAS).

Finally, the UK Department of Health advocates using patient-reported outcome measures (PROMs) to place individuals at the centre of their care. PROMs empower individuals to focus on their needs such as QoL or satisfaction.

Summary

QoL is a multidimensional concept including both subjective and objective aspects. Our understanding of the concept has widened from its original use in economic evaluations to recognising broad domains and the gap between present position and desired position related to these domains. Appropriate QoL scales are best evaluated based on the purpose of measurement and the existence of a clear theory or model on which they are based.

References and further reading

Antonovsky, A. (1979) *Health, Stress and Coping.* San Francisco: Jossey-Bass/Wiley.

Bethoux, F., Calmels, P. and Gautheron, V. (1999) Changes in the quality of life of hemiplegic stroke patients with time: a preliminary report. *American Journal of Physical Medicine and Rehabilitation* **78**, 19–23.

Bogden, R. and Taylor, S. (1975) *Introduction to Qualitative Research Methods.* Chichester: John Wiley & Sons Ltd.

Patrick, D. and Erickson, P. (1993) *Health Status and Health Policy: Quality of Life in Healthcare Evaluation and Resource Allocation.* Oxford: Oxford University Press.

Streiner, D.L. and Norman, G.R. (2008) *Health Measurement Scales. A Practical Guide to Their Development and Use,* 4th edn. Oxford: Oxford University Press.

Wywich, K. and Wolinsky, F. (2000) Identifying meaningful intra-individual change standards for health related quality of life measures. *Journal of Evaluation in Clinical Practice* **6**, 39–49.

59 The State-Trait Anxiety Inventory

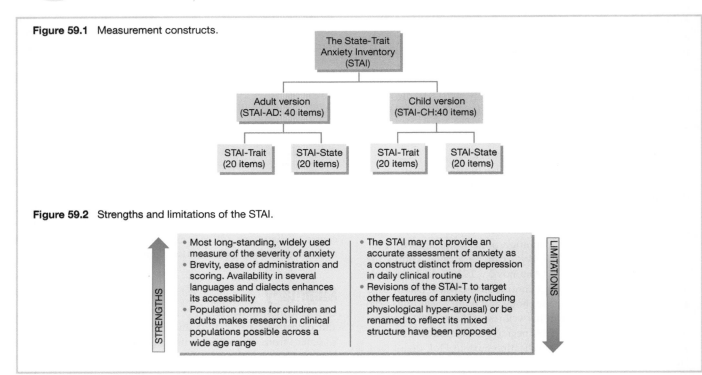

Figure 59.1 Measurement constructs.

The State-Trait
Anxiety Inventory
(STAI)

Adult version
(STAI-AD: 40 items)

Child version
(STAI-CH:40 items)

STAI-Trait
(20 items)

STAI-State
(20 items)

STAI-Trait
(20 items)

STAI-State
(20 items)

Figure 59.2 Strengths and limitations of the STAI.

STRENGTHS

- Most long-standing, widely used measure of the severity of anxiety
- Brevity, ease of administration and scoring. Availability in several languages and dialects enhances its accessibility
- Population norms for children and adults makes research in clinical populations possible across a wide age range

- The STAI may not provide an accurate assessment of anxiety as a construct distinct from depression in daily clinical routine
- Revisions of the STAI-T to target other features of anxiety (including physiological hyper-arousal) or be renamed to reflect its mixed structure have been proposed

LIMITATIONS

Purpose

The State-Trait Anxiety Inventory (STAI) (Spielberger *et al.*, 1983) is one of the most established and commonly used clinical scales for measuring the presence and severity of current symptoms of anxiety and a propensity to be anxious. The STAI has adult (STAI-AD) and child (STAI-CH) versions. The STAI distinguishes between state and trait anxiety. State anxiety is believed to fluctuate as a function of, and in response to, the stressors on an individual. An individual's level of state anxiety is high in circumstances perceived as threatening, irrespective of the presence of objective danger. Likewise, the person's level of state anxiety is low in non-stressful situations or in situations where an existing danger is not perceived as threatening. Conversely, trait anxiety refers to individual differences in the frequency and intensity with which anxiety manifests over time. Trait anxiety involves the activation of the autonomic nervous system and consists of feelings of worry, apprehension and tension. Trait anxiety is regarded as a relatively stable personality trait. People who score high in trait anxiety tend to perceive more situations as threatening or dangerous when compared with those who have lower trait anxiety scores and also tend to have higher state anxiety scores.

Content, number of terms and response scales

The STAI has 40 items designed to measure the *intensity* of the anxiety a person feels (STAI-State, or STAI-S subscale) and the *frequency* of feeling anxious (STAI-Trait, or STAI-T subscale) (Spielberger *et al.*, 1983) (Figure 59.1). The 20 STAI-S statements ask people to rate how they feel 'right now or at a particular period in time' (e.g. calm, tense) rated on a 4-point intensity scale, ranging from 'not at all' to 'very much so'. The 20 STAI-T statements describe 'how an individual generally feels' (e.g. confident) rated on a 4-point frequency scale, ranging from 'almost never' to 'almost always'. In order to reduce the influence of acquiescence on STAI responses, each subscale of the STAI form was constructed to include 10 items for which high ratings indicate high anxiety (anxiety-present, e.g. 'I am tense', 'I feel nervous and restless'), and 10 items written in a way opposite to what the scale is intended to measure (anxiety-absent, e.g. 'I am calm', 'I feel rested') (Spielberger *et al.*, 1983). Short versions of the STAI have been developed independently and psychometric properties of a few versions have been evaluated (Balsamo *et al.*, 2013).

Nursing and Healthcare Research at a Glance, First Edition. Alan Glasper and Colin Rees. © 2017 by John Wiley & Sons, Ltd. Published 2017 by John Wiley & Sons, Ltd.

The STAI can be obtained from the publisher, Mind Garden, 855 Oak Grove Avenue, Suite 215, Menlo Park, CA 94025, USA (http://www.mindgarden.com/145-state-trait-anxiety-inventory-for-adults).

Target population
- STAI-AD: ages 14 years and older with at least a sixth grade reading level comprehension.
- STAI-CH: ages 8–14 years with at least a fourth grade reading level comprehension.

Administration
The STAI-AD and STAI-CH can be administered in an individual or group setting. Specific instructions are provided for each of the STAI-S and STAI-T subscales. The STAI-CH may be used with younger children with average or above-average reading ability and with older children who are below average in reading ability.

Respondent burden
- STAI-AD: 10 minutes.
- STAI-CH: 8–20 minutes.

Translations/adaptations
As outlined in the Mind Garden website, the STAI has been translated and adapted in 46 languages.

Scoring
Item scores are summed to obtain subscale total scores. Nearly half the items are reverse scored (19 items of the total 40). Mind Garden has a service available to administer and score the STAI-AD/CH via a web-based interface available through http://www.mindgarden.com/state-trait-anxiety-inventory-for-children/308-staich-remote-online-survey-license.html.

Score interpretation
STAI subscale scores range from 20 to 80, with higher scores indicating greater anxiety. A cut-off point of 39–40 has been suggested to detect clinically significant symptoms for the STAI scale. A higher STAI-S cut-off score (44–51) is recommended in chronically ill patients with anxiety disorders, and at 53 in patients with mood disorders (Balsamo *et al.*, 2013).

Norms
- STAI-AD: norms are available for clinical patients, high school and college students, and working adults.
- STAI-CH: norm groups include fourth-, fifth- and sixth-grade elementary school children and were developed from two large samples in six different US schools. Norm tables for fourth- to sixth-grade children, reported by gender and grade level, are available.

Clinical use
- Psychological and health research.
- Clinical diagnosis and assessment of treatment efficacy.

- Assessment of clinical anxiety in medical, surgical, psychosomatic and psychiatric patients.

Psychometric properties

Reliability
A study on the reliability generalisation of the STAI reported excellent internal consistency for both the trait and state subscales ($\alpha = 0.89–0.91$) (Barnes *et al.*, 2002). The STAI-T is documented to have excellent test–retest reliability (average $r = 0.88$) at multiple time intervals, while the STAI-S is evidenced to have lower temporal stability (average $r = 0.70$).

Validity
To optimise content validity during tool development, most items of the STAI were selected from the Taylor Manifest Anxiety Scale and the Cattell and Scheier's Anxiety Scale Questionnaire based on high correlations (Spielberger *et al.*, 1983). Some studies on instrument dimensionality provide empirical support for a four-factor model of the STAI (consisting of state anxiety present and absent, trait anxiety present and absent) (Suzuki *et al.*, 2000), which is consistent with item polarity in the two subscales and of the view that state and trait anxiety is a unidimensional bipolar construct (Vautier and Pohl, 2009). Debate on the dimensionality of the STAI-T continues, with a bi-factor model comprising two first-order specific factors (anxiety and depression) and one first-order general factor (negative affect) proposed (Balsamo *et al.*, 2013). The hypothetical *anxiety* and *depression* factors seem to lack sufficient discriminant validity, due to the fact that they assess two partially different aspects of negative affect, more so than anxiety or depression in the strictest sense.

Strengths and limitations of the STAI
See Figure 59.2 for the strengths and limitations of the STAI. Further psychometric review of the short versions of the STAI is warranted.

References
Balsamo, M., Romanelli, R., Innamorati, M., Ciccarese, G., Carlucci, L. and Saggino, A. (2013) The State-Trait Anxiety Inventory: shadows and lights on its construct validity. *Journal of Psychopathology and Behavioral Assessment* **35**, 475–486.

Barnes, L.L.B., Harp, D. and Jung, W.S. (2002) Reliability generalization of scores on the Spielberger State-Trait Anxiety Inventory. *Educational and Psychological Measurement* **62**, 603–618.

Spielberger, C.D., Gorsuch, R.L., Lushene, R.E., Vagg, P.R. and Jacobs, G.A. (1983) *Manual for the State-Trait Anxiety Inventory*. Palo Alto, CA: Consulting Psychologists Press.

Suzuki, T., Tsukamoto, K. and Abe, K. (2000) Characteristic factor structures of the Japanese version of the State-Trait Anxiety Inventory: coexistence of positive–negative and state–trait factor structures. *Journal of Personality Assessment* **74**, 447–458.

Vautier, S. and Pohl, S. (2009) Do balanced scales assess bipolar constructs? The case of the STAI scales. *Psychological Assessment* **21**, 187–193.

60 Kelly's repertory grids

Figure 60.1 Constructs.

Illness	Wellness
• Nice	• Nasty

Fun	Dull
• Stimulating	• Someone poke me I'm nodding off

Figure 60.2 Elements.

Classic elements
- Wife/girlfriend
- Husband/boyfriend
- Father
- Mother
- Teacher you liked
- Teacher you disliked

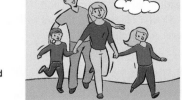

Figure 60.3 Elicited elements.

Visual method

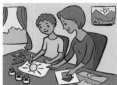

Laddering

Opposing construct

Examines why SOC is better, thereby identifying new constructs

Superordinate construct (SOC)

Figure 60.4 Matrix.

CONSTRUCT	Elements, e.g. mother	Elements, e.g. father	Elements, e.g. partner	Elements, e.g. good teacher	Elements, e.g. bad teacher	CONTRAST
1. Health						1. Illness
2. Thoughtful						2. Impulsive
3. Adults						3. Children
4. Boring						4. Interesting
5. Happy						5. Sad
6.						6.
7.						7.
8.						8.

Definitions

Kelly (1970) defined *personality* as our abstraction of the activity of a person and the generalisation of this to all matters of this relationship to other persons, known and unknown, as well as to anything else that may seem particularly valuable.

Background theory

George Kelly developed an extension of the Gestalt and cognitive theory of personality based on the assumption that all people behave as scientists and that we create and test hypotheses (personal constructs) to help us understand and predict our world. This led to the fundamental principle of *constructive alternativism* that underpins Kelly's Personal Construct Theory. Therefore to understand someone we need to know what their constructs are; most people have between seven and eight constructs. The theory is oriented towards the future – Kelly postulated that by showing people their constructs and any errors within them, we can attempt to alter them.

What is it?

The theory is used in a psychobiographical method to elicit the constructs. The repertory grid is a way of examining the individual's cognitive and perceptual dichotomous constructs developed by Kelly. Constructs are formed by our experiences, knowledge and observations. Kelly's repertory grid is an objective tool to elicit subjective material during an interview to generate a mental map of how subjects view the world. Figure 60.1 illustrates some examples of dichotomous constructs. The grid is a matrix of elements and constructs, and these are either provided by the investigator (depending on the purpose of the grid) or elicited by the individual or a mixture of both. Elements typically consist of five areas (e.g. introspective, close relationships, themes and roles).

Grid stages

Stage one elicits the elements and constructs, usually in the form of a semi-structured interview where individuals are asked to think about their lives and compare one element to another. Alternative methods include full context elicitation, where all the elements are used together, or triadic elicitation where three elements are examined at one time and the individual says how two are alike and one is different. An example of this is to ask an individual to consider three people and say how two are similar and one is different; these would then generate the two anchors for one construct. In the classic repertory grid the elements are people: your wife/girlfriend, husband/boyfriend, father, mother, teacher you like and teacher you dislike (Figure 60.2). There are also two further methods of eliciting constructs: the non-verbal elicitation, which uses pictures to stimulate ideas, and laddering, which uses the triadic method but then gets the individual to look more closely at the first construct and to identify why it is preferable, thereby generating new constructs from the original one to produce a superordinate construct (Figure 60.3).

Stage two examines how the constructs are applied to different elements to detect patterns in their responses. The constructs and elements are mapped onto the matrix deciding how or whether the construct applies to each element ranking them (Figure 60.4). Methods of ranking include Likert's, VAS (visual analogue scale) and direct weighting, where both extremes are anchored as best or worst possible options.

Advantages and disadvantages

Advantages

The process minimises bias in eliciting responses whilst using a flexible procedure.

Disadvantages

The procedure is not standardised and therefore the different forms of the grids generate different results. Supplied constructs maybe interpreted differently by each individual. The theory does not recognise the role of motivation within it.

Applications

The grids can be applied to any disease population and can also capture change over time. The grids have been used to determine quality of life within multiple scales including the Schedule of Individual Quality of Life. The grids were originally developed to be used within an interview but they can also be used in a computerised form. Other applications of the grids look to establish mother and children's interactions, religion, information technology and shopping habits.

Summary

Kelly's repertory grid technique is based on a relevant theory that directly translates into the grid technique and has been widely used in numerous applications over 60 years. An awareness of the pros and cons of the method should be considered when using the method. Fixed elements will improve standardisation and the psychometric properties but will detract from relevance to the individual. Therefore if you wish to capture information relevant to individuals, you should allow them to nominate the elements and constructs but should recognise its limited psychometric properties; conversely, if you use fixed elements, this improves the psychometric properties but limits individual relevance.

Reference and further reading

Buttle, J. (1985) Measuring food store image using Kelly repertory grid. *The Service Industries Journal* 5, 79–89.

Easterby Smith, M. (1980) The design, analysis and interpretation of repertory grids. *International Journal of Man–Machine Studies* 13, 3–24.

Kelly (1970) In: C. Monte (1995) *Beneath the Mask: An Introduction to Theories of Personality*. Orlando, FL: Harcourt Brace College.

Rawlinson, J. (1995) Some reflections on the use of repertory grid technique in studies of nurses and social workers. *Journal of Advanced Nursing* 21, 334–339.

Thunedborg, K., Allerup, P., Bech, P. and Joyce, C. (1993) Development of the repertory grid for measurement of individual quality of life in clinical trials. *International Journal of Methods in Psychiatric Research* 3, 45–56.

Critical incident technique

Figure 61.1   Critical incident technique.

The critical incident technique is a qualitative method of gathering data from participants about specific incidents in order to develop an understanding about the situation under study. CIT was developed by Flanagan (1954) who identified five steps.

Step 1: Determination of the general aims of the study
- Aim and research question
- Activity to focus on

Step 2: Development of plans and specifications
- Inclusion criteria to identify critical incidents
- Selection and training of researchers and participants
- Data collection proforma

Step 3: Collection of the data
- Individual or group interviews
- Written self-reports
- Direct observation
- Questionnaire

Step 4: Analysis of the data
- Inductive process
- Thematic content analysis
- Coding categories
- Inferences and conclusions

Step 5: Interpretation and reporting
- Findings disseminated to improve practice in relation to the activity studied

---

The critical incident technique (CIT) is a popular qualitative methodology originally developed to identify factors which enhanced the performance of United States Army Air Forces crews in the 1940s. Since it was first described by Flanagan (1954) it has been refined and developed. The technique is particularly useful in gathering data about the effectiveness or ineffectiveness of healthcare activities in clinical practice, education and management. CIT is a set of actions for gathering observations of people's behaviour in order to solve problems and develop principles. In the technique an incident is regarded as a discrete observable episode of activity from which inferences and predictions can be made. CIT does not consist of an inflexible set of rules; rather it is an adaptable set of principles which can be tailored to the activity being studied. Adhering to the set of procedures promotes objectivity leading to a complete picture of the situation from which hypotheses can be generated rather than a more subjective consideration of anecdotes from practice. There is also a dispute about whether CIT is a method or a methodology.

Terminology

There is debate about terminology in relation to CIT. Some researchers avoid use of the term 'critical incident' because in healthcare it is now synonymous with a crisis, error or negative event and use in audit. Alternative terms include 'significant', 'revelatory', 'dilemma', 'situation' and 'event'. Critical incident analysis (CIA) is widely used in healthcare education as a technique to foster reflective and experiential learning.

Five main steps of CIT (Figure 61.1)

Determination of the general aim of the study

Researchers agree an aim and research question for the study and the specific type of activity to focus on. A clear aim is central to a CIT study in order to elicit appropriate critical incidents from participants.

Development of plans and specifications for collecting factual incidents regarding the activity

Clear and specific rules regarding data collection need to be put in place to ensure objectivity. Because of the important methodological debate about what is and what is not a critical incident, it is recommended that inclusion criteria are devised; for example, the account of the incident could include what led up to the incident, a detailed description of the experience, the outcome, what made the action effective or ineffective and how the action could have been made more effective. Attention should be paid to the selection and training of researchers and participants. It is suggested that the sample size in a CIT study should focus on the number of critical incidents gathered rather than the number of participants; it is likely that the more complicated the activity being studied, the larger the number of incidents needed. Once plans and specifications are agreed,

a data collection proforma can be devised to include essential information to guide researchers and inform participants about the study (e.g. clarifying its aim and confidentiality issues).

Collection of the data

Incidents collected should be very specific and remarkably effective or ineffective because atypical events are more easily remembered. Various methods of data collection can be employed; for example, group interviews or one-to-one interviews which may be face to face or by telephone and may include probes and prompt questions. Other methods include written self-reports, direct observation and record forms, and questionnaires can be sent to a large number of people by post or online. An important factor which can affect the quality of the data collected is how recently and accurately incidents are recalled; ideally they should be recorded while the events are still fresh in the memory of the participant. It is suggested that the accuracy of reporting is evident in the accounts of incidents themselves: if detailed and precise information is given, it can be assumed that the account of the incident is accurate, while vague accounts suggest that information may be incorrect and the incident is poorly remembered. The richness of the data will be enhanced if researchers are skilled in eliciting precise accurate descriptions of events by using effective questioning techniques; a method that can improve the quality of interviewing is an interactive-relational approach that incorporates self-awareness, authenticity, attunement, personal characteristics and new relationship.

Analysis of the data

Data are analysed using an inductive process. Thematic content analysis involves classification of the critical incidents and identification of themes and sub-themes with comparative analysis between themes. Alternatively, data can be organised using coding categories. Inferences are made regarding how performance can be improved in the activity being studied based on the recorded incidents and conclusions are drawn.

Interpretation and reporting

The final stage involves discussion, interpretation, reporting and dissemination of the results of the study in order to improve practice.

Reference and further reading

Bradbury-Jones, C. and Tranter, S. (2008) Inconsistent use of the critical incident technique in nursing research. *Journal of Advanced Nursing* **64**, 399–407.

Cormack, D.F.S. (2000) The critical incident technique. In: D. Cormack (ed.) *The Research Process in Nursing*, 4th edn. Oxford: Blackwell Science.

Flanagan, J.C. (1954) The critical incident technique. *Psychological Bulletin* **51**, 327–358.

Schluter, J., Seaton, P. and Chaboyer, W. (2008) Critical incident technique: a user's guide for nurse researchers. *Journal of Advanced Nursing* **61**, 107–114.

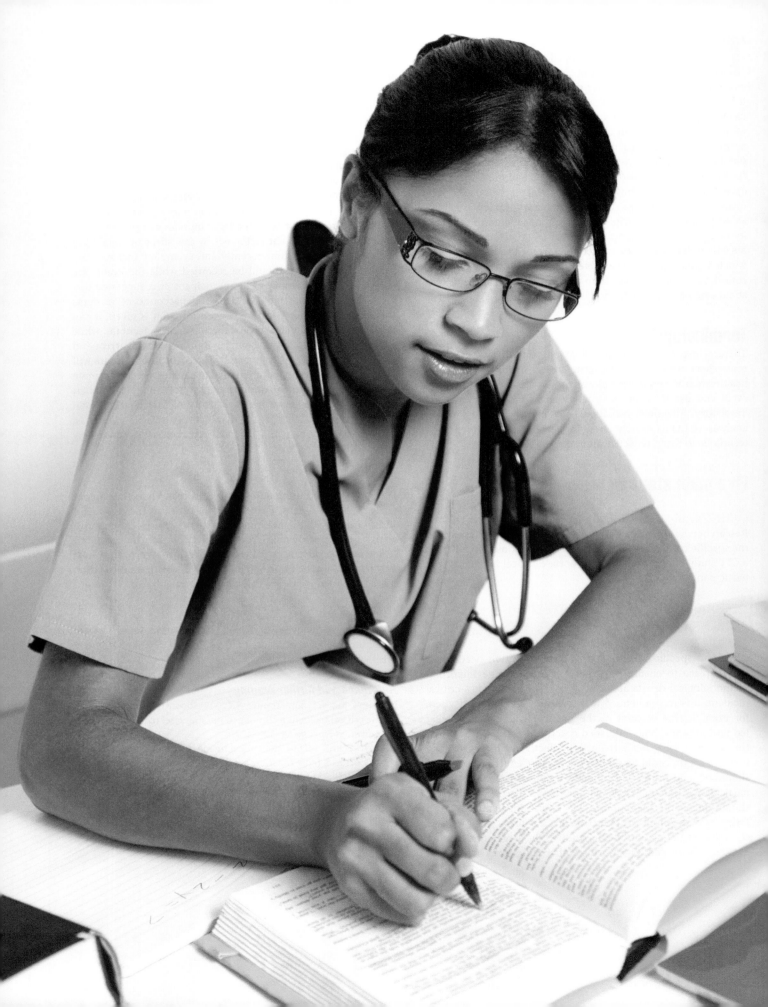

Conducting research with special groups

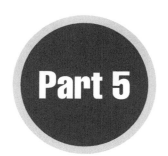

Part 5

Chapters

Conducting research with vulnerable groups

Figure 62.1 Which groups might be considered vulnerable?

Potentially, a number of groups of people might be considered vulnerable in the context of research but those groups often viewed in this way include:
- Children and young people
- People with mental health problems
- People with learning disabilities
- Women who are pregnant
- Older people
- People who are detained in some way (e.g. in prison)

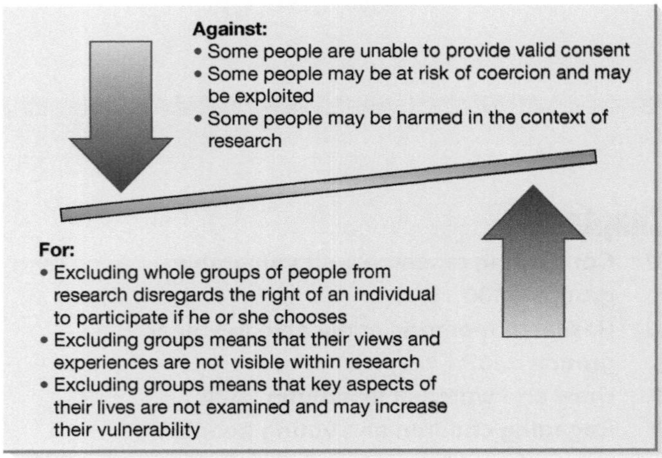

Figure 62.3 What are people vulnerable to?

- As history has demonstrated, some people may be vulnerable to coercion, exploitation and harm in the context of research
- Nonetheless, it is important that careful consideration is given to whether this is an inevitable consequence of them belonging to a specific group or whether it is due to inappropriate behaviour on the part of researchers
- It is important that researchers are aware of potential harms that can result from participation in research and that some groups of people may be at greater risk
- However, excluding them from research also places them at risk of marginalisation and exclusion
- The onus should therefore be on researchers to examine how they can best support the inclusion of people who may be vulnerable in research that is relevant to their lives

Figure 62.2 Arguments for and against the inclusion of 'vulnerable' groups in research.

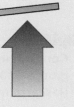

Against:
- Some people are unable to provide valid consent
- Some people may be at risk of coercion and may be exploited
- Some people may be harmed in the context of research

For:
- Excluding whole groups of people from research disregards the right of an individual to participate if he or she chooses
- Excluding groups means that their views and experiences are not visible within research
- Excluding groups means that key aspects of their lives are not examined and may increase their vulnerability

Figure 62.4 Supporting inclusion.

- Research should only be undertaken with people who might be considered vulnerable if it is relevant to their lives and experiences
- This may include research that focuses specifically on the situation of people who might be considered vulnerable (they are the key participants) and also wider research where they may benefit from participation
- Careful consideration needs to be given to how valid consent can best be obtained: this may include consideration of the format(s) in which participant information is provided, the timing of such information and who provides it. Usual ethical standards of stressing the voluntary nature of participation, the right to withdraw, confidentiality and identifying risks and benefits must be communicated but in ways that are accessible and understandable to potential participants
- Where someone is unable to provide valid consent (e.g. due to a lack of mental capacity), then legal requirements should be examined to determine whether participation may still be possible if key requirements are met
- Potential risks and benefits to participants must be identified and these should include the potential risk of being excluded from the research. The benefits should outweigh any risks and strategies should be in place to address any risks and their consequences

A number of groups of people might be considered to be vulnerable in the context of research and these include people with mental health problems, people with learning disabilities, children, pregnant women and people who are detained in some way, for example in prison (Figure 62.1). However, rather than just labelling such groups as 'vulnerable', it is important for researchers to consider what we mean by vulnerability in this context, whether such a label is helpful, and whether vulnerability can be reduced to enable participation in research (Figure 62.2).

What are people vulnerable to?

History unfortunately shows us that certain groups of people have been subjected to inhumane, harmful and even life-threatening treatment in the name of research. Moreover, their consent to participate in such activities has not been sought, they have not been fully informed about the nature of participation, or they have been in positions in which they are subject to coercion that they have been powerless to resist. It is not possible here to provide details of such research but readers wishing to learn more might usefully consult the Tuskegee Syphilis Study (http://www.cdc.gov/tuskegee/timeline.htm) and the Willowbrook Study (https://science.education.nih.gov/supplements/nih9/bioethics/guide/pdf/Master_5-4.pdf).

However, while the potential risks and harms of participation in research for some groups of people are recognised, there is also a growing awareness that harm can also arise from being excluded from research and that such exclusion can increase vulnerability (Figure 62.3).

The first risk arises from use of the term 'vulnerable groups' since this often means that people are grouped together on the basis of one or more personal characteristics. However, grouping people in such a way masks a wide range of variation in terms of personal capacities for understanding and participation. For example, people assigned to the group 'learning disabilities' could include those with only mild learning disabilities who live independently with no additional support and those with profound and multiple disabilities who require full support on a 24-hour basis in order to meet their needs. Therefore, while it would be challenging for some within this 'group' to understand information and consent to participate in research, for others consent would not be an issue if information were presented in formats that were accessible to them.

In addition, the terminology of 'vulnerable groups' can be challenging when considering the fluctuating nature of certain conditions. For example, someone with a serious mental health condition may not be able to provide valid consent at certain times when they are acutely ill but at other times their condition may be well managed.

It is also important to consider that certain research can only be conducted with groups who might be considered to be vulnerable. For example, if we want to know whether a particular therapy is effective for people with dementia, then we can only research this on people with dementia. Similarly, if we want to know whether the provision of healthcare in prisons meets the needs of prisoners, then we can only research this by seeking the views and experiences of prisoners. Indeed it has been recognised for some time that care for groups of people considered to be vulnerable will only improve when they are involved in research (Weaver Moore and Miller, 1999). Furthermore, it has been argued that excluding such groups from research can be unethical since it means that they are denied the potential benefits of participation (Alexander, 2010). The challenge for researchers is therefore to develop ways of researching that will support the inclusion of people who might be considered vulnerable while ensuring that ethical principles are upheld.

Promoting inclusion

The first issue to consider is whether the research can only be undertaken if people considered to be 'vulnerable' are included and examples of such research have been identified above. However, it may also be relevant to consider within wider research whether people who might be 'vulnerable' should have the right to participate if they so wish. For example, people with mental health problems or learning disabilities who also have cancer might wish to participate in a cancer trial that offers the hope of improved treatments for their cancer. In both situations it is important to consider how participation can best be facilitated where individuals wish (Figure 62.4).

A key issue is consent: full information regarding the nature of participation needs to be provided in ways accessible to potential participants. This will require attention to the use of language, format, timing and who presents the information. It may also be helpful to view consent as a process (rather than as a one-off event) and for continued consent to participate to be checked a number of times during the study. However, it is also important to recognise that some people may not be able to provide valid consent due to, for example, cognitive impairment. In such circumstances they may still wish to participate in a study and/or it may be beneficial to them and so it is important to consider whether the legal framework of the country in which you are researching permits such participation under certain specified circumstances.

The issue of potential harms and benefits is a further important consideration and this needs to include recognition of the potential harm of excluding certain groups from research. Nonetheless, all potential harms need to be considered and where these are greater for some groups of people then additional safeguards need to be put in place. All harms and benefits need to be communicated to potential participants, the benefits should outweigh the harms, and strategies should be in place to address any harms that occur. Using such an approach should support the participation in research of groups considered to be vulnerable, protecting their rights while also guarding against exclusion that can increase vulnerability.

References and further reading

Alexander, S.J. (2010) 'As long as it helps somebody': why vulnerable people participate in research. *International Journal of Palliative Nursing* **16**, 173–178.

Liamputtong, P. (2007) *Researching the Vulnerable*. London: Sage.

Weaver Moore, L. and Miller, M. (1999) Initiating research with doubly vulnerable populations. *Journal of Advanced Nursing* **30**, 1034–1040.

63 Research methods applicable to vulnerable groups

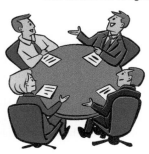

Figure 63.1 Focus Groups, see Gates and Waight (2007).

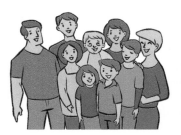

Figure 63.2 Participatory Research, see Northway (2000).

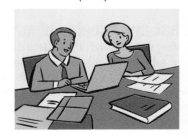

Figure 63.3 Multiple Methods, see Mafuba and Gates (2012).

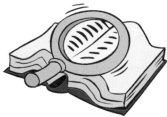

Figure 63.4 Historical, see Atkinson (2005).

Figure 63.5 Survey, see Emerson et al. (2005).

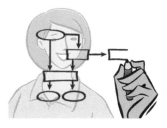

Figure 63.6 Experimental, see Willner et al. (2002).

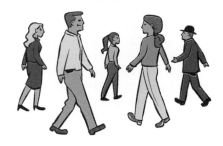

Figure 63.7 Ethnographic/Anthropological, see Edgerton (1967).

The range of methodological approaches for investigating aspects of learning disability (LD) healthcare is, in many ways, as varied as it is for all citizens, and all are based on philosophical and ontological assumptions (Figures 63.1–63.7).

Inclusive approaches

The role of people with LD within research has changed considerably over the past 20 years. Historically, people with LD have had research done to them: they have been the subject of the researcher, the studied, the analysed but never the participant (Dye *et al.*, 2004). Today, contemporary researchers try to make their research accessible and inclusive to people with LD. Since the development of the concept of participatory research (Northway,

2000) leading to emancipatory research (Hanley, 2005), a natural progression has been made to incorporate these principles into research with people with LD (Walmsley, 2004). The first of these approaches was first demonstrated by the use of personal narratives to illustrate life experience (Atkinson, 2005). This used an oral history approach that provided authentic accounts of people's lives, and placed them at the centre of the research. Extensive one-to-one interviews have also been used to study parenting by people with LD (Booth and Booth, 1996). Another approach to involving people with LD is that of engaging them as active consumer researchers (Feldner *et al.*, 2007). Increasingly, researchers are pairing up with people with LD to form research groups able to unite their strengths to respond to calls for research proposals from bodies commissioning such work.

Nursing and Healthcare Research at a Glance, First Edition. Alan Glasper and Colin Rees. © 2017 by John Wiley & Sons, Ltd. Published 2017 by John Wiley & Sons, Ltd.

Other qualitative approaches, not necessarily inclusive

Focus groups are a useful methodological approach for research with this client group (Gates and Waight, 2007). People with a shared interest (e.g. gender, age, ethnicity, religion, life experience, expertise) are brought together to discuss a particular issue. Anthropological studies are rare in the field of LD. Edgerton (1967) in his seminal work studied 55 people living in the Los Angeles area of the USA after their 'release' from the Pacific State Hospital. Through extensive interviews and observation he and his fieldworkers developed rich insights into their subjects, and reported on stigma in their lives, and how they seemingly cloaked themselves with competence that was more imaginary than real.

Quantitative methods

Notwithstanding these newer and perhaps more enlightened approaches to research methods for investigating aspects of LD healthcare, more traditional approaches are still used. These include quantitative approaches to generating knowledge that include observable relationships between independent and dependent variables. Such approaches include randomised controlled trials, an example being a controlled trial of the efficacy of a cognitive behavioural anger management group for adults with LD by Willner et al. (2002). Surveys may be used on this population. These are generally used on a large section of a particular population to collect large amounts of data, at a given point in time in order that statistical inferences can be made about the larger population being studied. They typically involve the use of polls, postal surveys, and telephone interviews and use questionnaires and interviewers; their use is rare in LD, with notable exceptions (Emerson et al., 2005).

Traversing the divides

One way of attempting to achieve fidelity to differing philosophical approaches to research is by adopting multiple methods. Multi-method, mixed methods, multiple methods and triangulation all refer to the concurrent or sequential use of more than one approach in a study at the methodological level (Mafuba and Gates, 2012).

Acquiescence

A classic challenge in the involvement of people with LD in research is that they may feel it is important to please the researcher, who may be perceived to be in a position of authority. This has led to claims that individuals may not answer questions truthfully, instead responding to questions in a certain way because they think that it is what the interviewer wants to hear.

Ethical issues

A classic paper on ethical and methodological issues by Stalker (1998) incorporates discussion on making choices, and on ways of involving people with LD. Also explored are dilemmas such as how to gain informed consent from people with profound impairment, the risk of intrusion when conducting research in people's own homes, along with dangers of raising expectations of continuing friendship after research has been concluded.

Summary

Researchers are responsible for making their research accessible and inclusive. However, it must be noted that it is not always possible to involve all people with LD, such as those with profound and multiples disabilities; also the methodological approach should clearly relate to the questions being asked.

References

Atkinson, D. (2005) Narratives and people with learning disabilities. In: G. Grant, P. Goward, M. Richardson and P. Ramcharan (eds) Learning Disability: A Life Cycle Approach to Valuing People, pp. 7–27. Maidenhead: Open University Press.

Booth, T. and Booth, W. (1996) Sounds of silence: narrative research with inarticulate subjects. Disability and Society 11, 55–69.

Dye, L., Hendy, S., Hare, D.J. and Burton, M. (2004) Capacity to consent to participate in research: a recontextualisation. British Journal of Learning Disabilities 32, 144–150.

Edgerton, R.B. (1967) The Cloak of Competence: Stigma in the Lives of the Mentally Retarded. Berkeley, CA: University of California Press.

Emerson, E., Mallam, S., Davies, I. and Spencer, K. (2005) Adults with Learning Difficulties in England 2003/4. Leeds: Health and Social Care Information Centre. Available at http://webarchive. nationalarchives.gov.uk/20130107105354/http://www.dh.gov.uk/en/Publicationsandstatistics/Publications/PublicationsStatistics/DH_4120033

Feldner, C., Gregory, C., Vakaria, A. et al. (2007) People with learning disabilities as consumer researchers: a case study. Learning Disability Today 7, 9–14.

Gates, B. and Waight, M. (2007) Reflections on conducting focus groups with people with learning disabilities: theoretical and practical issues. Journal of Research in Nursing 12, 111–126.

Hanley, B. (2005) Research as Empowerment? Report of a Series of Seminars Organised by the Toronto Group. York: Joseph Rowntree Foundation.

Mafuba, K. and Gates, B. (2012) Sequential multiple methods as a contemporary method in learning disability nursing practice research. Journal of Intellectual Disabilities 16, 287–296.

Northway, R. (2000) The relevance of participatory research in developing nursing's research and practice. Nurse Researcher 7, 40–52.

Stalker, K. (1998) Some ethical and methodological issues in research with people with learning difficulties. Disability and Society 13, 5–19.

Walmsley, J. (2004) Inclusive learning disability research: the (non disabled) researcher's role. British Journal of Learning Disabilities 32, 65–71.

Willner, P., Jones, J., Tams, R. and Green, G. (2002) A randomised controlled trial of the efficacy of a cognitive behavioural anger management group for adults with learning disabilities. Journal of Applied Research in Intellectual Disabilities 15, 224–235.

64 Draw and write/tell technique

Figure 64.1 The draw and write/tell technique (DWT).

The 'draw and write/draw and tell technique' can be used to elicit information (data) from children

Draw and write/draw and tell are two complementary qualitative research techniques which purport to more fully capture the 'voice' of the child than straightforward questioning or interviewing

In embellishing icons or drawings with metaphors or words it might be possible to glean information which children might find too difficult or complex to express or convert through the medium of the spoken word. When children draw pictures this improves their abilities to talk about their meaning

Stages of using the technique
- Gain consent (copy of protocol to parents)
- Plan scenarios that the children can make drawings of
- Prepare DWT proformas commensurate with the research question
- Prepare a pre-written protocol to ensure consistency of the approach
- Give each child a DWT proforma instrument and a pack of crayons/pencils/felt tip pens, etc .
- Check child understanding of the exercise
- Ask the children to embellish their drawing with words (for preliterate children /children with learning disabilities annotate their drawings with their words. It is important not to alter the child's words, i.e. no interpretation)
- Repeat for subsequent questions/topics
- Divide the results for the draw and write/draw and tell study into two categories, i.e. written words or metaphors and spoken words which were used by individual children to embellish their icons or drawings
- Transcribe the written comments from each of the drawings
- Separately transcribe the spoken comments where appropriate
- Use Riley's (1996) or similar technique of coding data using colour highlighter pens (or similar method) to delineate common themes
- Remember to give child a copy of their embellished drawing

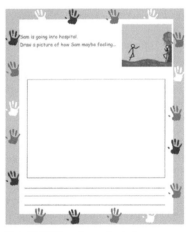

Sample DWT proforma topic 1

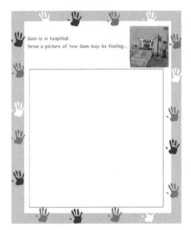

Sample DWT proforma topic 2

Draw, write/draw, and tell are two complementary qualitative research techniques that purport to more fully capture the 'voice' of the child than straightforward questioning or interviewing as in for example a focus group. The popularity of the technique as a legitimate methodology for reflecting the view of children is growing. In a critical appraisal of the methodology, Brackett-Milburn and McKie (1999) discuss its use as offering a number of opportunities from which to elicit children's views on a variety of topics, reflecting one of the technique's main claims of enabling children to participate. The authors suggest that the method offers a lens on the world of the child, which can reflect and illuminate their often hidden emotions. In embellishing icons or drawings with annotations, metaphors or words, it might be possible to glean information which children might find too difficult or complex to express or convert through the medium of the spoken word.

Early proponents of the technique were McWhirter *et al.* (2000) who used the it to seek children's views on safe sunbathing. They point out that only the written statements (from the child and adult scribes as appropriate) should be used by the researchers, with the drawings simply used to embellish the findings. However, Horstman and Bradding (2002) in employing the technique have used both the written words and the pictorial material to construct their dataset.

Example: using the technique to evaluate clown humour

To illustrate this technique, a published study by Weaver *et al.* (2007) will be referred to. In this study the draw and write/draw and tell technique (Figure 64.1) was used to elicit information from children about their experiences of receiving clown humour while a patient in hospital. In order to assess the efficacy of clown humour a group of children and their parents were asked for consent to participate in a two-part exercise using the draw and write/draw and tell technique which was conducted over the course of a day, one part before a clown encounter and the other after. It was hoped to explore children's perceptions of what children think about when faced with the prospect of an impending admission to hospital and, importantly, how that view of hospital might be influenced after a clown doctor performance. To capture the data, two draw and write scenarios were produced and face validity tested with a pilot group of 10 children (proforma 1 and 2). The children found no difficulties

in embellishing their drawings with words/metaphors and were able to talk to the investigator about their drawings.

The investigator followed a pre-written and piloted protocol to ensure consistency of approach and importantly there was no mention of clowns during the first component of the data collection using the draw and write proforma instrument. Individual children were asked to consider Sam, a boy or a girl in proforma 1, and were asked to draw and embellish with words (written or spoken) a picture of how Sam might be feeling before his admission to hospital.

The second part of the data collection was undertaken with the children after a clown performance later the same day. For the second stage of the data collection Sam is now in hospital (proforma 2) but significantly has just spent some time playing with the clown doctor. The children at this stage were asked to draw and embellish a picture about what helps children and young people best when they are in hospital. All children participating in the study were given a photocopy of their drawings to take home and a large colour postcard photograph of the clown doctor.

The written elements from the drawings and the spoken comments were separately transcribed and delineated for each child and Riley's (1996) technique of coding data was utilised to delineate common themes. The result of this study of clown humour using the technique shows that sick children believe it to be generally positive.

References

Brackett-Milburn, K. and McKie, L. (1999) A critical appraisal of the draw and write technique. *Health Education Research* **14**, 387–398.

Horstman, M. and Bradding, A. (2002) Helping children speak up in the health service. *European Journal of Oncology Nursing* **6**, 75–84.

McWhirter, J., Collins, M., Bryant, I., Wetton, N. and Newton Bishop, J. (2000) Evaluating 'Safe in the Sun': a curriculum programme for primary schools. *Health Education Research* **15**, 203–217.

Riley, J. (1996) *Getting the Most from Your Data. A Handbook of Practical Ideas on How to Analyse Qualitative Data.* Bristol: Technical and Educational Services Ltd.

Weaver, K., Prudhoe, G., Battrick, C. and Glasper, E.A. (2007) Sick children's perceptions of clown doctor humour. *Journal of Children's and Young People's Nursing* **1**, 359–365.

65 Engaging children and young people in research

Figure 65.1 The use of stickers and drawing helped this child to talk about her experience of the care she received from her support worker.

Figure 65.2 Use of arts-based approaches such as the use of collage can help young people express concepts such as their experience of pain.

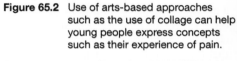

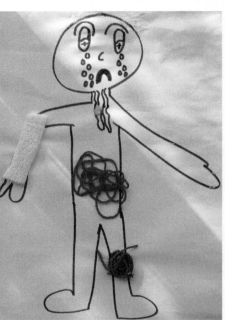

Figure 65.3 Empowerment can be facilitated through considering a range of factors relating to choice, control, methods and respect.

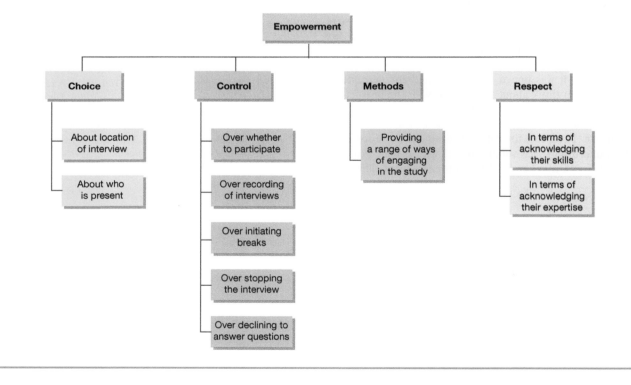

The shift to engagement

Research into children's and young people's health is essential to ensure that treatments, interventions and services meet their needs and are safe and effective and promote their health and well-being. The historical reluctance to undertake research on or with children – to 'protect' them from the perceived risks associated with research – has been superseded by a clearer understanding that robust, well-designed and ethical studies can bring enormous benefits to children's health. Children's health research now encompasses everything from randomised controlled trials of drugs and interventions through to qualitative research into children's views and preferences about the services they receive.

In recent years there has been a shift not just to recruiting children and young people into studies but also to ensuring that children and young people are centre-stage in research that affects their health and well-being.

The degree to which they are involved or engaged depends on a range of different factors, some of which are child-centred (e.g. age, capacity, willingness to engage) and some of which are research-centred (the type of study can either constrain or promote the possibilities for engagement). Engagement can involve actual participation in a study as well as identifying the research question, design of the study, undertaking data collection as a co-researcher, advising on communication, promoting public awareness of the study, supporting dissemination of outputs, and co-authoring papers.

When considering the terminology used there are distinct differences between 'consultation', 'involvement', 'participation' and 'engagement'. Sometimes used interchangeably, these terms reflect real differences in the level of partnership and control that young people have. The best studies are not tokenistic in how they involve children but are genuinely committed to working in partnership. Even as engagement of children and young people is becoming more deeply embedded, there are still some groups, such as children with disabilities, who tend to be at particular risk of exclusion.

Researchers need to engage with children and young people in ways that are consonant with the children's particular abilities, skills, interests and resources (Figures 65.1 and 65.2). This requires the researcher to be sensitive, reflexive and highly skilled in order to facilitate children's and young people's own perceptions, experiences and perspectives to be represented.

Special considerations

Engaging children and young people creates a number of special considerations in relation to three overlapping core elements: ethics, empowerment and methods.

Ethics

All research with children should be carried out to the highest clinical and ethical standards. Research involving children and young people as participants requires consideration of their particular abilities and competencies and the way in which disability or acute, chronic or life-limiting illness may compromise their communication and potential engagement.

The setting (e.g. ward, clinic, hospice, school or home) in which the study takes place needs to be taken into account as this will influence the child's or young person's participation. The researcher is responsible for ensuring that the child feels safe and comfortable.

As minors, children and young people under the age of 16 years are unable to provide legally binding consent to participate in research. Instead, informed consent must be sought from parents/legal representatives on their behalf. Children and young people can give their assent or can decline to take part. Their decision needs to be based on an adequate understanding and knowledge (e.g. why the research is being carried out, what it will involve, any benefits). Separate information sheets and assent and consent forms for children/young people and parents should be developed, providing age-appropriate information suitable for their psychological and intellectual maturity. Assent and consent are ongoing processes that should be maintained on a continuous basis by dialogue at each research encounter, observing for any non-verbal signs that may indicate unwillingness to continue.

Empowerment

The adult–child power imbalance is a major consideration but may be reduced by emphasising children's and young people's choices and control in the research process and creating opportunities for them to demonstrate their expertise (Figure 65.3).

Methods

Many participatory, child-centred, qualitative methods have been developed to facilitate children's and young people's engagement in communicating and interpreting their own experiences of health service provision. Core to successfully engaging children and young people is being respectful and taking into account their communicative ability and employing appropriate words and phrasing.

Most participatory methods aim to promote engagement through creating a relaxed atmosphere, decreasing anxiety, reducing feelings of self-consciousness, and being sensitive to the particular needs of children and young people. Methods should have resonance with their lives, preferences and daily activities. Using methods that do not rely on high levels of literacy creates a range of opportunities for engagement (e.g. drawing, photography, drama) and can be used alongside interviews, focus groups and nominal groups.

Further reading

Carter, B. (2009) Tick box for child? The ethical positioning of children as vulnerable, researchers as barbarians and reviewers as overly cautious. *International Journal of Nursing Studies* **46**, 858–864.

Carter, B. and Ford, K. (2013) Researching children's health experiences: the place for participatory, child-centered, arts-based approaches. *Research in Nursing and Health* **36**, 95–107.

Royal College of Paediatrics and Child Health (2012) *Turning the tide: harnessing the power of child health research*. A report by the RCPCH Commission on Child Health Research. Available at http://www.rcpch.ac.uk/harnessing-the-power-of-child-health-research (accessed 14 April 2014).

66 Photographic elicitation as a means of collecting data

Figure 66.1 Workshop 2.

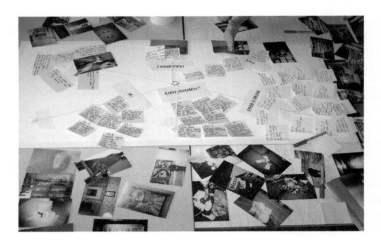

While numerous writers have offered guidance about the use of participatory techniques in visual-based research with children with varying degrees of success, there is less critical work surrounding the use of participant photography to facilitate consultation and qualitative health research. However, this should not put you off using this method as there is huge scope in using photographic images in consultation or research with young people as they can be a powerful medium through which, individually and collectively, young people can express their views across a wide range of the developmental continuum. So you can be confident in using photography in research as it is not a new technique.

Traditionally, photographs were taken by the researcher and interpreted by the participant; however, during the 1980s a more participatory type of photography was used to evoke a response or allow a participant to express a view (Harper, 1984). This is known as *photo-elicitation interview* (PEI), where a range of social scientists including nurses have used photographic images to evoke memories or enable participants to talk about difficult abstract concepts (Epstein *et al.*, 2006). This has been used effectively with children and young people (Figure 66.1).

Using photographic elicitation with children and young people

Preparation
- Disposable cameras (can be digital disposable) or iPad.
- Post-it notes and pens (optional flipchart paper).
- Elastic or string to pull photos together (optional).
- Suitable venue.

Example
Drawing on work by the author, Coad and Needham (2005) used photographs to elicit views about what it meant to be a young person aged 13–17 years living in Birmingham and Bristol, UK. The purpose in both areas was to explore (i) what young people believed about health and (ii) what preferences young people had for healthcare services.

In total, 62 young people were enrolled in a project where each was issued with a disposable camera and asked to take 24 photographs of their lives, with a particular focus on their health outcomes. We agreed as a team not to use mobile technology imagery as the budget was limited and we wanted to engage with large numbers of diverse young people. In total, access and recruitment included three secondary schools, one youth club, one child and adolescent mental health (CAMH) facility, one children's home and one health-based advisory group.

Two workshops took place. Workshop 1 helped familiarise the young people with the cameras, discussed issues of consent and agreed ground rules. After 2–4 weeks, photographs were collected by the research team for development prior to the focus group of Workshop 2, which enabled images to be pulled together and meanings explored, i.e. not only *what* the photograph represented but *why* it was taken. Workshop 2 commenced with the young people being given their own individual photographs and then in pairs they were invited to place the photographs of their choice haphazardly on the table. The photographic quality overall was excellent and included aspects of what they considered healthy living: 'healthy' food and drinks, sport activities, families, outdoor life and activities of living. In addition, there were photographs where the young people wanted to show 'unhealthy issues', such as junk food, cigarettes and rubbish. Less in number were photographs of health services, such as a local pharmacy, NHS drop-in/walk-in facilities, or healthcare facility such as a CAMH or general practitioner's surgery.

Young people were invited to arrange similar photographs on the floor or table and agree concepts as a pair. Members of the research team probed choices and concept mapping. The participants were asked to write this on a Post-it note (or the researchers offered to do the writing) and attach this to the photographs. In this way themes were assembled. Young people had a good knowledge of their own identity in terms of personal health and what made them healthy, such fresh fruit, water, vegetables and recreation. Equally, they understood that smoking, junk food and limited exercise were unhealthy. Although some young people did suggest a number of health services they knew to be places where 'sick people' visited, such as hospitals and the doctor's surgery, in the main healthy living featured in the workshop activity. It was also evident that the young people cared very much about the absence of, and accessibility to, health-based facilities and professionals. For example, a recurring theme surrounded the lack of 'health facilities' geared specifically to their needs. Thus, the photographs acted as a medium to enable the young people to make a record of their lives *through their own eyes*.

Conclusion
Using photographs can be interactive and effective in obtaining children and young people's views around health and healthcare services (Hanna *et al.*, 1995). One concern in the planning stages should be what guidance to give to children and young people in taking the photographs. While the aim might be about choice, as professionals and researchers we have to be safe. Children and young people's consent should be ascertained on an ongoing basis and using photographs is no exception. Feedback on the findings of any study is an important part of acknowledging the children's views, and can be done in a number of ways, including returning the photographs (or copies), positive verbal/written feedback, an organised event and personal certificates.

References
Coad, J. and Needham, J. (2005) Snapshot: an exploratory survey of young people's perceptions of health and healthy living using a photographic record. Heart of Birmingham (HoB)tPCT Report. Available at jane.coad@coventry.ac.uk

Epstein, I., Stevens, B., McKeever, P. and Baruchel, S. (2006) Photo elicitation interview (PEI): using photos to elicit children's perspectives. *International Journal of Qualitative Methods* 5(3), 1–11.

Hanna, K., Jacobs, P. and Guthrie, D. (1995) Exploring the concept of health among adolescents with diabetes using photography. *Journal of Pediatric Nursing* 10, 321–327.

Harper, D. (1984) Meaning and work: a study in photo elicitation. International *Journal of Visual Sociology* 2, 20–43.

67 Focus groups with children and young people

Figure 67.1 Moderators need to remember that children in a focus group are all different, have different experiences, characters, capacities and expectations. It takes skill to ensure that all the children feel safe and comfortable.

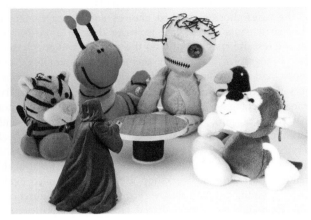

Figure 67.2 An example of a 'map' of children in a focus group and some key notes to support more detailed field notes. Maps like this can help make sense of the transcript.

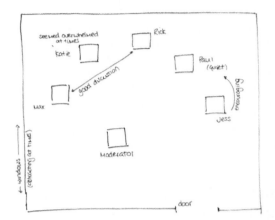

Figure 67.3 Setting out ground rules for behaviour during the focus group can be helpful for children. It can also help if children are given a flag or other object to signal they don't want to answer a question. It can be easier for a child to use an object than have to say 'no' or 'pass'.

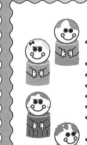

Group Rules

- If you're not sure of something let us know and we will explain
- Everyone has good ideas
- Everyone gets a turn to talk
- Take time to think before you talk
- We won't tell other people what you say
- Listen to what the other children are saying
- The group should be fun but nobody gets teased
- If you don't want to say anything you can wave the flag or just say 'pass'

Nursing and Healthcare Research at a Glance, First Edition. Alan Glasper and Colin Rees. © 2017 by John Wiley & Sons, Ltd. Published 2017 by John Wiley & Sons, Ltd.

Focus groups have been used in social science and health research with adults for many years and are now increasingly being used with children and young people. Focus groups need to be tailored to their cognitive, linguistic and psychosocial competencies and take into account pragmatic issues such as their concentration span, appropriate settings and pacing.

Focus groups allow children to explore, share, develop and discuss a particular topic with a selected group of other children and/or young people. They are particularly useful for generating information about their attitudes, thoughts, beliefs, values, perspectives and opinions. A focus group can generate multiple views, points of consensus and divergence, different stances, positions and meanings.

Focus groups can be used either as the sole method within a study or as part of a multi-method study. They are often used either at the start of the study (e.g. to help generate hypotheses or refine the focus for subsequent phases) or at the end of the study (e.g. to gain further insight into a topic).

Online (synchronous or asynchronous) focus groups offer young people the opportunity to participate in topics that may be too sensitive to be discussed in a face-to-face meeting. Although cyber-safety and other issues have to be carefully thought through, they are an interesting option to consider.

Selecting children to contribute

Generating robust data is dependent on the moderator making clear decisions about who to invite to the group. Focus groups with children need to have the right balance between enough participants to talk creatively about the topic area and not so many participants that the children have to wait too long to speak. A group of five to eight children is about right. Children are selected based on their experience, knowledge and skills associated with the topic area. The best groups are sufficiently heterogeneous to trigger interesting discussions between the children. The age range, gender and competence of the children and young people invited to a group must be carefully considered. While mixed age and gender groups can work well, careful thought should be given to whether separate groups (e.g. boys/girls only groups, younger/older children, experienced/less experienced children) is preferable.

The moderator, observer and helpers

The moderator is key to a successful focus group. The moderator requires excellent child-friendly communication skills, a high degree of emotional intelligence and patience. In particular, he or she needs to be skilled in initiating and sustaining the engagement of the children and young people (Figure 67.1). Although encouraging different perspectives is important, the moderator needs to be careful that this does not become too challenging, especially with young children. The moderator needs to ensure that every child has the opportunity to contribute and for them to know that their contribution is important. The moderator also needs to manage any disruptive behaviour. Unlike a one-to-one interview where the researcher can fully focus on the child they are interviewing, many things compete for their attention in a focus group. Working with an observer who can take field notes is vital (Figure 67.2). Focus groups with children often need additional helpers to be available to support the children (e.g. if

they become upset, need to be accompanied to the toilet or keep them company if they withdraw from the focus group).

Benefits and issues with focus groups

Focus groups are a time-efficient means of accessing the views of a group of children. However, they require careful preparation. Being invited to be part of a focus group can make children feel valued. Since focus groups rely on verbal interaction, low levels of written literacy do not impede children's participation.

If one child dominates a focus group, the other children can feel left out, anxious and upset. Focus groups require a level of energy and excitement to promote a lively exchange of ideas. Pacing the group, encouraging movement and engagement in activities can all help reduce the potential for children to get bored or distracted. The data generated from focus groups with children can be complicated to transcribe and analyse.

Conducting a focus group with children

The venue in which the meeting is held should be accessible, convenient (for the child and their parents), child-friendly and in a neutral setting. Scheduling the group needs to take into account schooling, exams and holidays. The children should be welcomed, made to feel comfortable and offered appropriate food and drink. At the start of the focus group, the moderator should clearly explain the ground rules, for example respecting each others' views, being clear that they can say 'pass' to questions they do not want to answer (Figure 67.3). The use of age- and topic-appropriate ice-breaker activities by the moderator can help the children to get to know each other and relax (e.g. creating their own name badge). Letting the children become familiar with the audio-recorder can also help them. Successful moderation requires the flexible use of a series of pre-prepared, open, child-oriented questions that are relevant to the competence and capacities of the participants. In principle these questions fall into three categories: opening (easy questions to help settle the children and get them engaged with the topic); exploring (questions that are more focused and which encourage thoughtful and more detailed discussion from the whole group); and exiting (questions clarifying understanding). Rather than simply asking the questions, the moderator may choose to use a range of different participatory and/or art-based activities (e.g. drawing, collage, puppets) as a means of triggering the children's responses. The moderator should ensure that they provide praise and check that the children are willing to continue at regular intervals. After thanking the children for their contributions, the moderator should create space and time to be available for them and their parents. Children value being given a certificate or a badge or a small present to acknowledge their contribution to the study.

Further reading

Carter, B. and Ford, K. (2013) Researching children's health experiences: the place for participatory, child-centered, arts-based approaches. *Research in Nursing and Health* **36**, 95–107.

Gibson, F. (2007) Conducting focus groups with children and young people: strategies for success. *Journal of Research in Nursing* **12**, 473–483.

Gibson, J.E. (2012) Interviews and focus groups with children: methods that match children's developing competencies. *Journal of Family Theory and Review* **4**, 148–159.

142

Part 5 Conducting research with special groups

68 Critical ethnography with children

Figure 68.1 Constructions of childhood.

Discontinuity and change
- Childhood is a modern phenomenon
- Increasing concern for the welfare and well-being of children over time

Continuity and evolution
- Concern for children has existed over centuries
- Children's activity and contribution always set by the context and needs of their family

Current status
- No agreed definition of childhood
- Universal concept that differentiates being a child from being an adult
- Age of majority different in different countries

Children as social agents
- Not merely reactive-adaptors
- Interact with, influence and shape the world in which they live
- Different but equal in their claim to rights and for their views to be heard
- Age is an inadequate organising framework

Figure 68.2 Ethnographic methods.

Reconnaissance
- Mapping out the research territory
- Reconceptualising research problems and questions with intended participants
- Establishing researcher position
- When, where and how to engage children
- Reflect on and acknowledge self-awareness, current beliefs and values regarding children
- Check what, whom and why you afford privilege to certain people/groups

Fieldwork
Participant or non-participant observer

(Fully Involved) ←——————→ (Not involved)

Field observations
Passive and active events
Spoken words and silences
Informal and formal interviews and conversations
Scrutiny of visual and audible artefacts
Contemporaneous field notes/impressions
Reflexivity

Analysis
- Inductive analysis
- Privileging children's voices
- Researcher as research instrument
- Managing 'in' difference
- Concept mapping

Figure 68.3 Scaffolding children's communication competence.

What helps
- Recognise and understand individual children's preference for communication
- Develop a rapport: children may think you know more than they do
- Elicit a free narrative: let the children tell you in their own words what they think/feel/know
- Use supportive utterances, comments, non-verbal affirmations
- Use probing open questions to check and clarify understanding
- Use closed probing questions

What hinders
- Tag questions: 'he's nice isn't he?'
- Repeating the same question more than twice
- Excluding children due to limited language skills, shyness or augmented communication needs

Figure 68.4 Engaging children in research activity.

DO
- Approach pre-existing groups of children: schools, sports clubs and activity clubs
  Remember: be inclusive
- Be prepared with a raft of games and craft activities suited to the children's interests and capabilities: let them choose
- Take your time: never rush children
- Keep promises, attend when you say you will, leave when children signal they have had enough (e.g. switching off digital recording device, turning or walking away)
- Give children as much control as possible, e.g. with digital recorders
- Ask children to design information sheets, posters and consent forms, etc.

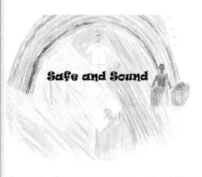

Example of study logo designed by children

Figure 68.5 Data analysis: example of early concept map.

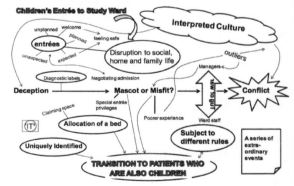

Nursing and Healthcare Research at a Glance, First Edition. Alan Glasper and Colin Rees. © 2017 by John Wiley & Sons, Ltd. Published 2017 by John Wiley & Sons, Ltd.

Children in research

Children as passive objects

The construction of childhood remains contested (Figure 68.1) with no universal definition. Research concerned with children during the mid twentieth century tended to focus on professional concerns for the benefit of public policy. Many researchers examined the relationship between physical and cognitive development and chronological age. The knowledge derived has been instrumental in improving the lives of some children but may have blighted the lives of others that fail to reach expected developmental milestones by a certain age. With a few notable exceptions, research into children's experiences had relied on deductive and predetermined instruments that fit adults' conceptual understandings. This was consistent with the dominant view that children are less knowledgeable than adults until they reach the age of majority (right to vote). These views are also evident in current structures and systems used to organise children's lives.

Children as active social agents

More recently, scholars from the New Sociology of Childhood have asserted that children are social agents (Figure 68.1). This has led to an upsurge in research activity with children as participants rather than objects. Outcomes demonstrate how children use their agency to influence their lives on a day-to-day basis, and that they have the capacity to derive subjective interpretations that often differ from those of adults. The impact of such research for the children involved is wide-reaching but includes improved safety, leadership for disabled children and a positive impact on living conditions. Research involving children means spending time with them in the places they ordinarily frequent. Ethnographic methods are fit for this purpose.

Ethnography

Traditional approaches

Ethnography is rooted in anthropology and rests on the assumption that people live their lives in social and cultural contexts. Ethnographers observe others as they go about their ordinary day-to-day lives, undertaking formal interviews, having informal conversations, and scrutinising visual and audible artefacts. Writing rich descriptions to communicate what has been gleaned and meanings derived from the final analysis follows. However, this approach can lead to apolitical accounts that are over-simplistic in which researchers assume a dominant and powerful position over those being researched.

Critical approaches

Social systems and structures frame people's lives and are co-created by those who at the same time experience and reproduce them. Researchers adopt critical standpoints to see beyond what seems 'to be' to consider what 'is' in the context of dominant, structural constraints from a particular perspective. It involves privileging the voice and accounts of those with least power or those considered oppressed. Critical research with children incorporates the need to discover and explore both tacit and a propositional knowledge in the context of structures that inform and influence the children's experiences. For instance, research undertaken with dying hospitalised children in the USA revealed how the children were aware of what was happening but engaged in 'mutual pretence' with adults.

Methods

Methods used in critical ethnographic research include a reconnaissance phase, fieldwork observations (along a continuum of participant to non-participant), informal and formal interviews, documentary analysis and scrutiny of artefacts associated with the field (Figure 68.2).

Reconnaissance

Reconnaissance can be used to work with children to assess their understanding of the research problems and questions. For example, one study undertaken with hospitalised initially focused on safety. Following reconnaissance work this was re-conceptualised to consider the influence of child–adult relations. The reconnaissance phase can also be used to establish boundaries and identify gatekeepers. It can also inform decisions regarding the level of participation the researcher wishes to adopt, what counts as 'voice' in research with children and how children's communicative competence may be scaffolded (Figure 68.3) and the exploration of engagement strategies such as play and craft activities (Figure 68.4).

Data collection

Sampling strategies focus on ensuring depth and insight rather than size. They should seek to be inclusive. Age, ability, linguistic impoverishment or the need for augmentative communication should not be used to discriminate against participation.

Fieldwork observations are the hallmark of ethnographic work as far more insight can be gained from asking people to explain their actions than observing or talking to them alone. In critical work, establishing the 'position' of the researcher is key. For instance, sitting next to children in their hospital beds was used by one researcher to signal that she was not part of the healthcare team. Likewise, children attending a school for those with special needs quickly identified that the adult was not part of the teaching staff. Still, in both examples the children were able to use the researchers' adult power to achieve their best interests. It is also essential that passive and active events, spoken words and silence are given equal attention.

Analysis

There is a plethora of guidance related to inductive analysis. What matters in critical research with children is that the voices of the children are privileged, and that differences between them are managed into rather than out of written accounts. Concept maps (Figure 68.5) provide a useful mechanism for demonstrating conceptual relationships derived from the analysis.

Further reading

Livesley, J. and Long, T. (2014) Communicating with children and young people in research In: V. Lambert, T. Long and D. Kelleher (eds) *Communication Skills for Children's Nurses*. London: McGraw Hill.

Atkinson, P., Coffey, A., Delamont, S., Lofland, J. and Lofland, L. (eds) (2010) *Handbook of Ethnography*. London: Sage.

69 Using pre-test post-test designs with children

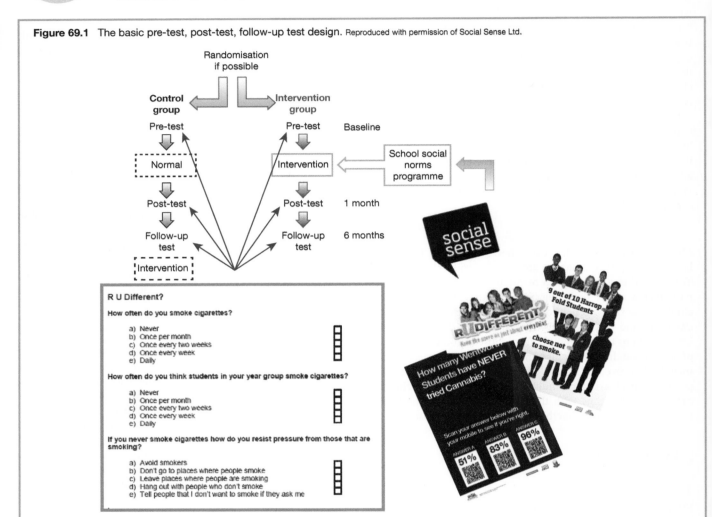

Figure 69.1 The basic pre-test, post-test, follow-up test design. Reproduced with permission of Social Sense Ltd.

One of the most commonly used designs in experimental research is to test a group at baseline for a particular attribute, to introduce an intervention, and then to measure the attribute again to see if a change has resulted. This is the most basic design and can be summarised like this: pre-test → intervention → post-test.

Increasing the rigour of the design

Threats to pre-test post-test studies

Test effects
It is possible that children will learn from the tests themselves, perhaps realising that they have a gap in knowledge which they address in various ways before the next test. Even without an intervention, their test score will increase at post-test.

Temporal effects
This relates to changes that would happen over time anyway. As young people grow older it becomes more likely that more of them will engage in risky behaviours as just a part of growing up. This may be seen to skew post-test scores.

Regression to the mean
This is a common phenomenon, linked to measurement error, in which extreme scores tend to ameliorate and move towards more average scores on further testing. The impact is that group scores are often closer together on post-test. A number of strategies can be adopted to minimise or remove these problems.

Control group
The strength of a true experiment lies in a number of factors, including the use of a control group and randomisation to groups.

Testing a single group before and after an intervention may show a difference in test scores, but there is no way to know if the change would have occurred regardless. One way to be more convinced that the intervention was directly linked to the change is to see what happens to test scores in another group at the same time, but without including the intervention.

This is shown in Figure 69.1. The control group of schoolchildren does the test but instead of an intervention this group received normal treatment or learning experiences. If the intervention group scores differ significantly more, it lends strength to the suggestion that the intervention was involved in the changes observed. However, it still does not demonstrate directly that the intervention *caused* the change.

Sometimes a control group is not possible for ethical or practical reasons, but the inclusion of a control group makes this design much stronger.

Randomisation
In any experiment, randomisation helps to minimise the likelihood of unintentional bias in arranging membership of control and intervention groups. It is possible to be ignorant of a particular characteristic and unintentionally load one group more than the other with this factor. Children in one class may all have been on a school trip and learned about how sewage is treated, while another class had yet to experience the visit.

Allocating these classes as a whole to intervention or control groups for a study of children's knowledge of environmental issues would unbalance the experiment.

Much of this *selection bias* is both unintentional and unknown. Randomisation helps to overcome this, but, again, it is not always possible. In a study of children's knowledge and attitude to asthma management, allocating children randomly within a school would lead to contamination, as children who receive the intervention would share its details with control group children, and the effect of the intervention would be less clear. In such cases, it may be necessary to allocate whole schools to control or intervention groups.

Multiple test times
Testing both groups on multiple occasions before and after the intervention (*interrupted time series*) helps to distinguish between intervention effects and the effect of underlying trends as the study progresses. It stabilises measurement after the intervention so that the lasting effect of the intervention can be seen. In a simpler design, this is often achieved with a single follow-up test. The length of time between post-test and follow-up test is a matter of judgement Too long a time period risks *maturation effects* as children naturally develop and become more knowledgeable and able. Too short a period may not capture long-term effects.

Baseline comparison
Analysis of the control and intervention groups at pre-test to ensure that there are no significant differences between them in key characteristics is important since any major differences may then be a plausible explanation of differences at post-test. Testing should be undertaken for both groups at the same time to reduce temporal and testing effect differences between groups.

Sharing the intervention
When the post-testing is complete, the intervention is often provided for the control group so that its members can also benefit.

Further reading
Dubuy, V., De Cocker, K., De Bourdeaudhuij, I. *et al.* (2014) Evaluation of a real world intervention using professional football players to promote a healthy diet and physical activity in children and adolescents from a lower socio-economic background: a controlled pretest–posttest design. *BMC Public Health* **14**, 457.

Dunn, W., Cox, J., Foster, L., Mische-Lawson, L. and Tanquary, J. (2012) Impact of a contextual intervention on child participation and parent competence among children with autism spectrum disorders: a pretest–posttest repeated-measures design. *American Journal of Occupational Therapy* **66**, 520–528.

Fives, A., Pursell, L., Heary, C., Nic Gabhainn, S. and Canavan, J. (2014) *Parenting support for every parent: a population-level evaluation of Triple P in Longford Westmeath. Summary Report.* Athlone: Longford Westmeath Parenting Partnership (LWPP). Available at http://www.childandfamilyresearch.ie/sites/www.childandfamilyresearch.ie/files/parenting_support-summary_report_inside_pgs_0.pdf

70 Conducting research with older adults

Figure 70.1 Older adults' involvement in research.

User Informant	• This can also be referred to as consultation • Provide views on the research from service user perspective
Expert Advisor	• This is referred to as collaboration • This involves overseeing running and conduct of the research project
Co-researcher	• Involvement in every aspect of research starting from research question development to dissemination of findings
Participant	• Relatively passive role • To participate in the research by means of sharing views on the given topic

Figure 70.2 Examples of research involving older adults.

Health service research	• Equity • Use of, and access to, services • Research related to service development and improvement • Research related to service evaluation
Health conditions specific	• Long-term health conditions such as diabetes, stroke, cancer • Falls • Healthy eating • Mental health • General health
Health need assessment	• Quality of life • Assistive technologies

Figure 70.3 Impact older adults' involvement in research.

Impact on older adults	Impact on research and researcher
• Increase in confidence	• Provide broader and practical perspective resulting in improved research design
• Learning to listen to other points of view	• Identification of issues that the researcher did not anticipate
• Increased awareness of social and political issues	• Better recruitment
• Increased ability to confront situation	• Facilitated consent process
• Meeting others in similar situation	• Facilitated dissemination of findings
• Involvement in other research activities/ projects (further opportunities)	
• Realisation that they can shape policies	

Figure 70.4 Barriers to involvement in research.

Communication
- Language issues (use of technical language and/or jargon)
- Uneasiness at working with non-English from other cultures (if relevant)

Commitment
- May not be able to commit to attend regular project meetings
- Ill health, medical conditions; hospital ppointments; physical frailty

Capability
- Lack of research skills
- Difficulties in expressing beliefs or opinions to others
- Lack of confidence

Capacity
- Lack of time
- Lack of resources

Old age can be defined from various perspectives (chronological, biological or sociocultural) and various terms are used to refer to this group, including older adults, old people, seniors, senior citizens, the elderly and elder. According to the World Health Organization (2014), an arbitrary age of 60–65 years (an age when most people retire, especially in developed countries) is used to define old age in most countries around the world. Research with older adults is becoming increasingly important as the population of older adults in the world is rising rapidly. It is estimated that by 2050, the world's population of people aged 60 and older will rise to 2 billion. Regardless of the difficulties in defining the terms 'old age' and 'older adults', it is an important group for those researchers who focus on the healthcare concerns of this population, often classed as 'hard to reach' and difficult to involve.

Involvement of older adults in research

There are various ways by which older adults can be involved in research, as shown in Figure 70.1. They can help researchers identify research priorities, develop research questions, discuss the research process, and interpret and disseminate findings to the relevant people. They can be involved in all or some stages of the research process (research design, data collection and analysis, dissemination of findings). Older adults are a major user group of health and social care and therefore it is their right to be involved in the research involving them as *service user informant* and to contribute to the planning and conduct of research. They can be part of the advisory group, providing *expert advice* about the subject area of the research. Older adults can participate as *co-researcher* in a research project. Older adults can also contribute to a research project as a *participant*. Some examples of research projects where older adults have been involved are shown in Figure 70.2. Involvement of older adults, like any other group, can have a very positive impact not only for older adults but also for the researchers (Figure 70.3).

Types of older adult research participant

From the perspective of conducting research with this group, older adults can be classified into two main groups: (i) those who are energetic, independent and autonomous; and (ii) those who are dependent, vulnerable and with impaired decision-making ability. The first group is no different from the usual adult population and therefore the same principles and practices governing research with adults are applicable. Barriers to involving this group in research are no different from those with research involving the usual adult population (Figure 70.4). This is the group that can be involved in all of the above-mentioned roles in any relevant research project. However, research involving the second group is more complex and requires the special attention of the research team. In this group there are many different issues which impact involvement/participation in research and pose a challenge to researchers. However, an awareness of the potential challenges can help researchers to plan their research more innovatively. In the following sections some of these challenges, and strategies to overcome them, are presented.

Ability to provide informed consent

Old age is associated with many physiological changes that result in visual problems, hearing loss, and cognitive impairment resulting in difficulties in understanding and retaining information. All these various issues affect the ability of older adults to comprehend the information and make an informed choice about whether or not to participate in a study.

Strategies

Older adults may need more time and help to make sense of the study to enable them to make an informed decision to participate in the study. Researchers need to ensure that they spend as much time as needed with the participants. Information sheets and consent forms should be written in simple and easy-to-understand language, possibly using bigger fonts and appropriately tailored to the needs of those with visual impairments. It may be helpful to produce a summarised version of the information sheet that contains only essential information related to the study.

Willingness to participate in the study

Although evidence suggests that older people generally identify their participation in research as a useful contribution to society, there are many factors that impinge on their willingness to participate in research. For instance, the presence of symptoms such as fatigue and pain may affect their motivation to participate. Dependency on others, mobility issues and transportation problems may also hinder their ability to participate. Many older adults live in care homes and this may make them more susceptible to coercive participation in research as a 'captive audience' and this obviously breaches confidentiality and privacy issues. This group may also feel reluctant to criticise healthcare professionals, thinking it may affect their care or feeling 'this is how things work'.

Role of significant others

Another very important factor that affects the involvement of older adults in research projects is the influence and involvement of significant others, including family members (for those living independently or in care settings) and staff members or carers (for those living in care settings) who act as gatekeepers. Often, older adults may themselves request the involvement of their children or a family member in the consent process. Likewise, in institutional settings, a further layer of gatekeeping is provided by staff members.

Strategies

Researchers may consider including this factor in the research process and may approach the potential participant and their family member at the same time to avoid duplication of effort and to save time. Separate information sheets about the study should be developed. Researchers conducting studies with older adults living in care homes need to be aware of the issues specific to these settings. Involvement of the staff in the research process, spending time understanding routine practices in the care setting, and building rapport with the participants as well as the staff may be helpful.

Reference

World Health Organization (2014) Definition of an older or elderly person. Available at http://www.who.int/healthinfo/survey/ageingdefnolder/en/index.html (accessed 30 July 2014).

71 Conducting surveys with people with learning disabilities

Figure 71.1 Conducting surveys with people with learning disabilities.

1. Develop a user-friendly information sheet for person with learning disabilities and their carer

2. Ensure the items/statements/questions are clear

3. Ensure the rating scale is clearly understood (smiley faces, tick boxes)

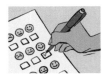

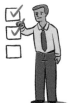

4. Work with a service user group to examine the face validity of the questionnaire

What is a survey

A survey is a data collection tool using questionnaires to gather information about individuals or groups of people, normally in a self-report format. Surveys are commonly used in a range of health and social care disciplines to collect information about attitudes, opinions, feelings, behaviours, etc. A range of questionnaires are commercially available to purchase and some can be downloaded free from the web.

Questionnaires

Most questionnaires have been developed and tested on representative samples that employ some form of rating scale to measure the individual's response: these are known as standardised questionnaires (i.e. they have strong reliability and validity).

Rating scales

All questionnaires have a list of items or items/statements/questions that the individual has to respond to using a rating scale. This can take the form of:
- yes/no responses;
- multiple choice, where the individual has to tick or circle one response;
- a Likert scale, where individuals indicate their agreement (strongly agree, agree, neutral, disagree, strongly disagree);
- visual analogue scale.

Nursing and Healthcare Research at a Glance, First Edition. Alan Glasper and Colin Rees. © 2017 by John Wiley & Sons, Ltd. Published 2017 by John Wiley & Sons, Ltd.

People with learning disabilities completing surveys

Many individuals with mild to moderate learning disability should be able to complete a survey/questionnaire (Figure 71.1). However, to ensure the person understands the items/statements/questions and also how to score the rating scale, some reasonable adjustments may need to be made. Words may need to be simplified and the rating scale made clearer. A family/paid carer or researcher could also read aloud the items/statements/questions. The rating scale could employ pictorial symbols to support the responses (i.e. smiley/sad faces, thumbs up/down, etc.).

In order to avoid response bias, namely the tendency among people with learning disabilities towards recency, suggestibility, confabulation and agreement, careful consideration to the types of questions that are asked is required. Cognisance needs to be given to the apparent limitations identified with 'either/or', 'yes/no', multiple choice and open-ended questions, and also to the avoidance of leading or abstract questions.

Barriers to completing surveys for people with learning disabilities

Some people with severe/profound learning disabilities with more severe cognitive impairment will have difficulties understanding both the items/statements/questions and how to complete the rating scale: they will be unable to read and write. Some people will not be able to communicate verbally and will depend on objects, symbols and/or signs. These can take the form of photographs, drawings or some of the commercially available symbol sets (i.e. Change, Makaton, Talking Mats). They will have to depend on a family/paid carer to complete the survey on their behalf: these individuals are sometimes called proxy informants. Although proxy informant reports can be helpful in providing factual information (e.g. demographic details, services used, behaviours, costs), these responses may not truly reflect the individuals' about attitudes, opinions and feelings.

Other barriers to engagement in surveys

In order to access people with learning disabilities to complete a survey, researchers have to obtain ethical approval. This involves engaging with gatekeepers (i.e. family/paid carers) to gain access to the adults with learning disabilities; sometimes this proves difficult as they assume the person cannot give consent (i.e. lack the capacity to consent) and are also unable to complete the questionnaires. These gatekeepers may also want to protect the person with learning disabilities from research and potential harm.

Hints for helping people with learning disabilities and their family/paid carers to engage in surveys

• Ensure both family/paid carers (the gatekeepers) and the person with learning disabilities have user-friendly information explaining the nature and purpose of the survey.

• Ensure the questionnaire is in an easy-read format with a clear rating scale.
• Short, straightforward, everyday words and sentences should be used which are less linguistically demanding.
• Questions may need to be repeated and rephrased if necessary. This strategy can help to reduce anxiety and develop rapport.
• Make the text bigger and use colour paper for different sections of the questionnaire.
• Ensure you have informed written/verbal consent from the adults with learning disabilities (aged 18 years plus) and assent from parents/guardian for children or young people with learning disabilities.
• For studies that involve a randomised controlled trial and the testing of an intervention, it is important that the person with learning disabilities and their family/paid carer understand what is involved and how the randomisation will work. Giving potential participants a DVD showing peers with learning disabilities explaining the study, the consent process and how each person is randomised into the experimental or control group will aid uptake in recruitment.
• Researchers should meet potential participants with learning disabilities and their family/paid carers before completing the survey if possible.

Conclusion

The UN Convention on the Rights of Persons with Disabilities Article 9 states that governments should take action to ensure accessibility, equal to that of the non-disabled population; this includes information and communications services and also surveys/questionnaires. The MRC Guidelines (2007, p. 4) state:

> Research involving adults who lack mental capacity to consent can lead to innovations in healthcare that can substantially improve their health and quality of life and that of others with similar conditions. It is therefore important that these adults are given the opportunity to participate in such research. To exclude them from any research would be discriminatory and would diminish their ability to participate as fully as possible in society.

Reference and further reading

Department of Health (2010) *Making written information easier to understand for people with learning disabilities. Guidance for people who commission or produce Easy Read information*, revised edition 2010. London: HMSO.
Medical Research Council (2007) *MRC Ethics Guide 2007. Medical Research Involving Adults Who Cannot Consent*. London: MRC.
Porter, J. & Lacey, P. (2005) *Researching Learning Difficulties: A Guide for Practitioners*. London: Sage Publications.

Conducting focus groups with people with learning disabilities

Figure 72.1 Focus groups involving people with learning disabilities.

1. Benefits of focus groups

- Enable issues to be explored from a range of perspectives
- Peer support
- Can be an effective way of increasing the active participation of people with learning disabilities in research

2. Possible challenges

- Enabling participation of people with severe and profound learning disabilities
- Maintaining the focus of the group on the key issues for discussion
- Facilitating group discussion and encouraging participants to reflect on, and discuss, the contributions of other group members

3. General considerations

- Whether to work with an existing group or to bring together a new group solely for research
- Size of group
- Where to hold the focus group
- Timing of session(s)
- How best to record discussion
- Payment of expenses and/or for participation

4. Preparation for focus groups

- Understanding the abilities and support needs of group members so that appropriate supports can be planned in advance
- Preparing a range of strategies that can be utilised during the focus group to encourage/support participation
- Making practical arrangements regarding travel and support

5. Possible challenges

- Some people may require the support of an advocate or supporter to enable their participation
- The role of the supporter needs to be agreed in advance and clearly understood
- Failure to do this can affect the data collected if the supporter influences the responses of the participants rather than supporting them to offer their own views

6. Conducting focus groups

- Establish ground rules
- Check consent
- Have a range of strategies available to promote participation
- Encourage participation of all group members
- Adopt a flexible approach
- Where possible provide a 'concrete' rather than abstract frame of reference to facilitate discussion
- Photographs and objects of reference can be helpful

The benefits and disadvantages of focus groups

Focus groups enable data to be gathered from a wide range of people in a relatively short period. However, perhaps the key strength of this approach lies in its ability to facilitate discussion: participants not only share their own views but they also listen to, discuss and reflect on the views of others, offering the potential for richer data (Figure 72.1).

Potential disadvantages can include difficulties with bringing a group together, with ensuring that everyone is able to contribute, and with exploring some topics in a group context. An additional challenge when using this approach with people with learning disabilities can be facilitating discussion within groups where some may have difficulties with both expressive and receptive language since it can be difficult to promote the reflection on other people's contributions that is central within focus groups. As a consequence some authors have suggested that this approach should be used only with people with mild learning disabilities, thus excluding those with more severe and profound disabilities (Kaehne and O'Connell, 2010). However, others have indicated that people with severe learning disabilities were included in their study (Gates and Waight, 2007).

Planning focus groups

Perhaps the first consideration is whether to access an existing group (such as a self-advocacy group) or whether to bring together a new group specifically for the purpose of the research. The former can lead to some groups being 'over researched' (Kaehne and O'Connell, 2010) but Llewellyn (2009) found that working with an existing group led to better discussion.

Where to hold meetings can be difficult: physical access, and the availability of transport and parking may need to be addressed. The timing of meetings can also present challenges since potential participants may have other competing activities or only be able to access support to attend at particular times. Whether people should be paid for their participation and/or expenses needs to be considered: while payment for their time provides recognition that their contribution is valued, some may be loath to accept payment due to any potential impact on their welfare benefits. Other ways of valuing contributions may therefore need to be found.

Some studies include a series of focus groups with the same group of people while others have one-off meetings with participants. Where there is a series of meetings then there is the opportunity to get to know participants and their support needs over a period of time but this is not the case with a one-off session. Therefore, in preparation, it is advisable to gather information regarding participants' strengths and support needs prior to the meeting so that the session can be planned accordingly and any additional support requirements accommodated.

Finally, it is important to carefully consider how the discussion will be structured. Gates and Waight (2007) found it helpful to have a range of strategies that could be used in each session and that providing a 'concrete' rather than an abstract frame of reference assisted participants to engage in discussion. For example, Northway *et al.* (2013) used photographs and objects of reference to promote and focus discussion.

Conducting focus groups

As with all focus groups the role of the facilitator is crucial in ensuring that the group runs smoothly and that data are collected. An additional challenge in focus groups involving people with learning disabilities is that some participants may require personal support to participate and the role of the supporter needs to be carefully considered. In her study, Llewellyn (2009) felt that some supporters influenced participant responses to the extent that they became 'secondary' participants and Kaehne and O'Connell (2010) suggest they may encourage participants to provide what are seen as desirable answers. It therefore needs to be stressed that the role is to support individuals to participate rather than to influence their responses and this needs to be reinforced at the beginning of each session (Llewellyn, 2009).

Each session needs to commence with checking consent, establishing ground rules and reminding people of the purpose of the session. Gates and Waight (2007) recommend that facilitators have an extensive 'methodological toolkit' and adopt a flexible approach since individuals and groups will respond differently to the same issues and questions. They also advocate including turn-taking activities since these ensure that all members of the group have the opportunity to participate. Skills are also required to tactfully restore focus to a discussion that has gone off on a different track while being sensitive to the fact that the other issues raised may be very important to those who are discussing them.

Within focus groups it can be difficult to ensure that all data are carefully recorded. Audio recordings are perhaps the most commonly used and here it is suggested that using two recording devices at different ends of the room may be helpful in picking up comments made to supporters that might not be clearly heard within the group (Gates and Waight, 2007). Consideration might also be given to the use of video recording since this would also enable other aspects of group dynamics to be recorded such as body language. Whichever method is chosen the consent of the group needs to be given and it is advisable to have a back-up plan, such as a flipchart that can be used to record key issues and themes should anyone in the group object to other forms of recording.

References

Gates, B. and Waight, M. (2007) Reflections on conducting focus groups with people with learning disabilities. *Journal of Research in Nursing* 12, 111–126.

Kaehne, A. and O'Connell, C. (2010) Focus groups with people with learning disabilities. *Journal of Intellectual Disabilities* 14, 133–145.

Llewellyn, P. (2009) Supporting people with intellectual disabilities to take part in focus groups: reflections on a research project. *Disability and Society* 24, 845–856.

Northway, R., Melsome, M., Flood, S., Bennett, D., Howarth, J. and Thomas, B. (2013) How do people with intellectual disabilities view abuse and abusers. *Journal of Intellectual Disabilities* 17, 361–375.

73 People with learning disabilities as co-researchers

Figure 73.1 Common concerns.

- People with learning disabilities as 'vulnerable' research subjects
- Capacity to consent
- Ability to provide the required data

Figure 73.2 Addressing these challenges.

- Vulnerability is not inevitable: consider what it is that people may be vulnerable to and then develop strategies to reduce vulnerability
- Make sure that in terms of consent you work within the legal framework of the country in which you are undertaking research
- Remember that capacity to consent can be influenced by how and when information is given to people
- Approach seeking consent as a process rather than as an event and check continued willingness to participate
- Rather than just considering traditional research approaches and data collection tools, think about how adjustments can be made to how information is to be gathered
- Present information in a range of formats suited to individual needs
- Avoid the use of jargon or (where it is necessary) make sure that explanations are provided in clear language
- As a general rule look for barriers that may prevent the participation of people with learning disabilities and develop strategies for overcoming such barriers

Figure 73.3 Some practical considerations.

- Accessibility: of both information and location of data collection
- Specific communication needs of participants and communication abilities of the researcher
- Transport (if data collection takes place at a venue the individual does not normally attend)
- The need for support (if the individual wants this)
- Whether individuals should be compensated for participation

Figure 73.4 Additional considerations when supporting people with learning disabilities to be researchers.

- The importance of working as a team and valuing everyone's contributions
- Training needs
- Flexibility and creativity to facilitate active involvement at all stages of the research process
- Support needs of researchers
- Issue of payment for work

Common concerns

Historically, people with learning disabilities have been afforded a very passive role in other people's research. Sometimes they were not even afforded the status of participant and if research focused on their lives and experiences, the views of families and carers were sought rather than the views of the individuals themselves. More recently this situation has changed and people with learning disabilities are taking a much more active role. Nonetheless, common concerns persist on the part of both researchers and ethics committees (Figure 73.1).

Rather than viewing these concerns as reasons not to include people with learning disabilities, it is important that they are seen as potential barriers to participation and as the basis for the development of strategies to promote inclusion (Figure 73.2). For example, history has demonstrated that people with learning disabilities have been vulnerable to coercion and exploitation in the context of research. However, this is not inevitable and attention to how information is provided to assist decision-making can have a significant impact on the capacity of an individual to consent to participation. It is essential that the safeguards afforded by the law are respected but adjustments to the process may be required: providing information in (for example) an easy-read format supported by pictorial information is more likely to assist someone with limited reading ability than a complex jargon-filled patient information leaflet. Similarly, rather than just viewing consent as a one-off event, it may be more appropriate to see it as a process in which understanding and continued willingness to participate are regularly checked. Some traditional data collection tools (such as self-completion questionnaires requiring free text responses) may not be appropriate for use with participants who have limited literacy. However, if researchers are clear regarding the core data they wish to collect, then alternative approaches can be considered. For example, might an interview be more appropriate? Could a simpler questionnaire be produced in an easy-read format?

There are some other practical concerns that also need to be considered when seeking to include people with learning disabilities as research participants (Figure 73.3). While support needs will vary from one individual to another, some common considerations include the need to determine both the communication needs of participants and the communication abilities of the researcher. For example, does an individual use a communication aid or sign language? If they do, does the researcher have the ability to sign? Where data collection takes place also needs to be carefully considered, particularly if it is going to take place at a venue the individual does not usually attend. Is it physically accessible and (if required) are there facilities for disabled people? Will the individual need personal support and/or transport to reach the venue? The issue of whether participants should be financially compensated for their time and (potential) inconvenience due to participation can be a difficult issue. Ethically it would not be appropriate if financial incentives encouraged individuals to take risks they would not normally take in order to receive the payment but at the same time it is important to recognise that there is a cost to them in terms of their time. This ethical dilemma is further complicated by the fact that payments above a certain threshold may lead to loss of welfare benefits, which can be detrimental to individuals. Ethical issues and other challenges must be identified, discussed and a clear rationale provided for decisions taken.

People with learning disabilities as researchers

In addition to taking a more active role as research participants, recent years have seen an increasing number of people with learning disabilities taking on the role of researcher. While all the above considerations may be relevant in this context, there are some further issues that need to be addressed (Figure 73.4). First, it is essential that attention is paid to team building and that it is recognised that while people will bring differing experience and expertise to the research project, all contributions are valued. All new researchers require training and support in order to develop in their role and therefore this applies to people with learning disabilities who become researchers. However, consideration needs to be given to the content, format and timing of such training. For example, it may need to be delivered in shorter sessions to accommodate attention spans and it may be better to provide training relevant to each stage of the process just before that stage is reached so that relevant learning is recent. Flexibility and creativity may be required in order to facilitate active participation and it may be necessary to try different ways of working before the most appropriate strategy can be identified. In addition, researchers with learning disabilities may require dedicated personal assistants to support them in their role (e.g. to assist with reading papers, inputting data, travelling to venues). This can increase the costs of research but this should not be viewed as a reason to exclude them from becoming researchers. Finally, the issue of payment for work also applies to people with learning disabilities who are researchers: it is important that they receive payment for their work but the impact on any welfare benefits also needs to be considered.

74 Undertaking research with family carers

Figure 74.1 Beauchamp and Childress's (2013) four principles.

Autonomy
Within this principle the decisions made by participants are valued and respected. It also relates to the consent of individuals to participate and ensuring they are supported to make informed decisions

Beneficence
According to this principle the research that is being undertaken should be of benefit to the participants and to society, and other carers, in general

Non-maleficence
This is where the researcher tries to avoid harm occurring, both physically and psychologically, to carers

Justice
This principle relates to being fair and demonstrating equality and respect for the rights of all participants>

Figure 74.2 Beneficence.

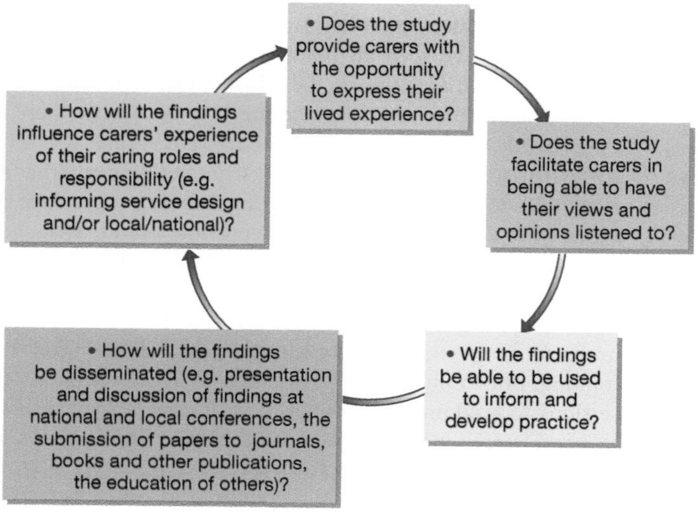

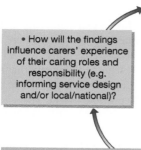

- Does the study provide carers with the opportunity to express their lived experience?
- How will the findings influence carers' experience of their caring roles and responsibility (e.g. informing service design and/or local/national)?
- Does the study facilitate carers in being able to have their views and opinions listened to?
- How will the findings be disseminated (e.g. presentation and discussion of findings at national and local conferences, the submission of papers to journals, books and other publications, the education of others)?
- Will the findings be able to be used to inform and develop practice?

Figure 74.3 Justice.

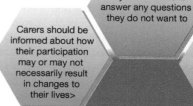

Advise carers that they do not have to answer any questions they do not want to

Length of interview should be dictated by the participants and their needs

Carers should be informed about how their participation may or may not necessarily result in changes to their lives>

Justice

Information given about any relevant complaints procedures

The wishes/decisions of carers should always be respected

Contact details should be given for other appropriate individuals for participants to contact should they have any concerns about the researcher or research

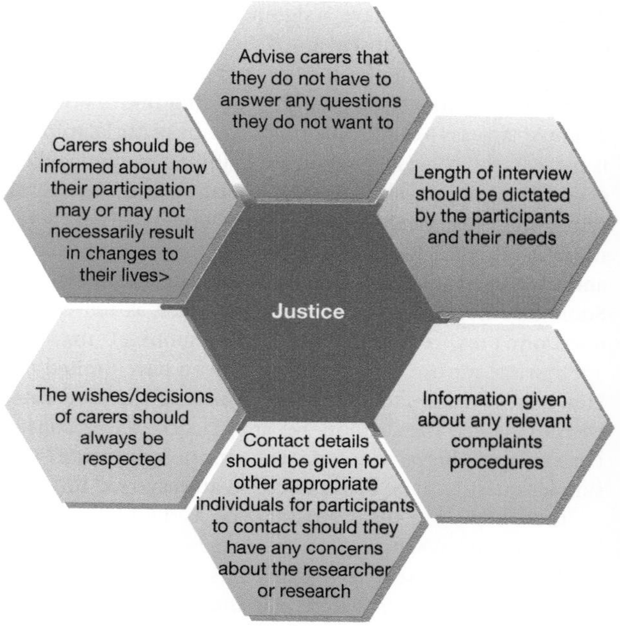

Figure 74.4 Non-maleficence.

Questions that need be answered are:

- Is there a risk of physical and/or emotional harm to carers by being involved in this study?

- Given their experiences, would being involved in the study cause them any further distress and/or raised emotions as a consequence of reflecting and discussing their experiences?

Figure 74.5 Maintaining confidentiality.

- All personal and other identifiable data need to be anonymised
- Passwords used for any information stored on computers
- Copies of any information with personal data should be stored safely in a locked cabinet
- Local data protection policies should be consulted and adhered to

In the UK it is estimated that about 2% of the population have a learning disability and approximately 60% of those who are adults live at home with their family (James, 2013a). In respect of care decisions and the planning of services, UK policies, strategies and legislation promote the involvement of people with learning disabilities and their families as much as possible (James, 2013b). Accordingly, family carers need to be recognised as valuable resources for their relative and also as key contributors to the development of knowledge and understanding about their needs and own caring experiences. In order to evidence and develop an appreciation of these experiences, research needs to be undertaken that provides carers with the opportunity to tell their stories and express their views and opinions. When undertaking this research, as with other types of research, it is important that consideration is given to the safeguarding and protection of the participants (Flick, 2006). In respect of family carers, this is of particular importance because they may have had quite challenging caring experiences with their relative and also in their relationships with services and professionals. It is imperative therefore that ethical issues are identified as part of the research planning process with approval sought and gained from relevant ethics committees. In order to consider the ethical aspects of undertaking research with family carers, Beauchamp and Childress's (2013) four principles can be used (Figure 74.1). Some examples of how researchers can consider these in respect of undertaking research with family carers will now be illustrated.

Autonomy

The initial contact made with possible carer participants could be via a letter that introduces the researcher and the topic. In order to ensure anonymity for the carer, this letter could be sent by a third or independent party. A response form and stamped addressed envelope could be included with the letter for return to the researcher in order to maintain carer anonymity in respect of others knowing about their involvement in the research.

Arrangements can be made to undertake an initial meeting with the family carer to introduce you as the researcher, review the information sheet, discuss the study in more depth and go through the issue of consent. If appropriate, the venue for meetings should be discussed and agreed with carers so that it provides confidentiality and does not cause unnecessary inconvenience or expenditure. Carers should be given the opportunity to ask questions and confirm that they understand the aim of the study before providing consent. They should also be informed that they are free to change their mind about being involved in the study at any time. Information about the data collection process, such as the recording of interviews and focus group participation, should be discussed and the wishes of participants always respected and catered for where possible. The approximate time commitment required from participants should be discussed in order for an informed decision to be made about participation.

Beneficence

Figure 74.2 shows the questions that could be asked to address this principle. It is important that carers are also provided with feedback in respect of the findings and/or recommendations made from the study.

Justice

This requires the researcher to avoid giving any preference to particular participants and placing the needs of the participants before that of himself or herself and the study. Examples of how this principle can be facilitated are shown in Figure 74.3.

It is imperative that it is made clear to carers what contribution they are being asked to make. This should be provided within an information sheet and verbally where appropriate. Should carers incur any financial costs, such as travelling costs, these need to be reimbursed. To minimise inconvenience and cost to participants the place of interview, where appropriate and possible, should be the decision of the participant. Information should be provided about how the findings/outcomes of the study will be used to inform others and what this might mean, for example helping to inform professionals of ways in which good support and relationships can be developed and facilitated.

Non-maleficence

In order to reduce potential harm and/or distress, it is important that participants are afforded time to discuss issues important to them and, if necessary, be provided with detailed information about support services, professional and/or voluntary, that are available for them to contact should they feel necessary (Figure 74.4). Limits to confidentiality also need to be discussed with carers when the study aims and its processes are being discussed with them (Figure 74.5). For example, if during the course of an interview there is reporting of abuse, which had not previously been reported, they need to be informed that you may have a professional responsibility to report these through the appropriate channels. Again, sources of support for carers need to be highlighted and reassurance provided.

A potential negative for participants could be when the researcher leaves the field of enquiry and they are left to carry on with their lives. To address this, advice should be given to participants about carer support groups and that if they need further support to contact their local learning disability services.

References

Beauchamp, T.L. and Childress, J.F. (2013) *Principles of Biomedical Ethics*, 7th edn. New York: Oxford University Press.

Flick, U. (2006) *An Introduction to Qualitative Research*, 3rd edn. London: Sage Publications.

James, N. (2013a) How families perceive the care-giving experience. *Learning Disability Practice* **16**, 32–37.

James, N. (2013b) The formal support experiences of family carers of people with an intellectual disability who also display challenging behaviour and/or mental health issues. What do carers say? *Journal of Intellectual Disabilities* **17**, 5–22.

75 Obtaining consent from vulnerable groups

Figure 75.1 The recruitment process.

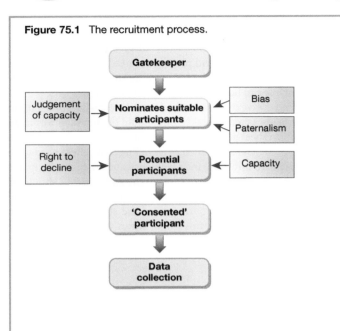

Figure 75.2 The requirements for valid consent.

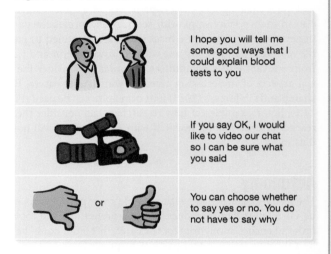

Figure 75.3 Accessible information.

People with a learning disability should be treated with the same dignity and respect as any other member of the community. However, when recruiting for research, attention should be given to the fact that people with a learning disability are considered a vulnerable population, and additional measures may be necessary to avoid any breach of their human rights. Concerns include doubt about their capacity to consent to research, the tendency of people with a learning disability to acquiesce to the wishes of others, and the unequal power relationship between researcher and participant. In this chapter the focus is on obtaining consent from research participants with a learning disability. However, in this context, it is important to consider both the process of recruitment and that of obtaining the participant's informed consent.

The recruitment process

It is common practice in learning disability research to utilise 'gatekeepers' to nominate and possibly identify suitable participants for a research study. For this reason, it is important to have a clear set of inclusion criteria that relate to potential participants. The use of gatekeepers is designed to ensure that participants considered as possibly vulnerable are not coerced into taking part in research. Examples of gatekeepers might include carers, health professionals, teachers or parents. Figure 75.1 illustrates a possible process for recruiting and obtaining consent and shows the issues that may arise, such as paternalism when gatekeepers may be over-protective of those in their care, or bias shown towards certain potential participants.

The requirements for informed consent

Three elements constitute informed consent: information, lack of coercion and competence (Figure 75.2).

Information

Information about taking part in the research (the participant information sheet) should be provided in a format that is accessible for a person with a learning disability (Figure 75.3). If a participant cannot understand the information given or disclosed, the consent will not be valid.

Lack of coercion

There must be no coercion on the part of the researcher. This is not straightforward due to the tendency of many people with a learning disability to want to please or to acquiesce to the demands of others. As mentioned, gatekeepers may be used in an effort to avoid undue pressure from researchers. However, this is not a simple process and careful consideration should be given to choice of gatekeeper (if any).

Capacity

The potential participant must have the capacity to consent to take part in the research. In the UK, the Mental Capacity Act (2000) includes a code of conduct for researchers wishing to conduct research involving people who may *lack* capacity. However, researchers should assume capacity unless proven

otherwise, and potential participants should receive support to enable them to make the decision whether or not to participate.

It should be noted that for a person to be judged as having capacity to make a decision, the following criteria must be fulfilled.
• Does the person have a general understanding of what decision they need to make and why they need to make it?
• Does the person have a general understanding of the likely consequences of making, or not making, this decision?
• Is the person able to understand, retain, use and weigh up the information relevant to this decision?
• Can the person communicate their decision (by talking, using sign language or any other means)?

Ways to ensure a rigorous consent process

It is important to have a clear set of inclusion criteria, and to communicate these effectively to any gatekeepers. For example, potential participants should be aged 18 years or over, with no active health problems.

Study information material in the form of participant information sheets should be tailored to the needs of the participant group. If necessary, advice should be taken from experts in the field, possibly speech therapists or learning disability specialist nurses. Participant information can be in any format; in most cases it will be written down, but audio-visual media could also be used to facilitate understanding or for those who cannot read. The use of images, symbols or photographs is common.

Having produced the participant information sheet, there should be evidence that the person understands the information given; this can often be confirmed (or otherwise) by asking the person to repeat the information back to you in their own words. It can be helpful during the consent process to invite the potential participant to bring a 'supporter' of their own choice (preferably someone who knows them well). The supporter can often confirm whether there is understanding both of the information and of the consequences of consenting to participate in the study.

Finally, the potential participant should be asked to communicate their decision, usually be signing the consent form, but if this is not possible, by expressing consent verbally.

Further reading

Cameron, L. and Murphy, J. (2007) Obtaining consent to participate in research: the issues involved in including people with a range of learning and communication disabilities. *British Journal of Learning Disabilities* 35, 113–120.

Department of Health (2009) Mental Capacity Act 2005 and consent for research. Available at http://webarchive.nationalarchives.gov.uk/20130107105354/http://www.dh.gov.uk/prod_consum_dh/groups/dh_digitalassets/documents/digitalasset/dh_079671.pdf

Nind, M. (2008) Conducting qualitative research with people with learning, communication and other disabilities: methodological challenges. ESRC National Centre for Research Methods Review Paper. Available at http://eprints.ncrm.ac.uk/491/ (accessed 9 February 2009).

76 Living lab approach

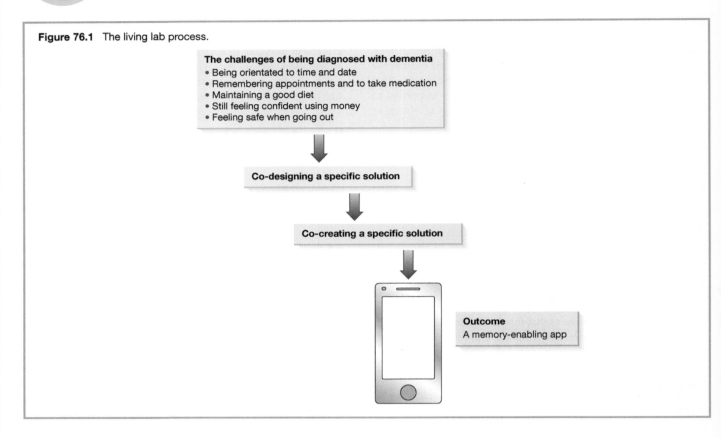

Figure 76.1 The living lab process.

The challenges of being diagnosed with dementia
- Being orientated to time and date
- Remembering appointments and to take medication
- Maintaining a good diet
- Still feeling confident using money
- Feeling safe when going out

Co-designing a specific solution

Co-creating a specific solution

Outcome
A memory-enabling app

Delivering effective and good-quality health and social care is a challenge that practitioners face on a daily basis. This challenge can be both at a macro level, being part of a wider service delivering care, and at a micro level, the practitioner delivering direct face-to-face care. As resources become scarce and care becomes more complex, the practitioner is required to develop and apply new and different solutions to these challenges, in other words 'innovate'. One way of openly innovating at a macro level and also ensuring useful and usable outcomes is to involve end users in the innovation process; one example of this is the Living Lab approach.

A Living Lab is a user-centric innovation milieu built on every-day practice and research, with an approach that facilitates user influence in open and distributed innovation processes engaging all relevant partners in real-life contexts, aiming to create sustainable values.

(Bergvall-Kåreborn & Ståhlbröst, 2010, p. 191)

A living lab focuses on utilising the knowledge and expertise that users bring to this collaborative process and in doing so shared learning takes place. This approach emerged from the information communication technology field but it is increasingly being applied to health and social care, such as in the development of new approaches for people living with dementia. As a pragmatic research approach it can be argued it is akin to the philosophical pragmatism of Richard Rorty, where ideas and practices are valued in terms of their 'usefulness, workability, and practicality'. At an application level it has the characteristics of action research, where there is a focus on developing 'practical knowing through a participatory process'.

Context: dementia

Demographic change across Europe indicate that people are living longer and the predicted consequences of this change is there will be an increase in the incidence of long-term conditions such as dementia. It is also predicted that these changes will have a significant socioeconomic impact, including a potentially adverse impact on good-quality service delivery and provision. Dementia as a long-term condition adversely affects cognitive functioning, emotional control, mood, social behaviour and activities of daily living. There are more than 800,000 people currently diagnosed with dementia in the UK, and it is forecast that the number of cases will triple by 2050.

The challenge

In response to this societal challenge, the UK Prime Minister launched the 'dementia challenge', which focused on delivering major improvements in dementia care and research by 2015. The challenge on dementia was designed to make a real difference to the lives of people living with dementia. There are three main areas of action:
1 driving improvements in health and care;
2 creating dementia-friendly communities;
3 improving dementia research.

Practical application

In terms of dementia research the innovate dementia project is a European (Interreg IVB) funded project that has the following aims (Woods *et al.*, 2013, p. 6).
• Evaluate how innovative approaches in dementia care are utilised across north-west Europe, highlighting best practice and future areas of research and development.
• Create collaborations that bring people living with dementia together with health and social care, academic and business ('triple helix' approach) to share and enhance each other's knowledge, expertise and performance.
• Influence the development of health innovation, new technologies and lifestyles to prevent the development of dementia and enable people to live well with dementia.
• Establish 'living labs' in order to test and evaluate innovative dementia care models.

Innovating

Bringing partners together in a triple helix arrangement creates the space and drive to innovate, explore and validate potential solutions to the challenge of living everyday with dementia

(Figure 76.1). This open innovation process is then structured by the living lab, which is dynamic as a structure and is driven by the real needs of people living with dementia. To provide a sense of consistency and to ensure it is fit for purpose for the work of the project, the definition for a living lab was further refined:

> A pragmatic research environment which openly engages all relevant partners with an emphasis on improving the real-life care of people living with dementia through the use of economically viable and sustainable innovations.
>
> *(Woods et al., 2013, pp. 13–14)*

This definition is also underpinned by the following principles:
• continuity
• openness
• realism
• empowerment of users
• spontaneity.

The work of this living lab focuses on innovation within the areas of intelligent lighting, nutrition and exercise, living environment and models of assistance. It is recognised within the project that the work of the living lab will only be successful if the proposed innovations reflect the real needs of people living with dementia. On this basis the strength of using a living lab approach is that it creates an environment where the real needs of people living with dementia are recognised and championed.

References and further reading

Bergvall-Kåreborn, B. & Ståhlbröst, A. (2010) 'Living Lab: an open and user-centric design approach. In: D. Haftor and A. Mirijamdotter (eds) *Information and Communication Technologies, Society and Human Beings: Theory and Framework*, pp. 190–206. Hershey, PA: IGI Global.

Reason, P. (2003) Pragmatist philosophy and action research: readings and conversation with Richard Rorty. *Action Research* **1**, 103–123.

Reason, P. and Bradbury, H. (eds) (2001b) *Handbook of Action Research: Participative Inquiry and Practice*. London: Sage Publications.

Weber, M.E.A. (2011) *Customer co-creation in innovations: a protocol for innovating with end users*. PhD thesis, Technische Universiteit Eindhoven.

Woods, L., Smith, G., Pendleton, J. and Parker, D. (2013) *Innovate Dementia Baseline Report: Shaping the Future for People Living with Dementia*. Liverpool: Liverpool John Moores University.

World Health Organization and Alzheimers Disease International (2012) *Dementia: A Public Health Priority*. Geneva: World Health Organization.

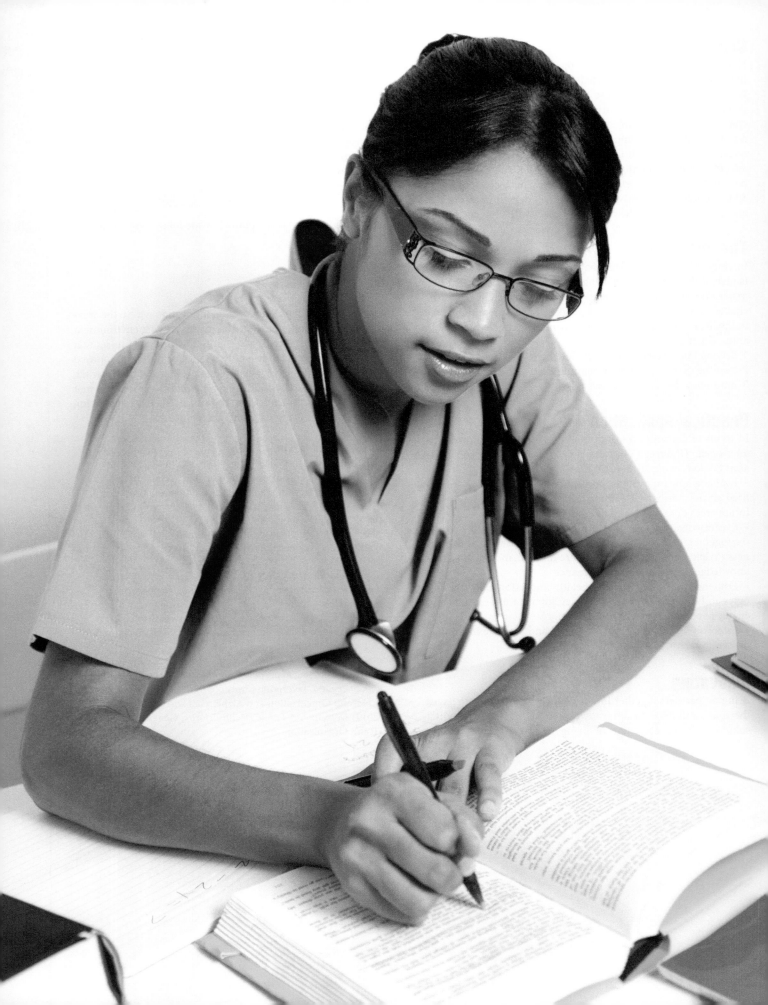

Historical research

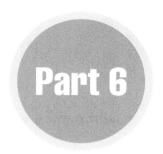

Part 6

Chapters

77 What is historiography?

Figure 77.1 What is historiography?

Definitions (Wallace and Gach, 2008)			
(i) The history of academic history	(ii) The philosophy, theory and methodology of history		
⬇	⬇	⬇	⬇
Situational	Context	Perspective	Frameworks

Situational	Where the researcher's work fits with other historian's findings
	Critical, but not over-critical approach to the work of other historians

Context	Past	Primary sources Events experienced at the time they were happening
	Contemporary	Risk of anachronism Benefit of being able to recognise the consequences of events

Perspective	The historian (context and biases)		Cyclical
	Narrative		Sequential
	Chronological	Thematic	

Frameworks	Theoretical frameworks (paradigms)	Implicit paradigms
	Marxism Psychoanalytic approaches Structuralism	Atheoretical historians

History enables us to understand the past and to appreciate, for example, the pioneering work achieved by nurses, doctors and scientists, coping without the scientific knowledge and technological advantages that we take for granted today. It also helps us to recognise which elements of the past have influenced subsequent events and to recognise change over time, while acknowledging that this does not necessarily always imply progress. The value of history is thus clear, but what of its nature?

Definitions

Historiography has two definitions: (i) the history of academic history and (ii) the philosophy, theory and methodology of history (Figure 77.1). However, there are overlapping elements to each definition.

The history of academic history

Carr (1990, p. 23) advised that it was apposite to 'study the historian before you begin to study the facts'. This maxim reminds

Nursing and Healthcare Research at a Glance, First Edition. Alan Glasper and Colin Rees. © 2017 by John Wiley & Sons, Ltd. Published 2017 by John Wiley & Sons, Ltd.

us to consider the biases and contexts from which historical data are analysed and interpreted. Such biases can hardly be avoided. As with other forms of qualitative research, the researcher's own influences are brought to bear on their findings, but in historical research this is seldom 'bracketed' or made apparent. It is therefore for the reader to consider what is known of the historian and to read his or her account with that awareness. For instance, David Irving, the discredited British historian who was jailed for 3 years for denying the Holocaust, would have interpreted wartime data very differently from an Auschwitz survivor. Similarly, school textbooks of history tend to present particular versions of events when informing their readers of the history of the British Isles or world history. Accounts often present Britain as the victor in wars or as instigators of industrial progress. Their accounts often neglect the other perspectives and overlook the social and personal effects that these events had on significant numbers of its population.

Philosophy, theory and methodology of history

Philosophy and methodology of history interact. According to Wallace and Gach (2008) the philosophy of history results from reflecting on historical methodology, whereas methodology is dependent on the demands of the subject matter and epistemology. There are some historians who consider themselves, or who are considered, atheoretical (i.e. they gather data and later theorise about it) while others conduct their research according to specific predetermined theoretical principles. Implicit within both these definitions are interconnected elements that may be termed 'situational', 'context', 'perspective' and 'frameworks'.

Situational

Part of the history research process requires researchers to situate their findings in the context of what has already been discovered and written about the topic. They should show where their interpretation of their findings supports, contradicts or embellishes the work of other historians. This should be done critically, but should not be over-critical, because previous researchers may well have paved the way for their colleagues who follow them.

Context

Our understanding of events will differ depending on whether we seek primary sources from those living at the time an event occurred or from our contemporary perspective (or any point in between). We may read diaries or newspaper columns of past events reported as they were happening, but it is important to remember that these, too, will represent the opinions and beliefs of those who wrote them. As with contemporary journalism, past newspapers would also have had political affiliations. Personal journals and diaries, depending on the time they were written, would have been written by the literate and would therefore have represented the social mores of the educated classes. We may read the medical notes of patients from more than 100 years ago, but we may seldom 'hear' the patients' own voices.

When we read secondary sources we will learn what historians have made of the primary sources available to them and their interpretations may differ from those who experienced the events, and from others who make or have made their own deductions from the material. The advantage to a more contemporary perspective is that the historian may be able to illuminate the consequences of the events which occurred with the benefit of hindsight. The risk is that these deductions may be made anachronistically without considering the period in which they occurred. It is easy to criticise the diet of our forebears without considering scarcity of food and local harvest failures, lack of refrigeration, transportation and international relationships with those from whom we imported goods for example.

Perspective

Much about the historian's perspective has already been discussed, and as researchers or readers of research we must be mindful of bias and context, but also of beliefs and narratives. Some historians hold with the philosophical view that events move in cycles (e.g. triumph or disaster, boom or bust) whereas others believe that progress occurs sequentially and change over time is usually an improvement over whatever preceded it. These perspectives affect a researcher's methodological approach where they claim to have one, and probably inadvertently where they claim they do not. Perspective will also affect the written narrative, with some organising their data chronologically and others choosing a thematic approach.

Frameworks

The beliefs, assumptions and perspectives a researcher has about the world and humanity will influence the theoretical frameworks or paradigms through which the research is conducted. Those who claim to be atheoretical, and not to work within an explicit framework or perspective, maintain rather that they collect and present the facts as they find them. As previously discussed, however, these historians are unlikely to be without beliefs or bias.

Fulbrook (2002) distinguishes several types of paradigm in historical research, including implicit paradigms (the likely province of atheoretical historians), perspectival paradigms, paradigms proper and pidgin paradigms. *Perspectival paradigms* are evident where researchers seek to identify and emphasise particular foci of study, for example political or economic aspects or the study of great men (kings, queens, politicians, explorers). *Paradigms proper* refers to belief systems which influence interpretation of, for example, political and economic events and processes and also affect the nature of the study. Examples include Marxism, psychoanalytical approaches and structuralism among many others. *Pidgin paradigms* tend to be eclectic and to borrow from other approaches.

Conclusion

History, then, for the researcher or reader requires an acknowledgement and awareness of all these factors in order to minimise bias and present, interpret or consider the 'facts' as authentically and reliably as possible.

References and further reading

Carr, E.H. (1990) *What is History?*, 2nd edn, pp. 7–30. London: Penguin Books.

Fulbrook, M. (2002) *Historical Theory*, pp. 31–50. London: Routledge.

McDowell, W.H. (2002) *Historical Research: A Guide*, pp. 3–14. London: Pearson Education.

Wallace, E.R. and Gach, J. (eds) (2008) *History of Psychiatry and Medical Psychology*, pp. 3–115. New York: Springer.

78 Source criticism

Figure 78.1 Source criticism is the process by which sources are assessed for their usefulness, trustworthiness, authenticity and representativeness.

Key question: What were the experiences of ANZAC nurses during the Gallipoli campaign during World War One?

1. The source is useful because it is written by an ANZAC nurse about her experiences

2. The source is an extract from a diary. It is a primary source

3. Matron Wilson created the source. She is authoritative in her account because she was on Lemnos Island

Extract from diary written by Matron Wilson, an ANZAC nurse, about her experience on Lemnos Island looking after soldier patients during the August 1915 offensive on Gallipoli

9 August – Found 150 patients lying on the ground – no equipment whatever … had no water to drink or wash.

10 August – Still no water … convoy arrived at night and used up all our private things, soap etc, tore up clothes [for bandages].

11 August – Convoy arrived – about 400 – no equipment whatever … Just laid the men on the ground and gave them a drink. Very many badly shattered, nearly all stretcher cases … Tents were erected over them as quickly as possible … All we can do is feed them and dress their wounds … A good many died … It is just too awful – one could never describe the scenes – could only wish all I knew to be killed outright.

Source: Grace Wilson, in Bassett, Guns and Brooches, p. 46
On Department of Veteran Affairs website Gallipoli and the Anzacs, 'Nurses at Gallipoli'
http://www.gallipoli.gov.au/nurses-at-gallipoli/nurses-experience.php

7. The extract humanises the well-documented causalities of the Gallipoli offensive through the eyes of a nurse.
For example, 'one … could only wish all I knew to be killed outright'

4. The source is date tagged in August 1915 at the height of the Gallipoli offensive

6. The source is largely opinionated in tone. Matron Wilson deplores the conditions on Lemnos Island for both the nurses and the soldier patients. While there are facts presented in the source, corroboration from other independent sources would be needed. It is also an extract, therefore incomplete

5. The primary purpose of the source is to privately record the events on Lemnos with personal reflection on the events. Matron Wilson eventually wrote a book describing the events so the secondary purpose was to gather data.
It is important to note that the source came from an ANZAC website. It must be noted that the source may have been chosen to fulfil an ANZAC agenda

Source criticism is an essential process for any style of research but particularly in historical research. Source criticism is the process by which sources are assessed for their usefulness, trustworthiness, authenticity and representativeness. For example, when writing about the Australian New Zealand Army Corps (ANZAC) nurses that were active during the Gallipoli campaign, it is important to ensure that the sources used are about or created by ANZAC nurses, present information which is accepted generally as correct, are from the correct time frame, and contain an agenda (Figure 78.1). A common ANZAC agenda is to emphasise the conditions of the battlefield to enhance the bravery of the soldier experience.

By evaluating sources, a historian can justify the inclusion or exclusion of a source from his or her research. Do not immediately discard a source just because it does not seem representative of the time. You may have found a doorway to new research, especially because the voices of nurses are largely underrepresented in the general historical record.

Process

Different historians have different techniques for evaluating sources. The process outlined in this section is just one method, but incorporates the questions historians ask about sources.

1 *Is the source useful?* Have a good look at the archival information with the source. What is the title? What is the attribution? Where did you find it? What information about the source's relevance can you identify? Have a quick scan of the content of the source. Is the information relevant to your study? Is the source worth evaluating further?

2 *What is the type of source?* Is it human, textual or an artefact? Is it a primary, secondary or tertiary source? What conclusions can you draw about the accuracy of the source from this information?

Remember: A primary source is a good source but not necessarily a better source. This is a common misconception.

3 *Who (or what) created the source?* Was the author or creator driving the policy or on the coalface of the event you are researching? What sort of authority does the creator have for making comment on the event?

4 *When was the source created?* Does the time the source was written help clarify, change or obscure the source's meaning?

5 *Why was the source created?* Does the source have an agenda? Was it created to elicit a reaction from the reader or simply describe events?

6 *Is the source factual?* Is the source an opinion? Are the claims made by the source supported within the source or by other independent sources? Is the account complete? Are there gaps or silences in the source that need to be filled? Why are the gaps and silences there?

7 *What is the tone of the source?* What language is used in the source? Is the language/image formal or informal? Is the language/image emotive? How is the reader positioned by the tone and/or language of the source?

Evaluation

Once you have answered these questions you will have a good idea of the value of the source to your research. The more you repeat this process, the more natural it will become as you peruse a variety of sources.

Further reading

Howell, M.C. and Prevenier, W. (2001) *From Reliable Sources: An Introduction to Historical Methods*. Ithaca, NY: Cornell University Press.

79 Critiquing historical research

Figure 79.1 The process for critiquing historical research.

Research question or topic: clarity and relevance
Researcher qualification and perspective? Researcher paradigm/theoretical tradition?

Primary data sources? Provenance of sources? Ethical approval where necessary	Secondary data sources?

Contextualisation of sources
Data analysis and interpretation
Historiographical contextualisation
Conclusions: believable and generalisable?

Primary sources: original textbooks

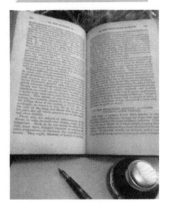

Primary sources: artefacts

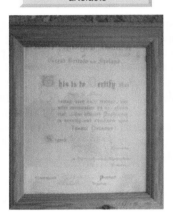

Primary sources: documentary data

Primary sources: photographs

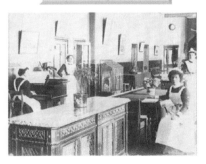

Secondary sources: contemporary textbooks, doctoral theses

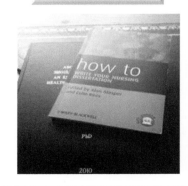

Nursing and Healthcare Research at a Glance, First Edition. Alan Glasper and Colin Rees. © 2017 by John Wiley & Sons, Ltd. Published 2017 by John Wiley & Sons, Ltd.

Historical research refers to the analysis of the past rather than research conducted many years ago. The former is the subject of this chapter, whereas the latter may provide a source of primary data for a historian. The use of historical research to contemporary healthcare is hotly debated, but without it we would be unable to bring experiences of the past to the analysis and potential resolution of current problems and would be in danger of repeating former mistakes or ineffective practices. It is essential to critique research of historical events just as rigorously as we would scientific studies (Figure 79.1).

The research question

It is important to ascertain whether the research question or topic is clearly articulated and relevant for the reader's purpose. You may have a general interest in the history of your profession, but if you are using historical research to answer a contemporary healthcare question, then its focus must be specific to your context.

The researcher

It is almost impossible to write unbiased history. Historians are likely to interpret data according to their demographic variables, including age, gender, sexual orientation, education, faith and politics. It is important to discover as much as possible about the historian in order to better contextualise their findings. Consider also whether the researcher is a qualified historian, an academic from another discipline or professional with an interest in history. Those who have not been trained in the historical tradition are possibly more likely to write from a biased perspective and to fail to contextualise their findings.

Some researchers consider the close reading, rigorous analysis, description, interpretation and critical discussion of primary sources sufficient for an empirical study, whereas others analyse their data and articulate their findings according to a particular paradigm or theoretical tradition (or perspective). Examples of paradigms include Marxism, psychoanalytic approaches and structuralism, whereas social, economic, political and feminist historical approaches are examples of perspectival paradigms along with the French *Annales* school and micro-history.

The sources

Data sources should be clearly identified. Some researchers collate and synthesise secondary sources written by others on the topic, but academic and amateur historians are more likely to conduct their own primary research drawing on original sources (or their facsimiles) as well as referring to research conducted by others which offers points for comparison.

Primary data sources

Examples include (i) manuscript sources such as administrative and clinical records, minutes of meetings, policies and procedures; and (ii) contemporary (to the historical period) published sources such as books, directories, journal articles, letters, magazines and newspapers, parliamentary papers and public general statutes. Historical patient records are subject to a 100-year exclusion clause, which means that researchers have to gain ethical and local permission to access more recent sources and reporting of findings have to respect confidentiality. In some

cases older records are contained in books which span a lengthy time period and overlap the exclusion period. These records may sometimes be made available to researchers if the more recent records can be obscured. Details of ethical permission and management of sensitive data should be reported in research articles. Administrative documents are subject to a 30-year exclusion and the ethical situation is the same for this time period.

Secondary data sources

These may include published and unpublished research written recently on the topic, including books, journal articles, dissertations, projects and theses.

Authentification of primary sources

It is not unusual for documentary evidence or artefacts to be faked so if you are undertaking your own research it is necessary to be certain that your sources are genuine. When critiquing research conducted by others look for evidence that primary sources were authenticated. Historical case books, for example, usually contain printed material with the name of the institution or a local manufacturer in typescript. Manufacturers' details can be verified by recourse to sources such as local directories (e.g. *Kelly's Directory*) found in the local history section of a public library or online (http://kellysdirectories.com/).

Analysis and interpretation

If researchers have used a particular paradigm or perspective to conduct their research, their analysis should be consistent with the methodological approach, explanations of which should be provided. Usually data are analysed in much the same way as with other types of research. Qualitative data are analysed using relevant approaches (e.g. thematic analysis) and quantitative data are analysed statistically. Where historical research differs is that the analytical findings must be interpreted according to the historical context. As an example, when considering the diet offered in a nineteenth-century pauper lunatic asylum it should be compared contemporaneously to the common alternatives such as workhouse diets or those available to the impoverished at home rather than to today's standards.

Historiographical context and research conclusions

Historian researchers should situate their findings in relation to similar or related research in the field, identifying their unique contribution and the extent to which their findings support or reject research conducted by others. Their conclusions should be clearly articulated and refer to supported illustrations from primary data. Historiography is considered in more detail in Chapter 76.

Further reading

Berkhofer, R.F. Jr (2008) *Fashioning History: Current Practices and Principles*. Basingstoke: Palgrave Macmillan.
Elton, G.R. (1979) *The Practice of History*, 9th impression. Sydney: Fontana.
Fulbrook, M. (2002) *Historical Theory*. London: Routledge.
Tosh, J. (2008) *Why History Matters*. Basingstoke: Palgrave Macmillan.

80 Oral tradition

Figure 80.1 Oral history is an approved method in historical nursing research that records the memories of nurses and patients as well as their history.

Stage 1
After finding the research topic you are interested in, assign it to a genre and decide on your theoretical approach. Clarify any ethical and legal considerations

Stage 2
Select your interviewees. To find them, ask your colleagues, advertise in print media, on boards or on social media

Stage 3
Select your interviewers. Do you have financial resources to pay for professionals? If you have to rely on friends, make sure they know how to conduct the interviews

Stage 4
Do your background research in literature, archives and libraries

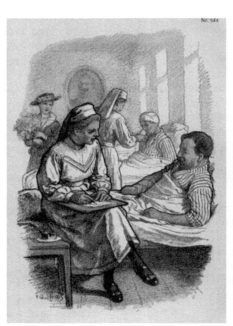

Stage 7
Present and publish your findings. Archive your records

Stage 6
Transcribe your records

Stage 5
Conduct the interviews. Make sure your recording devices work properly!

The artist who did the postcard was not determined despite careful research.
Copyrights are nevertheless protected. Please contact the author of this chapter.
The author wants to thank Naomi Barnes for proofreading the chapter.

Speaking, listening to and writing history

If you have constructed nursing care plans before, you have already taken the first step into oral history. Oral history is primarily about interest in people, the ability to listen and asking the right questions (Figure 80.1). Oral history projects mostly record the voices of the public, especially people from minorities and who are usually unheard and unseen in history's big picture. So, if you are interested in the history of nurses and patients, oral history might be your path of research.

Some things you should think about before starting the recorder

Usually, oral history projects are recorded on a recording devcie or audio tape. Make sure that your interviewees agree to be recorded. If you ask for sensitive information (e.g. traumatic experiences of patients), the interviewed person might feel uncomfortable with this and only agree to a written record. In this case, talk to your supervisor about whether she or he regards your project as 'proper' oral history.

Designing your project

Clarify what you are interested in. Your project could be topically based (subject-orientated), centred on one special person such as a former matron (life history), or the history of a whole community such as the sisters of a nurses' order (community history). Alternatively, you could research the history of a family of patients or nurses (family history). Assigning your project to a genre will help you to sharpen your research profile and prepare your central questions.

Grounded theory, feminism and other ideas

Having studied nursing you are probably familiar with grounded theory (GT). GT might be your method if you conduct your interviews without a theoretical framework and want to develop a new theory from your data. Quite a number of GT-based research projects use oral history.

Grounded theorists tend to conduct free-flowing interviews with no, or only a few, prepared questions. Nevertheless, context information is essential for working with the data. To complement your collection of data, you might want to have a look into *prosopography* works which, like GT, are also 'bottom-up' history but based on documents (e.g. Sue Hawkin's research about nurses at St George's Hospital in the nineteenth century).

Further theoretical questions could be sociological: whether your project is about the elite (e.g. matrons or nursing politicians) or non-elite (e.g. auxiliary nurses who, on the other hand, often belonged to the upper classes during the First World War); and whether feminism is an important context factor. As nursing has been a profession associated with womanhood, feminism is an important analytical basis to consider.

Planning your project

As soon as you have found the topic you are interested in, assigned it to a genre and are clear about your theoretical approach, you must select your interviewers (if you plan to do more interviews than you can manage on your own) and, most importantly, your interviewees. If you do not know your interviewees already, you can advertise in newspapers or on social media, through organisations or on the notice board.

Define the scope of your project. This will largely depend on your financial resources, your time frame and the number of interviewees.

Design your interview guide. If you are a GT disciple, you might not approve of such a guide. If this is the case, find out how to lead open interviews. If you use a guide, remember that it is not a dogma but a guideline and is flexible.

Do careful background preparation in libraries, archives and in secondary sources. (This might not be appropriate if you are a grounded theorist, as traditionally the contextualisation is done after the interviews.)

Remember that many successful oral history projects have been conducted by students and committed non-professionals who were interested in the history of their community or family.

Transcription, publication, archiving and responsibility

How you transcribe your records or video tapes will depend on your theoretical approach. Before you publish your material, make sure that your interviewees agree with the publication. This is especially important before you post a recording or video on the internet. Ask your university about interview and copyright regulations, and any data protection regulations which might concern the archiving of your records. Keep in mind that your interviewees open themselves to you. That makes you responsible for careful handling of information.

Key points

- Oral history is the recorded and self-told history of ordinary people who have not been heard yet.
- Oral history makes it possible for patients and nurses to tell their history.
- Oral history is an important expansion of medical history.

Further reading

Charlton, T.L., Myers, L.E. and Sharpless, R. (eds) (2007) *History of Oral History: Foundations and Methodology*. Lanham, MD: Altamira Press.
Perks, R. and Thomson, A. (eds) (2005) *The Oral History Reader*. London: Routledge.

Resources

Kingston and St George's Faculty of Health, Social Care and Education. Nurses' lives: the oral history of nurses. http://www.healthcare.ac.uk/nurses-lives-the-oral-history-of-nurses/
University of Manchester, UK Centre for the History of Nursing. Resource: Oral history. www.nursing.manchester.ac.uk/ukchnm/archives/oralhistory/

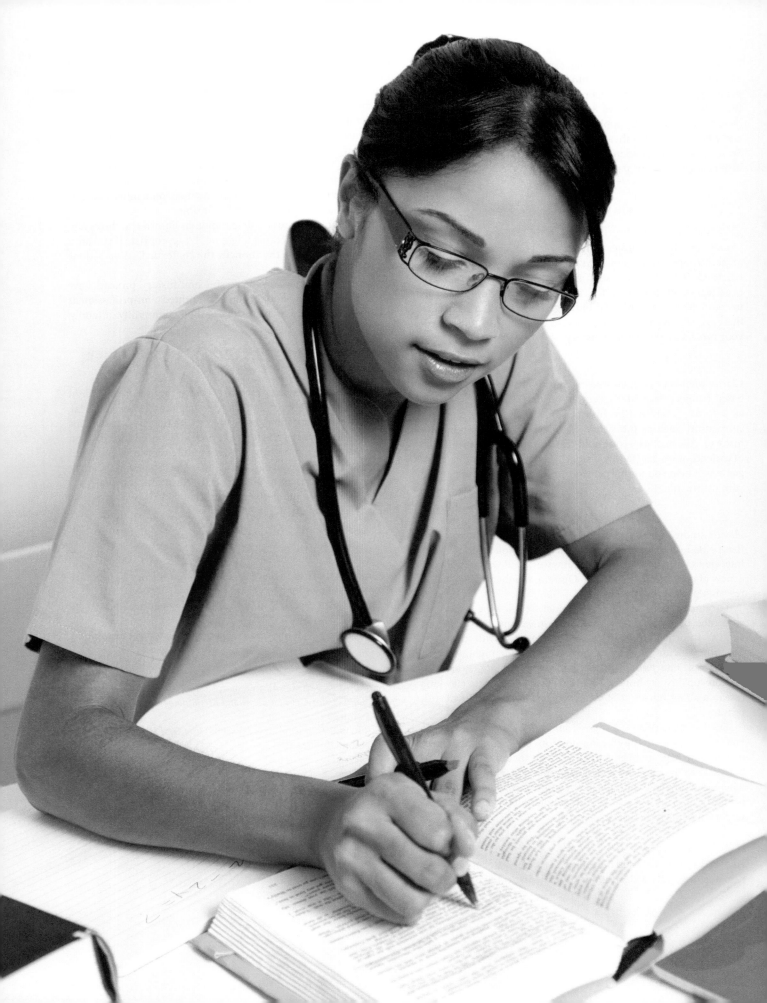

Educational research

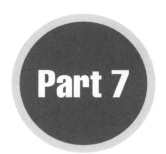
Part 7

Chapters

Secondary data analysis: analysing documents

Figure 81.1 Analysing documents.

Stage 1: General analysis of a policy or similar document

- Read document several times to gain familiarity with its form, content, intentions, and determine its target audience
- First and second readings: make annotations to note early impressions, queries and thoughts
- Determine the antecedents to the policy
- Note any novel words or esoteric usage of words not usually found within the subject
- Note the evidence base informing the document to determine its breadth and depth
- Determine the policies that have informed it or underpinned it
- Note contradictions and limitations of the policy

Presentation of the policy
- Layout?
- Readability?
- Clarity of purpose and directives?
- Tone?
- Charts or mainly narrative?

General overview of information
- Who wrote it?
- When was it written?
- What are the aims and objectives of the policy?
- What is the purpose of the policy?
- Why was the policy written (antecedents)?
- What political, social, public or other factors influenced its creation (antecedents)?
- Which professionals does it apply to?

Quality, review and monitoring
- What quality measures are embedded to ensure all get a high standard of service?
- Are the services the same for all?
- Is the policy culturally sensitive?
- Does it promote culturally sensitive services and practice?
- Who is accountable for the policy?
- Does the policy regulate practice and/or promote standardised best practice?
- Has it the potential to improve services and practice?
- Does the policy have the potential to reduce unwarranted variations in practice?
- When was the policy implemented?
- When, how and by whom will the policy be reviewed?
- Has the policy been revised?
- Is it mandatory or optional?
- Does the policy promote evidence-based practice?
- Does the policy protect the public from unsafe decision-making or practice?
- Is the evidence base relevant, contemporary and comprehensive?

Stage 2: Critiquing policy content

- Create new list of key words that capture the essence of the subject under examination and look for these in the document
- Search for these in the document and note any new words in another list
- Search for the second list of words in the document

Nursing and Healthcare Research at a Glance, First Edition. Alan Glasper and Colin Rees. © 2017 by John Wiley & Sons, Ltd. Published 2017 by John Wiley & Sons, Ltd.

The aim of this chapter is to outline the main principles of analysing documents collected for research purposes. A document is a written paper with information within it that may be factual or informative. It can be hard copy or electronic or other media. Analysis includes a study of the information in the form of words but can include or solely focus on images, symbols or graphics. The analysis takes into account the form, structure, style and space given to particular elements (see Stage 1 in Figure 81.1).

The term 'documentary analysis' can sometimes be confused with film studies, where students are required to analyse the content of film documentaries or other broadcast media. The collection of documents for research purposes constitutes secondary data. Secondary data is information composed, written or collated by someone other than the researcher of the study that it will be used by.

Documents can be examined using deductive approaches when theory is being tested or using inductive methods when an understanding emerging from the data (i.e. the content of the document) is being sought. This chapter deals with qualitative analysis of documents. For an account of how to conduct deductive or quantitative content analysis see Krippendorf (2013), who also provides guidance on qualitative content analysis.

Documents are commonly used in social research but nursing research has often included documents and their inclusion is increasingly becoming a requirement in most studies to ensure researchers collect contextual data. Researchers may intend to focus entirely on documents as this might be the only source of evidence. Researchers in nursing have largely focused on nursing records as a means to determine care given. For example, Tuffrey *et al.* (2007) examined community nurses' records to determine the end-of-life care given to children and their families. While there are limitations on using records (principally because records may not be an accurate representation of care given as they can be incomplete or too brief), they can nevertheless be used as data.

Methods and process

The analysis of a document is very similar to analysing the transcript of an interview (i.e. the audio recording of an interview that has been transcribed verbatim). However, there are some additional tasks to be completed when analysing a document, particularly as its creation has not been determined by the aims of the research or by the researcher. Stage 1 of Figure 81.1 describes what these are.

In addition to this, qualitative researchers analyse interview transcripts and documents using a process called coding the data. To begin the process they may develop a data extraction form, which might include key words from the study's aims and objectives, key words or terms arising from the literature review,

or other sources of prior knowledge. The same process can be followed for analysing documents. When instances of these key words or their meaning are found in the document, a shorthand for a particular code is highlighted on the document itself. In addition to this, researchers create tables or matrices where the codes are listed in a column, while in the next column the page and paragraph where the code is found in the data are noted. In the next column an extract of the actual data is inserted. Another column is usually added where researchers write their ideas, thoughts, notions, conceptualisations, cross-references to other codes, literature or hypotheses. Such frameworks help manage the analysis of large documents or qualitative data to allow the researcher to identify emerging themes.

Examples of inductive methods for analysing documents to determine health equity are described by Almond (2008) and Pinto *et al.* (2012). Sets of questions (open and closed) can be designed to facilitate analysis. Additionally, another set of words or questions arising from the general overview analysis and the learning gained from Stage 1 can be applied to the data and this is known as iterative analysis (see Stage 2 of Figure 81.1).

Conclusion

The inclusion of documents in research can provide contextual data and complement other data collected, or they can be the primary data source. There are some limitations of using secondary data, in that the documents being used are not usually originally developed or created for research purposes. The analysis of the information within the document (which may be words or graphics) and the appearance and structure of the document can be analysed using qualitative (inductive) or quantitative (deductive) approaches or indeed a combination of both. The purpose of the documentary analysis varies from research to research. In common with analysing interview transcripts or other qualitative data, coding frameworks and matrices can be created to manage and display the data and facilitate thematic analysis.

References

Almond, P. (2008) *A study of equity within health visiting postnatal depression policy and services.* Unpublished PhD thesis, University of Southampton.

Krippendorf, K. (2013) *Content Analysis: An Introduction to its Methodology*, 3rd edn. London: Sage.

Pinto, A.D., Manson, H., Pauly, B., Thanos, J., Parks, A. and Cox, A. (2012) Equity in public health standards: a qualitative document analysis of policies from two Canadian provinces. *International Journal for Equity in Health* 11, 28. doi: 10.1186/1475-9276-11-28

Tuffrey, C., Finley, F. and Lewis, M. (2007) The needs of children and their families at end of life: an analysis of community nursing practice. *International Journal of Palliative Nursing* **13**, 64–71.

82 Traditional annotation and coding

Figure 82.1 Traditional annotation and coding.

Defining levels of annotation
Words/text
• Basic word searches
Terminology
• Key words/tagging
• Information extraction based on a body of agreed knowledge
Annotation
• Using meta-information around an ontology to consider themes surrounding 'tasks', 'events' or 'clusters' of information
• Formal meaning and reasoning can be considered in relation to moments in time

Key points to consider when annotating video transcripts
• Clear ontology, rationale and methodology
• Well-defined class, attributes and roles that are being examined
• Clearly stated and defined coding system
• Consideration to ease of use, time management and multiple annotators to reduce bias
• Multimedia tools and annotation programs

An otology
A set of concepts and understanding relating to a world or situation

Concept or class
Ideas and classification of items within an ontology, e.g. a set of participants or patient group

Attributes
The properties or constituents of a class, e.g. individuals within the participant group

Roles
The relationship between ideas and their properties, e.g. between participants
Dyad = two participants

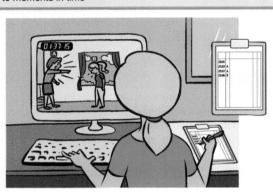

Tasks
A type of behaviour or verbal classification, e.g. what a participant might say in relation to a particular variable or experience. This might be related to a request or in response to a problem or task

Organising data and units of analysis: visual representation of themes within an ontology and their relationship to individual tasks

Behaviour: parent/main themes

Sub-themes relating to groups

Units/individual coded tasks or behaviours

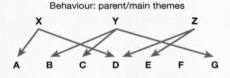

Annotation

Data in the modern world can be accessed from a vast number of resources, with both textural and visual content. One way of making sense of 'worlds' of information (an ontology), ideas and meanings can be by observing a 'snapshot' or defined instance in time or space. At the most basic level, this can be done by considering words and texts through a basic search, or by the more systematic system of key word searching and tagging, i.e. information retrieval defined by a body of knowledge.

Annotation of a document or transcripts of data such as video or surveillance recording requires more in-depth meta-information, knowledge and understanding of a particular ontology, in relation to reasoned themes and formal meanings. It may involve simple coding from observational methodology considering a particular behaviour or task, by an individual or team of annotators. High-level annotation informing multimedia tools and surveillance can also be formulated to consider longer time periods (see Chapters 83 and 85).

A research tool

All research methodology requires an informed, clearly defined question or hypothesis by which to define events, tasks or behaviours; the class and attributes of the participants/subject; and the different variables in behaviour that are to be analysed. These are defined by an ontology – a social theory that defines a particular world (Bryman, 2012).

Annotation and coding can be used to capture and evaluate qualitative data in a systematic and congruent way, and may be used in a variety of ways to support different types of research and research methodologies.

• Observational research: as part of a planned systematic observation of participants undertaking a particular task or demonstrating a behaviour. Transcripts or observation of video data, at timed intervals, can be used to analyse the relationship between independent and dependent variables.

• Content and thematic analysis, for example transcripts of focus groups and interviews, in grounded theory approaches to data collection and analysis.

• Secondary analysis of data collected or stored by other people, for example in critical incident analysis of video data, transcripts or stored online discussions.

• As part of mixed methodology: themes considering participant attributes, roles, tasks and interrelatedness might be considered in qualitative research methodology, while quantitative analysis of frequency and number of tasks or events may also be considered.

Coding

A coding system identifies meaningful units of analysis to be observed. This might include a particular phrase, type of task, or related set of words that form an idea. This may also inform hierarchies of codes, with different levels considering subsets of main themes.

• Open or initial coding: considering wide groupings and initial exploration of the dataset.

• Axial coding: considering the found themes and connections within the initial coding, and recoding in line with new themes.

• Selective coding: used to consider a main theme in more detail.

Complex algorithms and multimedia tools: data and units of analysis can be prioritised and arranged in relation to the difference in detail, and connections between datasets (see example in Figure 82.1). Algorithms can also be used to interpret data from advanced surveillance and annotation technology to identify basic interrelated data sources, for example matching facial recognition with a particular detected 'event' or activity.

Strengths

• Annotation enables the researcher to consider behaviour and use of language in detail and in context.

• It enables targeted analysis of large amounts of qualitative data and enables quantative analysis where appropriate.

• Systematic annotation based on an agreed ontology, with clearly identified coding systems, enables shared annotation, which also reduces bias.

Limitations

• Management and storage of large amounts of data.

• Potential bias and manipulation of meaning; more than one coder or annotator can ameliorate this to some extent.

• Time management: producing a transcript from video or audio recording and then coding it by hand is very time-consuming.

Ethical considerations

Consent, confidentiality and ethical approval are required for any data with regard to individuals or organisations. This must include the collection, storage, results and publication of data. This can be problematic with secondary data and approval for further analysis. Data must also not be stored for longer than required and must be disposed of appropriately (dated/timed).

Reference

Bryman, A. (2012) *Social Research Methods*, 4th edn. Oxford: Oxford University Press.

83 Video-view-point

Figure 83.1 BigSister interface which allows video to be aligned with several recorded commentaries. In addition to recording their commentary, the reviewer can mark the video by using left clicks to identify points of interest or the person they are talking about.

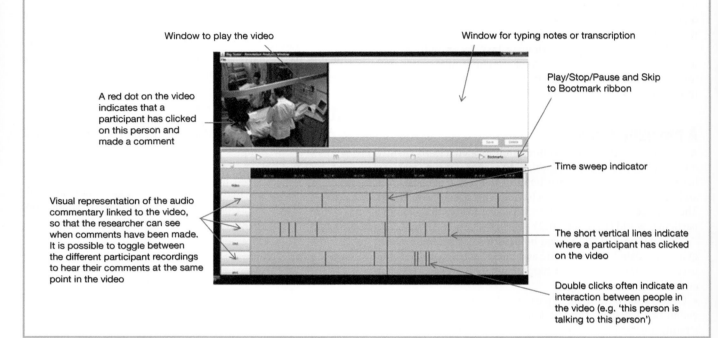

Window to play the video

Window for typing notes or transcription

A red dot on the video indicates that a participant has clicked on this person and made a comment

Play/Stop/Pause and Skip to Bootmark ribbon

Time sweep indicator

Visual representation of the audio commentary linked to the video, so that the researcher can see when comments have been made. It is possible to toggle between the different participant recordings to hear their comments at the same point in the video

The short vertical lines indicate where a participant has clicked on the video

Double clicks often indicate an interaction between people in the video (e.g. 'this person is talking to this person')

It is becoming increasingly common to video record activity. This may be initiated for a variety of reasons, such as safety, security, quality monitoring or as a teaching/learning strategy. From a research perspective this is a rich source of data which can be used to better understand the nature of interactions. Although technology has advanced and the infrastructure to collect video data has become widely accessible (e.g. CCTV, head-cams), the research tools for analysing these data are only just being developed. One of the biggest problems is the volume of data generated. It is possible to use traditional observational research methods to analyse video-captured data; however, many of these techniques rely on the spoken element of the video and overlook the 'unspoken' elements of behaviour. Video-View-Point has been developed to analyse video, particularly where the behaviour being studied cannot be easily described in words.

Preparation

Videos are loaded on to a technological tool that enables the recording of synchronised commentaries. Figure 83.1 illustrates the user interface of one such bespoke tool, BigSister, although this can also be achieved with commercially available eyetrackers and some computer-assisted qualitative data analysis software (CAQDAS) programs. These tools enable the video to be viewed and a synchronised 'Think Aloud' audio recording of the viewer's observations of the behaviours of interest. BigSister also allows the viewer to mark the video for examples of what the subjects are discussing or to 'point' at the person they are commenting about. The eyetrackers produce a visual representation of where the viewer's eyes were looking throughout the video, thereby producing a similar dataset to the point and click of BigSister.

Several different people can record their commentaries on the same video-recorded episode of behaviour. By collecting several different perspectives in this way, it is then possible to analyse the collated perspectives to gain a consensus view on the behaviours being studied.

Analysis

The first step in the Video-View-Point method of analysis is to draw up a log of the click marks on the interface. This log highlights where several of the observers have clicked at about the same time in the video. These 'interesting' episodes can then be looked at more closely, identifying whether the comments relate to the same person or event. The ability to focus the interpretative effort on these 'interesting' areas means that the task becomes more manageable. In practice, these interesting areas account for about 30% of the total video recorded. The episodes of the video can be used to illustrate the points being made, and the comments from each of the participants can be collated to provide a 'rich' description of the relevant behaviours.

Some of the behaviours we would like to study are collectively understood, but difficult to put into words. An example of this is nurse competence. A nurse can watch another nurse's practice and decide relatively quickly whether they have 'got it' or not. Describing what 'it' is or what they notice that allows them to make that judgement is not easy to put into words. The next step of the analysis is to categorise the comments as either *signifier comments* or *signified comments*. These categories are taken from the field of structural linguistics.
• Signifier: those which describe the activity, e.g. the nurse touched the patient's hand.
• Signified: those which provide insight into the perceived meaning, e.g. that nurse seems to have put it all together.
When the signifier comments are taken in conjunction with the videoed episode, greater depth of understanding can be gained about the collectively understood behaviours. For example, eight participants watched a video of students managing a cardiac arrest simulation. Seven of the observers made signified comments about the student who was picking up the pillow from the floor. The students who appeared to be doing the more technically important roles – airway management, getting equipment from the cardiac arrest trolley – were not commented upon. It became clear that the expectation was that the students should be able to follow the instructions they had been given. The student who was demonstrating an understanding of the bigger picture was more interesting in relation to competence.

In summary, Video-View-Point is a hybrid methodological approach that uses the advantages afforded by new technology.

Further reading

de Saussure, F. (2011) *Course in General Linguistics*, translated by W. Basking, eds P. Meisel and H. Saussy. New York: Columbia University Press.

Monger, E.J. (2014) *'Video-View-Point': video analysis to reveal tacit indicators of student nurse competence*. PhD thesis, Faculty of Health Sciences, University of Southampton.

Van Someren, M.W., Barnard, Y.F. and Sandberg, J.A.C. (1994) *The Think Aloud Method: A Practical Guide to Modelling Cognitive Processes*. London: Academic Press.

84 Ethnography and healthcare education

Figure 84.1 Ethnography and healthcare education.

- What can you observe?

- What is your impression of what you see?

- Who are the people? What are they doing? Why?

- What can be seen?

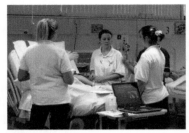
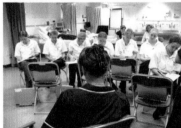
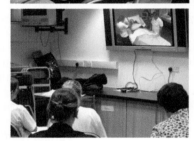

- What signs, insignia are present and what do they mean?

- How would you write this up?

- How can you analyse these 'still moments'?

- What questions would you pose to the participants if you were to talk to them/ interview them after the above incidents?

The main features of conducting ethnographic research in healthcare settings have been described by Savage (2006). Ethnography, when applied to the context of healthcare education, is particularly interested in the cultural overtones or implications that relate to the 'world' of learning professional practice, including the study of the institutions within which the learning occurs. Educational ethnography is interested in how these issues inform our understandings of education and training processes, including the socialisation of staff and students and their impact on or relationship to clients (Figure 84.1). For a useful guide to ethnography in medical education, see Reeves *et al.* (2013).

Educational ethnography

Ethnographic studies have a rich history in healthcare education. The in-depth exploration of the learning context, when complemented by 'thick descriptions' of actions, behaviours and reported intents, provides real insights into the daily world of the participants, identifying the factors that influence their learning and its nature. Seminal examples include Kansas medical student cultures (Becker *et al.*, 1976); the occupational socialisation and rituals of survival in British student nurses as they 'worked and learnt' as apprentices in the 1970s (Melia, 1987); the development of registered nurses from novice to expert status (Benner, 1984); and, more recently, how core educational concepts, intuition (Gobbi, 2009, 2012) and reflection are understood by teachers and students (Bulman *et al.*, 2014). The educational ethnographer considers the:

- curriculum (the explicit and hidden curriculum and their artefacts);
- ways of learning used by learners (formal and informal);
- strategies and behaviours of teachers/supervisors;
- impact of the client on educational interactions and learning;
- organisational and local educational cultures;
- student and professional behaviours and learning within the academic and practice environments.

Data collection and analysis

Chapter 36 summarised the usual methods of ethnographic data collection. In educational ethnography the documentary or text data usually comprises the institutional policies, curricula materials, student work, teacher feedback, student–teacher interactions and any regulatory specifications. Interviews and focus groups not only elicit the experiences of the educational stakeholders and service users, but also portray and, from an interpretive paradigm, evaluate the educational outcomes, processes and structures within a strategic context. The educational ethnographer observes relationships and behaviours between and among staff, students, clients, managers and stakeholders. Attention is paid to formal and informal communication and power structures, daily practices, organisational symbols and ways of talking. Of particular interest is evidence of any paradoxical messages, tensions and signs of transition between places, roles and relationships in the field. Triangulation is crucial to educational ethnography as the different participants may reveal different perspectives.

Challenges and problems

Access and recruitment are often challenging, as the researcher's presence may be perceived to be threatening, intrusive or, in clinical terms, a safety risk. Student education should not be compromised during the research. Four groups are at risk of harm, anonymity, conflict of interest, coercion and confidentiality in an educational study, namely the learners or students, their teachers or supervisors, clients or lay people who may be present, and researchers themselves. Table 84.1 outlines some problems that can be encountered and proposes a few key actions.

Table 84.1

Issues	Actions
1 Observing problematic educational or clinical practice. Managing disclosures	1 Have a strategy and procedures for consent, reporting and action
2 Resolving a conflict of loyalties: researcher versus practitioner versus educator	2 Have clear boundaries and mechanisms for debriefing/support
3 Record keeping	3 Maintain a reflective research log/diary. Be mindful of confidential conversations and personal information
4 How to maintain relationships and present yourself in the field	4 Ensure a good induction. Develop good communication skills
5 Is the participant giving the whole story or not?	5 Seek triangulation and reflect on the participants' motivation

References

Becker, H.S., Geer, B., Hughes E.C. and Strauss, A.S. (1976) *Boys in White: Student Culture in Medical School.* Piscataway, NJ: Transaction Publishers.

Benner, P. (1984) *From Novice to Expert: Excellence and Power in Clinical Nursing Practice.* Menlo Park, CA: Addison-Wesley.

Bulman, C., Lathlean, J. and Gobbi, M. (2014) The process of teaching and learning about reflection: research insights from professional nurse education. *Studies in Higher Education* **39**, 1219–1236.

Gobbi, M. (2009) Learning nursing in the workplace community: the generation of professional capital. In: A. Le May (ed.) *Communities of Practice in Health and Social Care*, pp. 66–82. Oxford: Wiley-Blackwell.

Gobbi, M. (2012) 'The hidden curriculum': learning the tacit and embodied nature of nursing practice. In: V. Cook, C. Daly and M. Newman (eds) *Work-based Learning in Clinical Settings: Insights from Socio-cultural Perspectives*, pp. 103–124. Oxford: Radcliffe Medical.

Melia, K. (1987) *Learning and Working: The Occupational Socialization of Nurses.* London: Tavistock Publications.

Reeves, S., Peller, J., Goldman, J. and Kitto, S. (2013) Ethnography in qualitative educational research: AMEE Guide no. 80. *Medical Teacher* **35**, e1365–e1379.

Savage, J. (2006) Ethnographic evidence: the value of applied ethnography in health care. *Journal of Research in Nursing* **11**, 383–393.

85 Semantic annotation of skills-based sessions

Figure 85.1 Semantic annotation includes the collection of a wide range of digital annotations collected from people and devices within a skills-based lab. These annotations are time-stamped and can confirm to pre-designed ontologies to facilitate reflection, analysis and more complex inference.

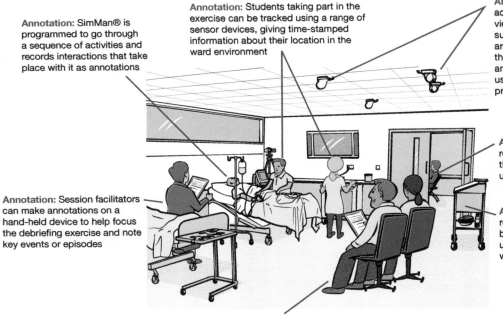

Annotation: SimMan® is programmed to go through a sequence of activities and records interactions that take place with it as annotations

Annotation: Students taking part in the exercise can be tracked using a range of sensor devices, giving time-stamped information about their location in the ward environment

Annotation: Video cameras record the activity of the session from multiple viewpoints and capture audio through suspended microphones. The videos are time-stamped to help synchronise the footage with the annotations captured and video analysis techniques can be used to identify objects within the video, providing additional annotations

Annotation: Session facilitators can make annotations on a hand-held device to help focus the debriefing exercise and note key events or episodes

Annotation: Observers in the control room can make annotations of what they see in the video feed in an unobstrusive way

Annotation: Moveable objects in the room such as medicine trolleys can be tracked using sensors to help understand how equipment is used within the space of the ward

Annotation: Students can observe their peers taking part in the exercise and make annotations on hand-held devices prompting critical reflection

Figure 85.2 Annotations overlaid on the video to support reflexive learning.

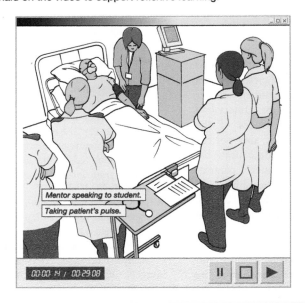

Mentor speaking to student.

Taking patient's pulse.

00:00:14 / 00:29:08

imulations are used to promote the acquisition of practical skills as well as decision-making, team working, communication and problem-solving. The laboratory can mimic the reality of ward life in both its behaviours and resources, such as equipment, clinical charts, wall displays and phones (Figure 85.1). The students are given a plethora of tasks and the computerised mannequins can be programmed to alter their parameters to a point of significant deterioration when emergency responses would be required.

Audio and video together present highly detailed capture of an activity, but because reviewing a recording can be as time-consuming as the original activity and annotating a video by hand can be an intensive and laborious process, alternative strategies need to be adopted. One approach is to make annotations 'live' during the teaching session. Although this is unlikely to be a comprehensive record of events and can preclude full engagement in the activity itself, ubiquitous computing technologies and techniques provide us with an additional mechanism to capture annotations on events that take place in the clinical skills laboratory and from sources that have a low impact on the participants.

Data gathering

As illustrated in Figure 85.1, annotations can be captured from a wide range of sources, both manually from observing students, facilitators or remote assessors, or automatically from simulation mannequins, sensing devices such as indoor location systems, or analysis of the video feed itself. All these annotations can be time-stamped to enable them to be synchronised with the video stream and to provide a chronological sequence of events. Annotations can be free-form, or perhaps based on a predefined ontology, such as year one competencies.

Analysis and reflection

• The annotation process itself, and resulting data, can augment skills-based teaching activities in a range of ways.

• Peer observation of fellow students can promote more active engagement with an observed session and focus attention on specific aspects of the activity, for example students may be asked to make annotations around infection control.
• The annotations can form a useful index into the videos of the session for the purposes of debriefing sessions, both allowing the rapid jump to particular moments, and also focusing attention on specific types of activity.
• The annotations can be used to provide a textual commentary on the session video for reflective activities by those students taking part in the session (Figure 85.2).
• The annotated sessions can become an object for study for those constructing and facilitating the session to help identify issues with pacing, direction of activity and organisation of the physical space.
• The annotations from multiple sessions can form a dataset that allows reflection on the cohort as a whole in terms of what learning objectives or perhaps what competencies students are finding it difficult to achieve.
• If used appropriately, annotations can form part of the assessment of student work as a record of activities undertaken and competencies demonstrated.
• Inferences can be made across the annotations to identify particular patterns, such as an undue delay in performing a sequence of activities, or poor infection control management through lack of hand washing between touching patients.

Further reading

Gobbi, M., Monger, E., Weal, M.J., Michaelides, D.T., McDonald, J.W. and DeRoure, D.C. (2012) The challenges of developing and evaluating complex care scenarios using simulation in nursing education. *Journal of Research in Nursing* **17**, 329–345.

Weal, M.J., Michaelides, D.T., Page, K.R., De Roure, D.C., Monger, E. and Gobbi, M. (2012) Semantic annotation of ubiquitous learning environments. *IEEE Transactions on Learning Technologies* **5**, 143–156.

86 Actor network theory

Actor network theory (ANT) is not a research method but a methodology, a way of conceiving and theorising research. The main method used by ANT is ethnography – close description of a 'naturally occurring' local culture, such as a surgical team at work, derived from fieldwork, sometimes enhanced by video and by 'insider' accounts that may be autobiographical (auto-ethnography). Bruno Latour (2007) describes how 'the social' is constructed through the formation of expanding networks or 'work-nets'. Networks are formed from alliances between persons, material artefacts and ideas, collectively called 'actors' or 'actants'.

• For data collection, ANT researchers look for an entry point into a local culture that signals a controversy, contradiction or fault-line and 'dig where they stand' (closely observe the controversy).
• Research focuses on ontologies (experiences and meanings) rather than epistemologies (theories).
• Data analysis focuses on how networks are initiated, stabilised and expanded, to hold 'objects' with multiple meanings such as different ontological readings of the same illness.
• Networks expand through translations involving mediators: communications, use of instruments and production of ideas that lead to innovations. Intermediaries are translators that fail to lead to innovation, causing crystallisation or collapse of a network.
• Data reporting draws on narrative descriptions rather than explanations, preferring baroque style to include attention to detail and refusing to 'cook' raw data through sterile analysis and selective reporting.

Auto-ethnography

ANT assumes that 'the social' is not given but is in constant dynamic production through networking. ANT research sets out to map how the social is achieved and expanded but, in doing so, adds to the production of the social. The research method that ANT usually draws on is ethnography (literally 'writing out a culture'), involving fieldwork in naturally occurring' environments – visiting a culture for extended periods and closely noting what people do and say. ANT's interest is in local cultures such as clinical work in a particular hospital. An 'outside' ethnographer is interested in how people 'perform' the culture: socialisation into common practices; becoming experts or outcasts; gaining an identity; and actively changing the culture. Fieldwork may be augmented by video analysis, interview and focus groups. 'Insider' ethnography involves description by a member of a culture, often an auto-ethnographic or autobiographical account. Where traditional ethnographers aim for objective accounts, postmodern ethnographers see accounts as necessarily biased social constructions and forms of fiction. Ethnographers make the familiar strange.

ANT process

ANT draws on ethnography for data collection, but is a conceptual framework for data analysis and synthesis. As the descriptor suggests, ANT focuses on 'actors', 'networks' and 'theory'. 'Actors' include three interacting worlds: persons, material artefacts (e.g. instruments, computers, tools) and languages (concepts, symbols and ideas), also referred to as 'actants'. ANT sees persons, artefacts and ideas as equal constituents, offering 'radical symmetry'. The ascription of kinds of agency to material artefacts is a controversial element of ANT.

ANT sees learning as the initiation, stabilisation and widening of potentially ever-expansive networks, also called 'work-nets', because maintaining productive associations between actors requires labour. A surgical team working around a patient forms a network or work-net through generative associations between clinicians, instruments and ideas. A wider network is formed as the surgical team engages with ward, anaesthetic, recovery, surgical sterilisation, pathology and radiography/radiology teams. A well-formed work-net offers a safety net for both patient care and safety and practitioner satisfaction and well-being.

ANT researchers look at how networks are formed and how robust they become. The quality of networks depends on the formation of strong alliances between persons, artefacts and ideas. In turn, alliances are facilitated by 'translations' between actors such as communication and effective use of instruments. Successful translations need 'mediators', exchange agents promoting innovation or reformulation. Translations involving 'intermediaries' include information exchange without innovation, development or expansion, where at best the network is stabilised, and at worst it crystallises, fails to expand and eventually collapses. In effective networks, mediators far outweigh intermediaries.

In tracking the dynamics of networks/work-nets, ANT researchers are sensitive to controversies, contradictions and fault-lines that are already evident in a culture, such as the introduction of a new practice or protocol in healthcare, or the presence of 'black boxes', i.e. habitual behaviours that are not critically examined. Researchers focus on ontologies rather than epistemologies – experiences and meanings rather than theory. It is typical for ANT research to expose how a single object, such as a medical treatment, is given differing meanings across practitioners. How are these ontological differences held within a network that aims to expand?

ANT researchers value good descriptions over explanations. Ethnography invites quality narratives, and ANT research accounts typically involve detailed, even baroque descriptions. Recognising limits provided by feasibility, ANT suggests 'digging where you stand' as entry into fieldwork, but the exit is often through a bird's eye view of a terrain. In preferring appreciation and meaning to explanation and rationalisation, ANT researchers like their data 'rare' rather than 'cooked', presented as compelling realistic narratives rather than adapted as themes, codes and taxonomies.

A health warning

Designing a research project with ANT in mind requires intensive preparatory work including ethics approval. ANT-inspired ethnographies can be deepened considerably through alignment with collaborative research processes – researching with rather than on people – adding complexity to the research. It helps enormously to design research with teams composed of 'insiders' (usually clinicians) and 'outsiders' (usually social scientists). Finally, ANT researchers tend to suspend a priori assumptions about the field of research and tolerate, even relish, messy local social contexts, suspending the compulsion to clean up data through sterile analysis and selective reporting.

Reference and further reading

Bleakley, A. (2012) The proof is in the pudding: putting actor-network-theory to work in medical education. *Medical Teacher* **34**, 462–467.

Latour, B. (2007) *Reassembling the Social: An Introduction to Actor-Network-Theory*. Oxford: Oxford University Press.

Mol, A. (2002) *The Body Multiple: Ontology in Medical Practice*. Durham, NC: Duke University Press.

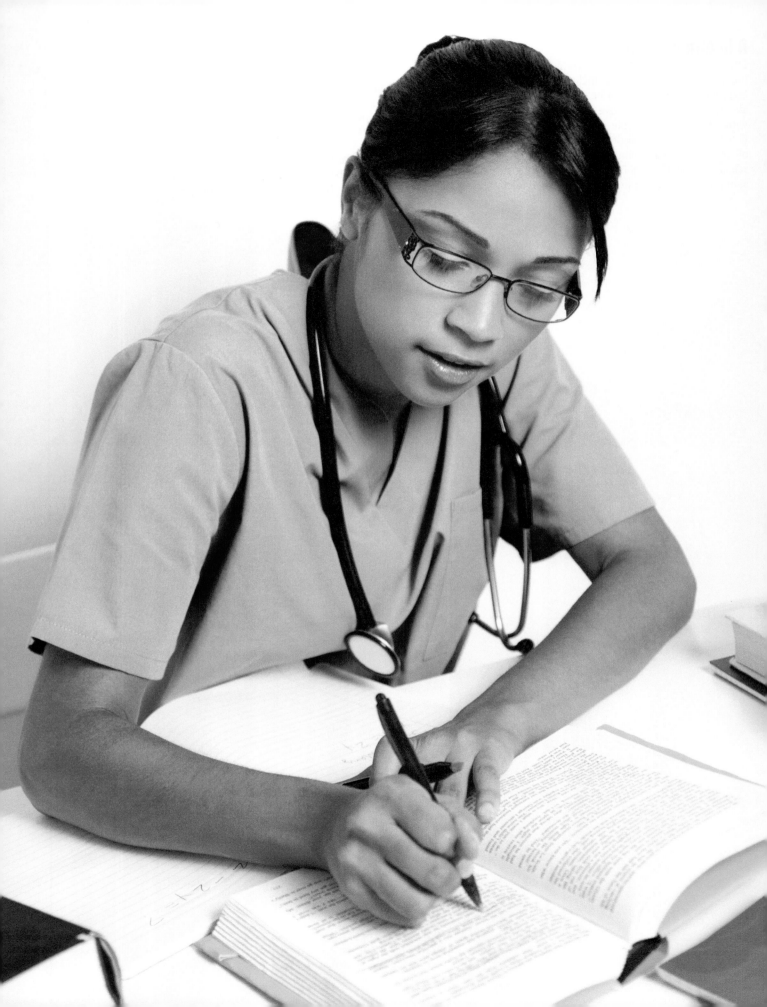

Appendices

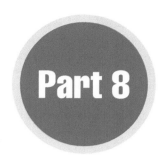

Part 8

Appendix 1: Sampling

We are familiar with the notion of a sample in everyday life. When we are in receipt of samples of products from supermarkets or in the mail, we hope that if we went on to purchase whatever we have sampled this would be a close representation of the product purchased. In research, the idea of a sample and the notion of representativeness are the same.

The challenges of sampling

While sampling appears simple at the conceptual level, it can pose a number of challenges in application and getting it wrong can adversely affect the entire research project. Where numbers involved are potentially large, it may not be possible or feasible to include every member of the relevant population and a subset of a larger population (or sample frame) needs to be selected for study. However, researchers need to know that the sample selected is representative of the larger population. When a sample is not representative it may be difficult to assert that the standards of validity, trustworthiness and rigour (Rolfe, 2006) have been adequately met.

The qualitative–quantitative quandary

It often makes little sense to discuss whether qualitative research is completely distinctive and separate from quantitative research as this can be misleading because not all research methodologies fit neatly into one or the other paradigms. Perhaps best seen as being on a continuum, the two paradigms often reflect the differing aims of the research: on the one hand, to directly perceive and measure the world and, on the other, to offer a more or less subjective interpretation of it.

Participant selection in qualitative research is just as important as in the more positivist quantitative research methods and the adequacy of participant numbers involves careful judgements; too few may risk inadequate depth and breadth, but too many may produce vast amounts of superficial or unwieldy data. Who

and how many participants in a qualitative research study will depend to a greater or lesser degree on 'what you want to know, the purpose of the inquiry, what's at stake, what will be useful, and what will have trustworthiness' (with its associated criteria of dependability, transferability and confirmability needing to be met) (Graneheim and Lundman, 2004). In qualitative research the key participant selection principles usually centre on a relatively small number of participants being purposefully selected and studied intensively to generate rich, dense, focused information on the research question to provide a convincing account of the phenomenon. Their selection is conceptually driven by the theoretical framework and is commonly sequential rather than predetermined. Stopping recruitment of participants and/or information gathering in qualitative research is guided by the principles of adequacy and appropriateness as well as analytical redundancy, whereby one or many more will not make further contributions or provide additional insights (Sobal, 2001). In all cases a rationale and accountability for the selected sampling strategies will need to be presented and defended (Tuckett, 2004). Tuckett's paper incidentally provides a good account of the complexities of the sampling process and potential sampling pitfalls, by taking the reader slowly through the sampling problems involved in his own research into the meaning of truth-telling in nursing homes providing care for older people.

Samples can be broadly divided into two categories: probability and non-probability samples.

Probability sampling

Numerous probability samples exist and include the following.
• Simple random samples: every individual in a population has the same probability of selection and thus considered to be highly representative (Figure A1.1).

Figure A1.1

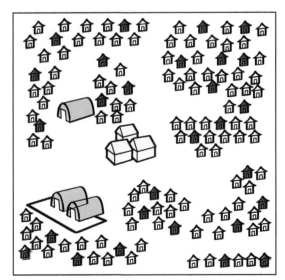

Simple random samples: every individual in a population has the same probability of selection and are thus considered to be highly representative

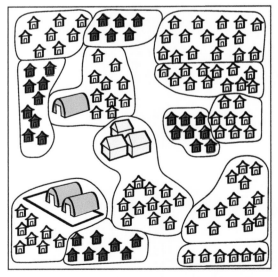

Cluster samples: often used where clusters are naturally occurring. Here you could draw a sample by randomly selecting geographic clusters within the study area, identifying all the village huts in each selected cluster, and randomly selecting a sample from the identified huts in each cluster

Nursing and Healthcare Research at a Glance, First Edition. Alan Glasper and Colin Rees. © 2017 by John Wiley & Sons, Ltd. Published 2017 by John Wiley & Sons, Ltd.

- Stratified random samples: achieved by dividing the population into subgroups (or strata) based on one or more essential characteristics and selecting random samples from each stratum. This requires that the researcher has sufficient understanding of the population proportion for one or more of the selected essential characteristics.
- Systematic random samples: involves a system being employed to select the sample from the frame. The use of a systematic sample requires an assessment of the likelihood of the existence of a pattern in the data in the sample frame.
- Cluster samples: often used where clusters are naturally occurring. Random selection of clusters and then random selection within each selected cluster constitutes a random sample (Figure A1.1).

Non-probability sampling

Non-probability samples are less useful for inference than probability samples because the conclusions that can be reached through statistical analysis of non-probability samples are sample specific and the results obtained may not be representative of the larger population.

Sample size

An essential aspect of planning any empirical study is to decide how many participants would need to be included. The smaller the sample size, the greater the chance that the investigator fails to detect important effects on the outcome(s) under study, or may estimate effects too imprecisely. In statistical terms, the power of the test may be inadequate. On the other hand, studies that are larger than necessary are an ineffective use of resources. The likelihood of missing an important difference (and making a Type II error) decreases as the sample gets larger. The larger the sample, the lower the risk of Type II errors and the greater the power. Very large samples are often required to detect small differences in the effects (or outcomes) of a particular intervention.

Researchers often recruit the help of statisticians and the use of extensive tables for calculating the number of participants for a given level of power (and vice versa). However, these procedures should be regarded only as providing a rough estimate of the required sample size, as they are based on approximate estimates of the parameters, subjective decisions about the size of an effect, and the use of approximate formulae/tables.

References

Graneheim, U. and Lundman, B. (2004) Qualitative content analysis in nursing research: concepts, procedures and measures to achieve trustworthiness. *Nurse Education Today* **24**, 105–112.

Rolfe, G. (2006) Validity, trustworthiness and rigour: quality and the idea of qualitative research. *Journal of Advanced Nursing* **53**, 304–310.

Sobal, J. (2001) Sample extensiveness in qualitative nutrition education research. *Journal of Nutrition Education* **33**, 184–192.

Tuckett, A.G. (2004) Qualitative research sampling: the very real complexities. *Nurse Researcher* **12**, 47–61.

Appendix 2: Calculating the required sample size

Statistical power

In research trials researchers want to know how many subjects will be required in order to be reasonably certain that the trial will give the correct result. Underlying this concern is the possibility that their data may lead them to make one of two types of error.

• Type 1 error: the conclusion that there is a difference between treatments or interventions when in fact none exists.

• Type 2 error: the conclusion that there is no difference between treatments or interventions when in fact one does exist.

All researchers want to minimise the probability of a Type 1 error while avoiding a Type 2 error. The probability of avoiding a Type 2 error, i.e. the probability of identifying an effect if one exists, is known as *statistical power*. Research trials are therefore planned in a way that ensures sufficient statistical power while reducing the probability of a Type I error to a minimum. The minimum acceptable level of statistical power is around 80%.

How are statistical power and sample size related and calculated?

For any given statistical test the statistical power equation relates five factors:

• statistical power;
• the specified level of statistical significance;
• the true difference in outcome measures;
• the variability in the outcome measures;
• the sample size.

Where four of these are known the fifth can be computed. Specifically, where the expected treatment difference in outcome is known or hypothesised, the standard deviation of the outcome is known or estimated and the level of probability defining statistical significance is set, then it is possible to calculate the sample size required to achieve the required level of statistical power. Alternatively, the available power can be calculated for a given sample size.

Statistical power equations exist for each data type and the comparison being made. While the equations are complex, published tables and online calculators are available.

Other aspects of sample size calculation

In postal surveys the required sample size is the *number of responses received,* not the number of questionnaires mailed or distributed. To achieve the required sample size, therefore, it is important to adjust the sample size upwards in order to allow for a less than 100% response. As an example, where the response rate to the survey is only 40% and the required sample size is 200, then the number to be circulated is calculated as 200/0.4 = 500. An equivalent adjustment is needed in a trial or cohort where loss to follow-up is expected.

Where outcome is measured using a measurement scale with less than perfect reliability, some adjustment is also needed. For example, for a scale with reliability 0.8, a calculated sample size of 240 needs to be increased to 300 (i.e. 240/0.8).

Appendix 3: Estimating population means

The effect of sampling in estimating population parameters

For reasons of cost and difficulty in access, researchers draw samples from populations rather than working with the whole population. However, even though the sampling process involves a representative subset of the population, the effect of *sampling error* is to introduce a level of uncertainty into the estimation process. Even where identical sampling procedures are followed, no two surveys produce identical results, essentially because they reflect the responses of different members of the population. In order to present meaningful findings, researchers therefore compute the sample size required to achieve an acceptable level of precision in their findings and report their findings with 95% confidence intervals.

How much do samples vary?

Researchers want to know the level of variation they should expect in their findings. Since it is known that the sampling error is normally distributed, some basic mathematics applied to the normal distribution shows that this variation is related directly to the variability in the population as a whole and inversely to the square root of the sample size.

For example, a survey of daily calorie intake would provide an estimate of both the mean and the standard deviation in the population as a whole. The algebra referred to above then indicates that if the sample size were to be quadrupled, then the standard deviation of the sample estimate (known as the standard error) would be decreased by half.

Reporting sample estimates using 95% confidence intervals

The survey data produces two items of information: an estimate of the population mean and the standard error of this estimate. Since the error is normally distributed, a statement can be made about how the survey estimates relate to the true mean for the population. However, the key point is that the uncertainty being described does not relate to the population but to the sample. The conclusions must therefore be expressed in terms of how often the sample-based estimate comes close to the true population value of the mean. The correct interpretation is that 95% of surveys will provide an estimate of the population mean that is within 1.96 standard errors of the true mean.

Appendix 4: Research data management

If you are collecting or generating data for a research project, then you should consider how the data will be managed during the lifetime of the project and once the project has been completed. In addition, when applying to a funding body you may be required to create a data management plan (Figure A4.1). This appendix considers some of the elements involved in managing your data.

Data management planning

A number of funding bodies now request that a data management plan (DMP) is submitted as part of any funding bid. A DMP identifies how data will be created, stored, shared and preserved and will allow you to plan all aspects of your project in advance.

Funding bodies will usually supply a template to aid creation of your DMP. The responsibility of creating a DMP lies with researchers but your organisation can provide guidance, infrastructure and support staff to help with many areas of data management planning. Even if a DMP is not required, then it is still useful to create one, as it will give you a plan of how to manage your data and potentially help to improve the success of the project.

Storage and backup of data

Always ensure that you have a plan in place for storing and backing up your data. This protects against hardware failure, software faults, malware infection, power failure and human error. Backup files can be kept on a networked filestore or offline on portable hard drive, tape or recordable CD/DVD. Physical media should be moved to another location for safekeeping.

When you develop your backup plan, consider how often you will make backups of your data and where data will be stored. It is tempting to make a backup of your work and then no further backups but you need to consider making regular backups, depending on what additions and changes have been made to the data since the previous backup.

Consult with your organisation on their backup policy. Networked filestore is likely to be the most appropriate solution, particularly if it is enterprise class infrastructure hosted in a secure data centre with offsite backups. You should check with your organisation if there any limitations on what type of data can be stored on networked filestore (e.g. patient identifiable data).

You should consider what volumes of data you will generate and if you are using network filestore, find out in advance from your organisation what storage space is available and if necessary build in any filestore costs to funding applications.

If you are transporting data on portable media or use a laptop computer, you should always encrypt the device. In the event of the device being lost or stolen, then it will be much more difficult for anyone to gain access to the data. If you intend using encrypted devices, then you must ensure that you keep a secure note of the encryption key. If you forget or lose the key, then it will be impossible to access your data as the whole point of encryption is to prevent unauthorised access.

You may wish to consider using a cloud storage service to store data but you should consider if it is appropriate for your data to be held on such services. Your organisation will be able to advise.

Sharing of data

You should consider how you will share your data with collaborators, internal to your organisation and externally. Sharing data externally can help enhance your research profile, promote your research, may be a requirement of your funder and of your organisation, and could help secure future funding. Data sharing is encouraged by all UK funding councils.

Anonymisation of data

Before you store or share data, you may need to anonymise the data so that individuals, organisations and businesses cannot be identified. Personal data should never be disclosed from research information unless specific consent has been given, preferably in writing. You should plan how you will anonymise data as anonymisation can be time-consuming and ultimately costly.

Documenting data

Documenting data should be considered when creating, organising and managing data and is particularly important for data preservation.

Formatting data

Ensure that you consider the file formats you are saving or creating data in. Data can be at risk if software or hardware becomes obsolete. Many software packages offer backwards compatibility and can import data created in previous versions of software; however, there is risk that software cannot be read correctly.

Retention and destruction of data

Consider how long you are going to retain your data, how it is going to be retained and, very importantly, how you are going to destroy the data. When you delete data from a hard drive, the data is not fully deleted and can be recovered very easily. There is software available which will allow data to be securely deleted that would make it very difficult for it to be restored. Your organisation will be able to advise on secure data deletion.

Further reading

UK Data Archive, http://www.data-archive.ac.uk/
Data Curation Centre, http://www.dcc.ac.uk/

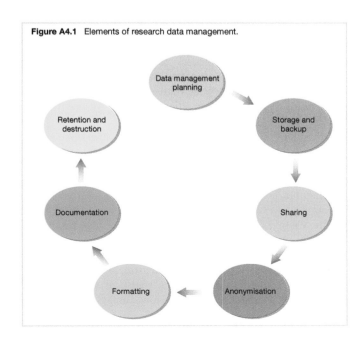

Figure A4.1 Elements of research data management.

Appendix 5: Types of data

In quantitative research, items of information (data) occur in different forms or *data types*, all of which may be observed or measured directly or indirectly.

• *Interval data* are physical measurements.

• *Ordinal data* take the form of ordered categories such as levels of symptom severity.

• *Nominal data* take the form of unordered categories, for example as used to describe marital status.

Items of data of any type may be referred to as *variables* or *items*. A fourth and less common data type is ratio data that arises from the comparison of two interval variables.

Identifying the correct data type is an essential step in planning data collection and in the choice of methods for data analysis.

Interval data

Interval data is collected from physical measurements such as height, weight or blood pressure. It is also referred to as *continuous data*. Interval data are the only type of data for which arithmetic procedures can be applied and can be summarised using descriptive statistics or compared in the form of ratios.

Ordinal data

Ordinal data is obtained when assessments are *ranked* into ordered categories. Examples include symptom severity or age groups. While the groupings are ordered, they may not be comparable in size. It follows that if ordered groups are labelled 1, 2, 3, etc. it does not make sense to apply arithmetic methods. Ordinal data may be summarised in terms of *frequency counts*, percentages and descriptive statistics based on ranking such as the *median*, the *interquartile range and the mode* but not the mean and standard deviation. Ordinal data is sometimes referred to as *discontinuous data*.

By definition, the coding of ordered responses to items or questions comprising quality of life or similar questionnaires or measurement scales is ordinal in form. Despite this, it is common practice to add together the resulting scores on each item to obtain a total score. Where this is done the total score should itself be considered ordinal. Where published work treats the total as an interval variable and reports means and standard deviations, there should be some justification in the text. Status as ordinal or interval has implications for the choice of method of analysis.

Nominal data

Nominal data are obtained from the coding of unordered categories; for example, coding of marital status or occupation would produce nominal data. At data entry the codes assigned to represent each category may be numeric (1, 2, 3, etc.) but again it is not appropriate to calculate means or standard deviations. The data are summarised using frequency counts, percentages and the mode.

Appendix 6: Data requirement planning

Research hypotheses, data requirement and methods of analysis

In quantitative research, the research hypotheses define the outcome measure(s), the overall data requirement, the sources of the data and the timing and methods used to collect data. In particular this seeks to eliminate effects that may bias findings. This includes a clear definition of the sources of the data, of the data sources (who or what is to be measured), and how and when the measurements are to be made. In turn, the outcomes to be reported largely define the scope and method of data analysis.

Data management

Researchers need to identify their precise data requirement and ensure that their data remain safe. Collecting too much data or insufficient data or failing to keep the data safe and private undermines the research process and is unethical.

Primary and secondary data sources

Primary data sources are those identified in the research proposal in the sense that they are a perfect match to the research hypothesis in question. They give a direct measure of outcome on a clearly defined population at a specified point in time. Where such primary sources are not available or is for some reason inaccessible, researchers may identify alternative or secondary sources of data. These may be in the form of existing datasets or in some form of proxy measure. For financial or other reasons there may be no alternative to this approach but it does introduce the possibility of bias, for example where definitions have changed over time or where earlier selection criteria are not a perfect match for the new research.

How much data is needed?

Sample size calculations based on the research hypotheses are used to determine the required sample size for the research.

Planned and secondary analyses

The planned or primary analysis of the data is that which tests the original research hypotheses. In a randomised controlled trial this involves comparing treatment effects; in a cohort study it involves identifying factors associated with the primary outcome(s). Additional planned analyses may assess other variables that may be associated with outcome.

Secondary or unplanned analyses are used to assess additional factors that may be associated with outcome. The results of such analyses need to be interpreted and presented with caution. It may be that the method of measurement or the method of case selection introduces some source of bias, for example in terms of overall health status or demographic profile. Changes in treatment or management may mean that data on historical cases are not comparable to more recent data and may bias outcomes.

The Bonferroni correction, an adjustment to the level of probability required to demonstrate statistical significance, is applied where a large number of unplanned analyses is proposed.

Appendix 7: Descriptive statistics

Descriptive statistics

In any set of data the values are seen to vary. Descriptive statistics are used to describe the data in terms of the mid-point and of the variability around the mid-point.

• *Measures of location* or *central tendency* describe the mid-point of the data.
• *Measures of dispersion* describe the spread or variability of the data around the mid-point.

Descriptive statistics based on a *sample* drawn from a *population* provide *estimates* of *true* population values or *parameters*.

As well as describing or estimating population parameters, descriptive statistics are used in *hypothesis testing* and other forms of statistical inference such as regression analysis.

Measures of location or central tendency

• The *mean* is the average value of the dataset. It is calculated as the sum of the data points divided by the number of data points.
• The *median* is the middle value of the range, so 50% of data values are less than the median and 50% greater than the median.
• The *mode* is the most common data value in the dataset.

Measures of dispersion

The *minimum* value is the lowest value in the dataset. The *maximum* is the highest value in the dataset. The *range* is the difference between the minimum and maximum.

The *standard deviation* and *variance* are the most common measures of dispersion. The variance is the mean squared difference between each data point and the mean and the standard deviation is the square root of the variance. Since the standard deviation is in the same units as the original data, it is the most important measure of how widely the data are spread on either side of the mean. Distributions with a small standard deviation have a narrow range; distributions with large standard deviations have a wide range.

Where 'data are skewed rather than symmetrically distributed around the mean, percentiles provide a more appropriate measure of dispersion.

• *Centiles* or *percentiles* (100 in total) each identify 1% of the distribution across the range.
• The *median* is the 50th percentile.
• Similarly, *quartiles* mark 25%, 50% and 75% of the range; *deciles* mark 10%, 20%, 30%, etc. across the range; *quintiles* mark 20%, 40%, 60%, etc. across the range; and *terciles* mark 33.3% and 66.7% across the range.

Appendix 8: Frequency distribution

Frequency and population distributions

Researchers often present their data in the form of frequency distributions. This may be in the form of a histogram for age or a bar chart or pie chart for marital status. In each of these the height of a bar or the area of a chart reflects the numbers of individuals within the specific grouping. For large samples such charts reflect the distribution for the population as a whole. Among these population-based frequency distributions a number of similarly shaped distributions are recognised. These include the normal, Poisson and binomial distributions.

The normal distribution

It is a common feature of physical measurements that there are relatively few extreme values at either end of the range and many values located in the middle of the range. Where the spread is symmetrical around the mid-point (mean) of the distribution, the data are said to be normally distributed. Typical examples include measures of height and weight.

The shape of the normal distribution is defined by a mathematical formula based only on the mean and the standard deviation, the parameters of the normal distribution. This formula is then used to calculate the percentage of the distribution that lies within defined distance from the mean. For example, some 95% of values lie within two standard deviations of the mean. The same applies to all the percentiles of the normal distribution.

• *Application 1*: neonatal weight for age and similar charts rely on the features of the normal distribution to track the growth of a child relative to a range of percentiles describing the range of values expected in the early years of life.
• *Application 2*: in estimating population parameters, for example in survey work, sampling error is understood to be normally distributed, so allowing the calculation of 95% confidence intervals for estimates of population parameters.
• *Application 3*: because it is so common, many statistical tests are based on the assumption of normally distributed data.

Other common data distributions

The *Poisson distribution* describes the frequencies or counts of random unrelated events in a given time period. Examples include the number of accidents per year on a defined stretch of road, the number of letters received in a day and the number of people requiring hospitalisation in a day. As with the normal distribution, the mean defines the mid-point but the distribution is skewed. The variance is equal to the mean and the standard deviation is equal to the square root of the variance. Other recognised distributions include the *binomial*, *multinomial*, *U-shaped*, *uniform* and *exponential*.

Appendix 9: Hypothesis testing and statistical significance

Null and alternative hypotheses

In quantitative research assessing alternative forms of treatment or intervention, researchers define a measurable outcome and design their research in a way that ensures an unbiased comparison can be made between interventions. Through the process of hypothesis testing they then assess their data in the context of two alternative understandings (hypotheses) of what the data may show. Most commonly these take the following forms.

- *Null hypothesis*: there is no difference between the interventions.
- *Alternative hypothesis*: either that a difference exists or that one intervention is more effective than the other (also known as *non-directional* and *directional* alternatives).

The hypothesis test then proceeds by assuming that the null hypothesis is true.

Statistical significance

To decide if the data are consistent with the assumption that the null hypothesis is true, the researcher wants to know how likely it is (the probability that) the observed difference between treatments could have arisen by chance. The methods used to compute this probability depend on the type of data being compared, its distribution and the type of comparison being made (see Appendix 10).

The chosen test is then applied to the data and reports the level of probability associated with the observed difference under the assumption that the null hypothesis is true. This is assessed by comparison with the level of probability defining *statistical significance*. Most commonly this is a probability of 0.05 (5%).

Drawing a conclusion

If the null hypothesis is true, then large differences will be rare and have small probabilities; in other words, low reported probabilities suggest the null hypothesis may be inappropriate. Specifically, probabilities less than the level defining statistical significance lead to the rejection of the null hypothesis and acceptance of the alternative. Such differences are said to be statistically significant at the 5% or 1% level, as appropriate, and reported in the form $P < 0.05$ or $P < 0.01$. Conversely, probabilities greater than the level defining statistical significance lead to acceptance of the null hypothesis and the conclusion of no difference between treatments.

Other points to note

Hypothesis testing is a probability-based procedure. It does not demonstrate causality. The statement of findings needs to make this clear by stating the level of statistical significance that has been applied.

As in repeated tosses of a coin, extreme results do occur by chance. In hypothesis testing this may mean that two forms of error may occur.

- A *Type I error* occurs when the data suggest a difference exists but in reality there is no real difference.
- A *Type II error* occurs when the data suggest there is no difference when in fact a real difference does exist.

The only way to demonstrate that either a Type I or a Type II error has occurred is to repeat the research. Meta-analysis of combined findings then benefits from larger numbers and reduces the probability of both Type I and Type II errors occurring.

Appendix 10: Choosing the right test

Factors to be considered

In hypothesis testing it is essential to choose the right statistical test. The choice of test depends on six factors.

1 How many variables are involved, one, two or three or more?
2 What data types are involved?
3 Do the data follow a normal or other recognised distribution?
4 Are dependent and independent variables identified within the data?
5 What is the nature of the relationship between variables?
6 What is the sample size?

With this information to hand, Tables A10.1, A10.2 and A10.3 provide a guide to selection of some basic tests. A number of web-based resources are available covering a much wider range of data types and relationships between variables.

Table A10.1 Tests involving two variables.

Variable type	Paired assessments	Independent assessments
Both variables nominal	McNemar test	Fisher's exact test or chi-squared test
Both variables ordinal (or interval data requiring non-parametric methods)	Sign test Wilcoxon signed-rank test	Mann–Whitney U test
Both variables interval data qualifying for parametric methods	Student's paired *t*-test	Student's independent *t*-test

Table A10.2 Tests involving three or more groups.

Variable type	Paired assessments	Independent assessments
Both variables nominal	Cochran's Q	Chi-squared test
Both variables ordinal (or interval data requiring non-parametric methods)	Friedman test (ANOVA of ranks)	Kruskal–Wallis test
Both variables interval data qualifying for parametric methods	Repeated measures analysis of variance	Analysis of variance

Table A10.3 Measures of correlation or association.

Variable type	Paired assessments
Both variables nominal	Contingency coefficient
Both variables ordinal (or interval data requiring non-parametric methods)	Spearman's rank order correlation coefficient (rho)
Both variables interval data qualifying for parametric methods	Pearson's product-moment correlation coefficient (*r*)

Appendix 11: Non-parametric tests

When to use non-parametric tests

Non-parametric tests are tests of statistical significance applied where data do not meet the requirements for parametric tests.

• When data do not meet the distributional requirements for parametric tests, for example the normal, Poisson and binomial distributions. Sometimes data can be transformed into a known form, for example log-transformed data may be normally distributed. When comparing means with sample sizes greater than 30, the central limit theorem allows this rule to be relaxed. The *Kolmogorov–Smirnov* and *Shapiro–Wilks* tests are used to test that data are normally distributed.

• When data within groups have different variances.

• When data are collected using a measurement scale where questions are assessed by responses such as 'Strongly disagree', 'Disagree', 'Agree', 'Strongly Agree' coded as numbers 0–3 or 1–4. This is ordinal rather than interval data so it is inappropriate to apply the arithmetic methods of parametric tests.

Examples of non-parametric tests and their use

• The *sign test* is used to assess whether a sample-based summary statistic, usually the median, differs from a known population value.

• The *Mann–Whitney U test* is the non-parametric equivalent of the Student independent samples *t*-test, a test for differences in the mean between two independent groups.

• The *Kruskal–Wallis test* is used to compare two or more groups and is the non-parametric equivalent of a one-way analysis of variance.

• The *Wilcoxon signed rank test* is the non-parametric equivalent of the Student paired samples *t*-test and is used to test hypotheses concerning differences between paired assessments. In the one-sample case, the comparison is with a specified mean value for the population.

• The *McNemar test* is a non-parametric test of nominal data in 2×2 tables in which matched data pairs are compared for the presence or absence of some characteristic of interest, including the presence of a symptom before and after some intervention.

• The *Friedman test* is equivalent to the one-way analysis of variance with repeated measures, most commonly across time.

• The *log-rank test* is a test of difference between survival rates.

Appendix 12: Student's *t*-test

Student's *t*-tests are used to assess differences between two means in the context of independent or paired assessments. They are designed for use where the standard deviation in the population is unknown and has to be estimated from the sample data. The precision of the estimate depends on the sample size, so it is a feature of *t*-tests that they are always reported for a specified number of *degrees of freedom*, which is the sample size adjusted downwards by 1 within each group to allow for the estimation of the standard deviation.

There are two separate tests, one used to compare the means of independent samples and one to compare the means of paired samples. Each requires the null and alternative hypotheses that are a feature of all hypothesis testing and works by calculating a value of the *t* statistic. For the available degrees of freedom, the range and shape of the *t* distribution is known, so the *P*-value or statistical significance can be reported.

Since the *t* distribution is sensitive to the number of degrees of freedom or sample size, values of the *t* statistic based on small samples require more extreme values in order to demonstrate statistical significance. In contrast, for larger sample sizes (more degrees of freedom), estimates are more precise and the critical value of the *t* statistic is correspondingly less demanding. As sample sizes increase, the *t* distribution becomes closer to the normal distribution.

Student's independent *t*-test

This test is used to assess the statistical significance of differences between means in two independent groups. It requires normally distributed data and equal variances in each group, though where variances differ the alternative (Satterthwaite) approach to computing the pooled variance is adopted. The degrees of freedom are calculated as the total group size less 2, making an adjustment for the estimation of the standard deviation within each group.

Student's paired *t*-test

This test is used to assess the statistical significance of differences between means of paired assessments. Such data arise from repeat assessments of the same subjects or from assessments of matched cases and controls. The test requires that the data are normally distributed.

The paired test examines the differences between paired assessments and tests for a difference significantly different from 0. The degrees of freedom are calculated as the number of paired assessments less 1, again making an adjustment for the estimation of the standard deviation from the available data.

Appendix 13: Analysis of variance

Analysis of variance (ANOVA) is the method used to analyse data from a wide range of experimental designs used in randomised controlled trials. These research designs may become very complex, with multiple treatments or interventions each defined at several levels. Among human subjects, the necessary level of control can be difficult to achieve, so simpler designs are preferred and results are interpreted with more caution.

ANOVA works by computing and comparing the difference or variation between treatment groups with the variation within treatment groups. Within each group all subjects receive the same treatment so the variability reflects only random variation in response. The variation between groups provides an estimate of the treatment effect. Comparing the between-group variation with the within-group variation therefore gives an estimate of the treatment effect. If between-group and within-group variation are similar, then there is no treatment effect. Between-group variation greater than within-group variation suggests there is a treatment effect. The extent of the treatment effect is reported in the F statistic and the related probability identifying statistically significant treatment effects.

Forms of analysis of variance and related terminology

• The analysis procedure is tailored to a mathematical *model* that for each subject identifies the treatment effects that may affect each subject's outcome.
• *One-way analysis of variance* is the simplest model, where outcome is dependent only on how subjects respond to a single treatment or intervention.
• *Two-way analysis of variance* is used for the more complex research design where outcome is dependent on how subjects respond to a combination of two treatments or interventions. (Similarly, three-way and more complex designs.)
• Additional *interaction effects* may be added to the two-way or more complex models where it is expected that the response to one treatment may vary according to the level of other treatment(s).
• *Factorial designs* are used to assess response to multiple treatments each defined at two or more levels and the complex interactions between them.

In all these, the research design is carefully managed to ensure that the separate treatment and interaction effects can be assessed using ANOVA, which compares appropriate between-group and within-group variation.

Further analyses and research design

• For each treatment, *post-hoc testing* may be used to compare and assess the effect of different treatment levels or dosage. For unplanned comparisons, the *Bon-Ferroni method* may be applied.
• *Repeated measure designs*: where research designs involve repeated assessments over time, the repeated measures on each subject are correlated. This requires an adjustment be applied in assessing the reported levels of statistical significance. Depending on the level of correlation the Huynh–Feldt, Greenhouse–Geisser or lower bound adjustments are applied.
• In *crossed* designs (as described above), the number of treatment groups matches the number of treatment combinations. In *nested* designs, the levels of one or more treatments may be nested within the levels of another. In this situation the levels of one treatment are said to be *confounded* within the levels of another. ANOVA methods can still be used to assess treatment effects, but a more complex comparison has to be made in order to overcome the confounding.
• In *crossover designs* subjects receive all treatments in turn.

Appendix 14: Tabulating data and the chi-squared test

Summarising data in tables

Presenting data in tables is a convenient way to summarise data from two ordinal or nominal variables, for example data on age group and severity of symptoms. These are also known as *contingency tables* or *cross-tabulations* since they summarise all possible outcomes.

	Low	Normal	Total
Younger	21	15	36
Older	16	2	18
Total	37	17	54

The *columns* of the table divide study participants according to some physical measure (columns) and age (rows). Each *cell* of the table gives the count of participants with the specific combination of the physical measure and age group.

Comparing the rows or columns of a table

The value of tabulating data is that it becomes possible to make comparisons between groups, for example answering the research question 'Is the physical measure associated with age group?' Comparisons are best made using percentages, so row percentages could be added to the table.

	Low	Normal	Total
Younger	21 (58%)	15 (42%)	36
Older	16 (89%)	2 (11%)	18
Total	37	17	54

The table now tells us that 89% of older patients had a low score for the physical measure compared with 58% in the younger age group, suggesting that the low measurements are somehow associated with age. To draw a conclusion, the researcher wants to assess the strength of the evidence: how likely is it that this result has arisen by chance? This requires a statistical test, the *chi-squared test*.

Applying the chi-squared test

Based on the assumption (null hypothesis) of no association, the chi-squared test procedure calculates the value of the test statistic and an associated probability. High probabilities suggest the outcome has occurred by chance, small probabilities suggesting an association exists. The value of the chi-squared test statistic for this example is 5.194 with 1 degree of freedom. The associated probability is less than 0.05, so it would be reported that there is evidence of a statistically significant association between age group and the physical measurement ($P < 0.05$).

The range of possible values for the chi-squared test statistic varies according to the number of rows and columns in the table. Chi-squared statistics are therefore always reported with the number of degrees of freedom. These are calculated as the (number of table rows − 1) × (number of table columns − 1); hence, 1 degree of freedom in the example above.

Alternative tests

- For small numbers (less than 100 data items) the calculation of the chi-squared statistic should include a continuity correction. Where the numbers are less than 40, Fisher's exact test should be applied.
- Chi-squared computed using the *likelihood ratio method*.
- Test of *differences between proportions*: apply the chi-squared test as described here.
- The *contingency coefficient* is a measure of association between variables in a 2 × 2 table calculated as the square root of the chi-squared value divided by the sample size and is denoted by the Greek symbol φ (phi).

Other test statistics calculated from data presented in 2 × 2 tables include the following.

- *Relative risks*: the probability of an outcome event in the experimental group compared with the probability in the control group. Where relative risk is less than 1.0, the event is less likely in the experimental group. Where relative risk is greater than 1.0, the event is more likely in the experimental group.
- *Sensitivity*, *specificity* and *positive* or *negative predictive value* (PPV, NPV) are used to compare a screening test to a standard method.
- *Cohen's kappa* and *weighted kappa* are used to assess inter-rater reliability by comparing observed agreement against agreement expected by chance.
- *Cramer's V* is an alternative measure of association between nominal variables in a contingency table.
- *Kendall's tau* is a measure of rank correlation.
- *Goodman and Kruskal's gamma* is a measure based on the difference between concordant pairs and discordant pairs.
- *McNemar's test* is a paired sample sign test.

Appendix 15: Correlation

What is correlation?

Correlation is a measure of association between variables. The statistical concept matches common usage in, for example, the positive correlation between the level of exercise and the level of perspiration and the negative correlation between the ambient temperature and the weight of clothing worn.

Statistical definition and characteristics

In statistical usage, correlation is a measure of the *linear association* between two variables, hence a *bivariate correlation*.

• Correlation is computed as a number in the range −1 to +1.
• Where the values of two interval variables increase together there is a *positive correlation*, i.e. a correlation greater than 0.0.
• A correlation of 1.0 is said to be *perfect positive correlation*.
• Where one of the interval variables increases as the other decreases there is a *negative correlation*, i.e. a correlation less than 0.0.
• A correlation of −1.0 is said to be *perfect negative correlation*. Two unrelated interval variables have a correlation of zero (0.0), each variable changing in a way that is independent of the other.
• The most widely used statistical measure of correlation is the *Pearson product moment correlation coefficient*, denoted by the letter *r* in publications.

• Correlations are *symmetrical*, the correlation between variables *x* and *y* being identical to the correlation between variables *y* and *x*.
• Correlations are also interpreted as the *proportion of variation* in one variable that is explained by the associated variable.

Limitations

• The Pearson correlation coefficient can only be calculated for interval data. The alternative Spearman rank order correlation is calculated for ordinal data.
• The correlation coefficient is valid only where there is a simple linear relationship between variables: across the whole range of values a change in one variable is associated with an equivalent change in the other.
• In addition, both variables should be normally distributed with equal variances, no outliers, minimal measurement error and unrestricted data from the full range of possible values.

Statistical tests of correlation

Available tests assess whether a correlation is significantly different from zero and whether two correlations differ.

Appendix 16: Measuring and interpreting correlation

In undertaking research, researchers are often interested in trying to find linear relationships (correlations) between two or more variables. Correlation measures how strongly two variables are related to each other. For example, as a researcher I might be interested in whether there is a relationship between the amount of time spent studying this textbook and the reader's knowledge and understanding of healthcare research.

Scientists measure the strength of a correlation by using a number called a *correlational coefficient*, which indicates the size and direction of the relationship between two variables. The number ranges from −1 to +1. If two variables (like the older your car gets, the more money you spend on repairs) have a correlation above zero (e.g. +0.76), then you have a positive correlation: as the car increases in age, the higher the annual cost of repairs. If the number is below zero (e.g. −0.42), then you have a negative correlation and when one variable goes up the other goes down (like winter and ice cream sales or sales of sunglasses). If two variables have a correlation of zero, then they have *no* relationship with each other. The closer the numbers to either +1 or −1, the stronger the correlation. The significance test for a correlation coefficient is directly related to the sample size. In general, if the sample size is small, the correlation coefficient has to be large (close to −1 or +1) for the correlation to be significant.

Although these values indicate the size and direction of the relationship between variables, this does *not* imply that one causes the other. For example, a student's exam performance may go down as anxiety about exams increases, but we cannot say that anxiety causes bad exam performance.

Returning to the earlier example of ice cream sales, a local ice cream vendor keeps track of how much ice cream he or she sells versus the temperature on that day. Table A16.1 illustrates the figures obtained for 12 consecutive days. We can graphically display the similarity (or otherwise) of the relationship between the two variables (i.e. ice cream sales and temperature) being measured. Figure A16.1 shows how that data looks when entered in a scatterplot and tells us several things about the data, such as whether a relationship exists and what kind of relationship it is. The pattern of the data would suggest that a positive relationship exists.

Bivariate correlation

Having taken a close look at the data, we can conduct the correlation analysis. There are two types of correlation: bivariate

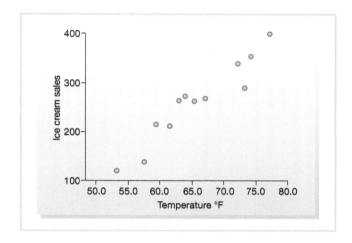

Figure A16.1 Scatterplot showing the relationship between ice cream sales and temperature.

and partial. A bivariate is a correlation between two variables (as described earlier), whereas a partial correlation looks at the relationship between two variables while controlling the effect of one or more additional variables. Pearson's product moment correlation coefficient and Spearman's rank correlation coefficient are examples of bivariate correlation coefficients (Field, 2009). Spearman's rank correlation coefficient (ρ or r_s) is regarded as the non-parametric equivalent to Pearson's product moment correlation coefficient. Spearman's rank correlation coefficient is calculated if neither variable is distributed normally or if one of the variables is discrete (e.g. the number of decayed, missing or filled missing teeth) or is measured on an ordinal scale (e.g. a depression rating score). Other non-parametric correlation coefficients also exist, including Kendall's rank correlation coefficient (denoted by τ).

In Figure A16.2 a straight line has been added that best represents the relationship between the two variables. We can easily see that warmer weather leads to more ice cream sales; the relationship is good but not perfect. In fact the correlation coefficient is 0.95. Research papers report correlational coefficients with regard to how big they are and what their significance value was, so in our case we are able to report that there was a significant relationship between the registered outside temperature and the

Table A16.1 Data collected on number of ice cream purchases and daily temperature.

Temperature (°F)	Ice cream sales
57.5	140
61.5	212
53.4	120
59.4	216
65.3	264
72	340
67	268
77	400
74	354
64	274
73	290
63	265

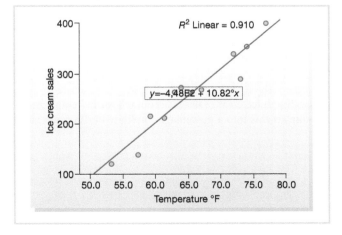

Figure A16.2 Scatterplot showing the relationship between ice cream sales and temperature following linear regression (line added).

Figure A16.3 How correlation coefficients are reported.

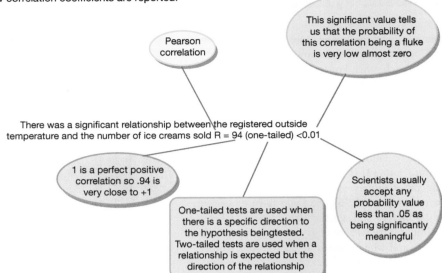

number of ice creams sold: $r = 0.94$, P (one-tailed) <0.01. Figure A16.3 explains each of the different elements.

Regression models

Regression models provide scientists with mean of fitting a predictive model to the data obtained and explain how an outcome variable (e.g. ice cream sales) varies for different values of one or more explanatory (or independent) variables (e.g. temperature). Different types of outcome variable require different forms of regression model. Simple linear regression, multiple linear regression, logistic regression and ordinal logistic regression are among the common types included in research reports. Simple linear regression, as used in our case, provides a measure of the nature of the linear association between two variables (i.e. the gradient of the straight line drawn through the points in Figure A16.2) and permits the prediction of an outcome variable given the value of an explanatory variable (Sedgwick, 2014). Multiple regression is simply an extension of the fundamental principles of simple regression but incorporates several predictors that are entered into a model to assess which predictors contribute substantially to the model's ability to predict the outcome. Field (2009) provides a user-friendly account of regression modelling, while Kasza and Wolfe (2014) provide a review of a number of different regression models as applied in respiratory health research.

Having run a simple regression analysis on the data, Table A16.2 provides values of R and R^2. The R value of 0.95 represents the simple correlation between temperature and ice cream sales. Although we cannot make direct conclusions about causality, we can take the correlation coefficient further by squaring it (known as the coefficient of determination or R^2), which is a measure of the amount of variability in one variable that is explained by the other. The R^2 value in this case is 0.91, which tells us how variability in ice cream sales is accounted for by temperature. If we convert this into a percentage (multiply by 100), we can say

Table A16.2 Regression model summary.

Model	R	R^2	Adjusted R^2	Standard error of the estimate
1	0.954[a]	0.910	0.901	25.884

[a] Predictors: (constant), temperature.

Table A16.3 ANOVA.

Model		Sum of squares	d.f.	Mean square	F	Significance
1	Regression	67533.021	1	67533.021	100.797	0.000[b]
	Residual	6699.896	10	669.990		
	Total	74232.917	11			

[a] Dependent variable: sales.
[b] Predictors: (constant), temperature.

that temperature accounts for 91% of the variability in ice cream sales.

The accompanying ANOVA (Table A16.3) includes two key pieces of information: the F ratio and the significance of that ratio. From the table we can see that $F = 100.79$, which is significant at $P < 0.001$. This result means that there is less than 0.1% chance than an F ratio of this size would happen by chance alone. In brief, the regression model overall predicts ice cream sales really well.

References

Field, A.P. (2009) *Discovering Statistics Using SPSS*, 3rd edn. London: Sage.

Kasza, J. and Wolfe, R. (2014) Interpretation of commonly used statistical regression models. *Respirology* **19**, 14–21.

Sedgwick, P. (2014). Spearman's rank correlation coefficient. *British Medical Journal* **349**, g7327.

Appendix 17: Simple linear regression

Regression analysis describes how an *outcome* or *dependent* variable changes in response to changes in a *predictor*, *explanatory* or *independent* variable.

Simple linear regression is the basic form of regression in which the rate of change in a measure of outcome is related to unit change (a change of 1.0) in a predictor variable. Typical examples include the relationship between bone density and age or between symptom severity and delay in diagnosis and start of treatment.

To quantify such relationships, simple linear regression computes the average rate of change in outcome for a change of 1.0 in the predictor variable. This is known as the *regression coefficient*. When the data are plotted on a chart, this indicates the *slope* of the regression line. In addition, the analysis also reports *95% confidence intervals* for the regression coefficient, whether the regression coefficient is statistically different from zero, and a statistic (R^2) which is the *proportion of variation* in the outcome explained by the predictor variable.

The method of analysis used to compute the regression coefficient is known as the *method of least squares*, the resulting slope of the regression line being that which minimises the squared difference between the observed values and the values predicted by the regression.

Other terminology related to regression: interpolation and extrapolation

These are best explained using an example. When the rate of change in bone density with age is known, the expected bone density for a given age can be estimated. When the age is within the range of ages used to compute the regression coefficient, this is known as *interpolation*. When the age is outside the range used to compute the regression coefficient, this is known as *extrapolation*. Extrapolation requires a cautious approach as it involves the assumption that the observed relationship extends beyond the range of available data. This may not be the case.

Correlation or regression?

Both correlation and regression measure association between variables. The important difference is that correlations are symmetrical, not taking into account the status of dependent or independent variables. Correlation assumes a linear relationship between variables, whereas regression analysis can be extended to assess more complex relationships between two or more variables. It also reports the rate of change in the predicted variable in response to one or more predictor variables.

More on regression

- Data need to be normally distributed or transformed to normal by applying a log-transformation.
- Data must be interval in form, otherwise the method of least squares is inappropriate.
- Outlying data points may have a disproportionate effect on the analysis. They need to be identified and checked, but it may be appropriate to exclude them from the analysis.
- *Missing values* may be dealt with by omitting subjects, by omitting variables, or by setting a default value.
- The differences between *observed values* and *predicted values* are known as *residuals*.
- *Multiple regression* is used to assess the predictive value of more than one predictor variable.
- *Stepwise regression* identifies variables that are statistically significant predictors, the best predictive model.

Appendix 18: Meta-analysis

Combining research findings

It is a common experience of researchers that their findings are suggestive of some effect but require much large numbers in order to be of real significance.

The method of meta-analysis is used by researchers to identify and combine similar research studies with a shared measure of outcome in the hope that the combined samples from multiple studies may demonstrate a statistically significant effect that was not evident from some or all of the individual studies. Typically, results of meta-analyses are presented as part of a systematic review of the literature.

Systematic reviews

Researchers use systematic reviews to collate and assess the accumulated weight of evidence concerning the effect of some treatment or intervention. Such reviews follow rigorous research procedures to identify and collate research findings, focusing on studies which themselves followed the most rigorous research designs, specifically randomised controlled trials as the gold standard, plus the findings from earlier systematic reviews. The design and execution of each trial is closely evaluated and only trials maintaining the highest standards are included. This process provides the researcher with a core of comparable and reliable trials from which results can be compared and/or combined.

Meta-analysis is the process used to compare and make sense of the results of a series of independent studies that assess a common treatment using identical or equivalent measures of outcome. By setting strict inclusion and exclusion criteria the approach brings together comparable studies, irrespective of their sample sizes, and uses a standardised approach to report a combined finding. Results are presented in a funnel plot.

Drawing conclusions

Meta-analysis extends hypothesis testing across multiple related studies with the possibility of generalisation across the populations represented. It therefore maximises the available sample size and statistical power and produces the most precise estimate of treatment effects or outcome. Findings may be summarised using a forest plot, which presents odds ratios or relative risks plus 95% confidence intervals for each study and in total.

Limitations

Since studies vary in size and may represent different populations, combining results can be problematic. Larger sample sizes should give greater precision, so should carry greater weight as should studies with more outcome events, while studies reporting greater variation in the effect should carry less weight.

Some meta-analyses include analysis of findings within subgroups that are of special interest. This may relate to a selection of studies, for example on the basis of rigour, or oriented to characteristics of patients. There may therefore be concern that this goes beyond the original research objectives and a potential source of bias. Other statistical methods are available to compute the effect size from combined studies.

Appendix 19: Propensity score matching

Propensity score matching (PSM) is a method for causal inference from observational studies (Figure A19.1). In medical research, causal inferences are typically drawn from randomised controlled trials; however, sometimes randomisation is not feasible for ethical or budgetary reasons (Rubin, 2007), which makes it acceptable to estimate treatment effects from observational studies.

A typical experiment assigns two or more groups of individuals to different treatments, for example a novel intervention versus usual care as control. The assignment can be part of regular care processes without randomisation (as natural experiment) or as part of an experiment with randomisation as in a randomised controlled trial. The randomisation primarily serves the purpose of avoiding selection bias. Selection bias in this context means that individuals receiving the novel intervention are different from individuals receiving usual care, which can ultimately lead to biased estimates of the treatment effect. This biased assignment could happen in a non-randomised experiment where the care provider consciously or unconsciously assigns participants with certain characteristics to either the treatment or the control group

Figure A19.1 Propensity score matching (PSM) is an analytical technique for estimating causal treatment effects from observational data.

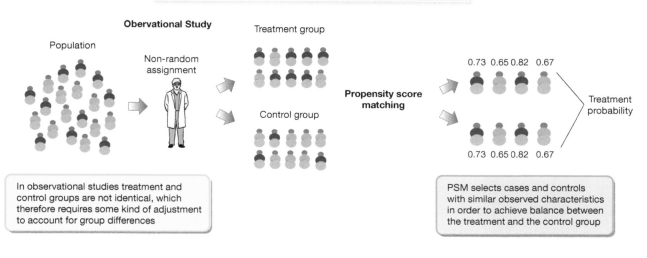

Randomised Controlled Trial

Population — Random assignment — Treatment group / Control group

Ideally, treatment effects are derived from large randomised controlled trials. However sometimes randomisation is not feasible and data from an observational study is used to assess the effectiveness of an intervention

Key characteristic of the random assignment of participants is the balance of observed and unobserved characteristics in the treatment and the control group

EXAMPLE

The Magnet programme recognises hospitals for excellent nursing care. It is a hospital-level intervention and an interventional study would require to (i) randomly assign patients to a Magnet hospital or a non-Magnet hospital in close proximity with identical hospital characteristics or (ii) to randomly 'assign' Magnet recognition to hospitals for a cluster randomised trial. Both options are not feasible, which makes an observational study the approach of choice. In an observational study we could compare publicly reported patient satisfaction data and hypothesise that patients in Magnet hospitals are more satisfied with the care provided than patients from non-Magnet hospitals. Because hospital (e.g. bed size, ownership status) and patient (e.g. age, severity) characteristics differ between Magnet and non-Magnet hospitals, we cannot directly compare patient satisfaction. PSM helps to select hospitals with similar characteristics in both groups. The propensity score is the probability of a given hospital to be in the treatment group. The probability is calculated with a logistic regression model and is determined by observed characteristics of the hospitals. When hospitals have been selected for the comparison, the balance (similar distribution of characteristics between treatment and control group) is the main criterion to assess if PSM has been successful. In this example, we would hope to find a similar number of university hospitals as well as a similar mean age of patients or case mix index (CMI) in the two groups of hospitals (Table A19.1).

Table A19.1 Hospital characteristics before and after PSM.

			Before PSM	After PSM
Treatment		Age	54	54
	% University hospital		35	35
		CMI	1.54	1.54
Control		Age	62	55
	% University hospital		18	32
		CMI	1.12	1.53

Obervational Study

Population — Non-random assignment — Treatment group / Control group

Propensity score matching

0.73 0.65 0.82 0.67

0.73 0.65 0.82 0.67

Treatment probability

In observational studies treatment and control groups are not identical, which therefore requires some kind of adjustment to account for group differences

PSM selects cases and controls with similar observed characteristics in order to achieve balance between the treatment and the control group so that the baseline characteristics in both groups are not alike. The advantage of randomisation is to evenly assign participants to the treatment and the control group so that characteristics in both groups are balanced. This balance is not just achieved for observed characteristics but also for unmeasured or unknown characteristics, which gives randomised experiments the fundamental advantage over non-randomised experiments and all observational designs.

Basics of propensity score matching

In order to address selection bias in observational studies, researchers usually account for differences in baseline characteristics with stratification or linear/logistic regression methods. Regression analysis is used to directly predict the outcome accounting for observed differences in characteristics in both groups and to determine if the treatment had a significant impact. PSM also employs logistic regression, but with the aim of determining the probability or 'propensity' of the participants to be in the treatment or control group. The propensity score is then used to match participants from the treatment to the control group (or vice versa). There are several matching methods (e.g. 'nearest neighbour') that ultimately achieve the same goal: to create two groups that share the same baseline characteristics.

Balance

The similarity of the treatment and the control group in the context of PSM is called *balance* and is the prime indicator for successful PSM. There has been some methodological debate on how to measure balance. The most obvious approach (and known from randomised controlled trials) of testing for significant differences between groups has been criticised for being arbitrary and primarily dependent on the sample size. Austin (2009) has therefore suggested utilising the standardised mean difference (SMD), which ranges from 0 to 100. A difference of less than 10 is considered to be in balance.

Regression versus PSM

Although in principle one could expect similar results from a regression analysis alone, there are some distinct advantages of PSM. Austin (2011) describes four practical reasons for choosing PSM over regression analysis alone.

1 Unlike regression analysis, which relies on fairly abstract measures of fit, the assessment of covariate balance in treatment and control group in PSM is straightforward.

2 The modelling of the propensity score can be conducted independently of the outcome assessment and therefore gives some

protection to fit the model to the desired outcome, a danger inherent to regression analysis.

3 If the outcome is a rare event, sample size requirements for regression analysis quickly increase with the number of covariates. PSM offers more flexibility in these situations.

4 PSM allows a more explicit assessment of the overlap between baseline characteristics of treatment or control group, which can be unnoticed in regression analysis, leading to a comparison of individuals or organisations that are not alike.

Hidden bias

The validity of all observational studies is threatened by unobserved but associated variables with the outcome. Although PSM provides a transparent framework for the analysis of observational data in estimating causal effects, it may still lead to biased results because of unobserved variables. Although there is no complete solution for this problem (*hidden bias assessment*), Rosenbaum (1991) provides an approach for estimating what strength an unobserved variable would need to have in order to change the conclusions, for example that a significant difference becomes non-significant. This type of sensitivity analysis therefore gives an indication of how robust the results are.

Conclusions

- It is not always possible to employ randomised controlled trials.
- PSM provides a transparent framework for estimating treatment effects.
- Validity of PSM still depends on the completeness of observed characteristics.
- Hidden bias assessment provides an indication of how robust the results are.

References

Austin, P.C. (2009) Balance diagnostics for comparing the distribution of baseline covariates between treatment groups in propensity-score matched samples. *Statistics in Medicine* **28**, 3083–3107.

Austin, P.C. (2011) An introduction to propensity score methods for reducing the effects of confounding in observational studies. *Multivariate Behavioral Research* **46**, 399–424.

Rosenbaum, P.R. (1991) Discussing hidden bias in observational studies. *Annals of Internal Medicine* **115**, 901–905.

Rubin, D.B. (2007) The design versus the analysis of observational studies for causal effects: parallels with the design of randomized trials. *Statistics in Medicine* **26**, 20–36.

Appendix 20: Mokken scaling

What is Mokken scaling?

Mokken scaling is a method of item response theory (IRT) (Watson *et al.*, 2012). IRT is a set of methods concerned with analysing the properties of individual items in questionnaires and is often compared with methods such as factor analysis. Both methods are capable of selecting groups of related items from large pools of items: factors in the case of factor analysis and scales in the case of IRT. However, only in IRT methods can the relative contribution of the items in the scale to measurement of the latent trait (what is being measured) be established properly. In other words, when we obtain a score on a latent trait (e.g. depression), then we can know which items have contributed to that score and, uniquely in IRT methods, in what order.

Mokken scaling is a non-parametric form of IRT; this means that it makes fewer assumptions than other forms of IRT and tends to retain more items in scales. Specifically, it makes fewer assumptions about the precise relationship between how items respond to what is being measured and the probability of obtaining that measurement, something that is described by the item characteristic curve (ICC).

Is Mokken scaling useful?

Yes. Mokken scaling has been very useful in developing clinical scales and in providing new insights about established scales. For example, Mokken scaling was used to develop the Edinburgh Feeding Evaluation in Dementia (EdFED) scale (Watson, 1996) which shows that feeding difficulty in older people with dementia follows a pattern and that feeding difficulties are cumulative, moving from a general refusal to eat to an inability to swallow food and just letting it fall out of the mouth. The pattern is very similar across different samples and even across international boundaries. A scale to measure activities of daily living (ADL), the Townsend scale, has also been shown to have cumulative properties using Mokken scaling and, in demonstrating this, the utility of the scale has been improved such that it can be seen that some fairly mild impairments in ADL in community-dwelling older people actually lies on a continuum with more severe impairment and could herald the development of more severe loss of independence and disability. Mokken scaling can also be used to improve such scales by adding further items to the scales and investigating whether or not they also scale alongside the other items or whether they indicate separate dimensions of disability.

How do you carry out Mokken scaling?

Mokken scaling is a multivariate statistical method and conducting it requires a computer program. Most commonly, Mokken scaling practitioners use the online publicly available statistical package *R*, within which there is a package 'mokken' (van der Ark, 2007). Unfortunately, *R* is not Windows compatible and could not be described as being user-friendly, requiring to be programmed and the syntax is not obvious to the uninitiated. Nevertheless, it is worth persevering and for anyone who is interested in getting started I have provided the basic syntax to convert SPSS files to *R*, to save and upload files and to run the essential analyses required for Mokken scaling at http://mokkenscaling.blogspot.co.uk/ (see Figures A20.1–A20.3).

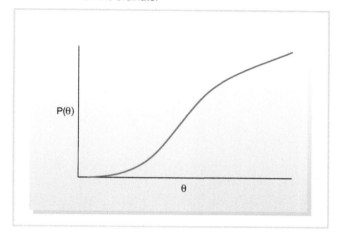

Figure A20.1 An item characteristic curve (ICC) where, as the score on the latent trait (θ) increases, so does the probability of a positive response to the items on the ordinate.

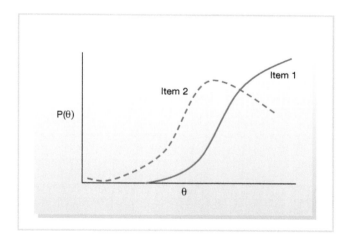

Figure A20.2 Two items, with Item 1 which is monotone and Item 2 which is not.

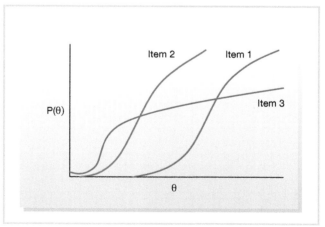

Figure A20.3 Three items, with items 1 and 2 not intersecting and item 3 which intersects items 1 and 2.

References and further reading

Mokken, R.J. and Lewis, C. (1982) A nonparametric approach to the analysis of dichotomous item responses. *Applied Psychological Measurement* **6**, 417–430.

van der Ark, L.A. (2007) Mokken scale analysis in R. *Journal of Statistical Software* **20**, 1–19.

Watson, R. (1996) Mokken scaling procedure (MSP) applied to feeding difficulty in elderly people with dementia. *International Journal of Nursing Studies* **33**, 385–393.

Watson, R., van der Ark, L.A., Lin, L.-C., Fieo, R., Deary, I.J. and Meijer, R.R. (2012) Item response theory: how Mokken scaling can be used in clinical practice. *Journal of Clinical Nursing* **21**, 2736–2746.

Index

Nursing and Healthcare Research at a Glance, First Edition. Alan Glasper and Colin Rees. © 2017 by John Wiley & Sons, Ltd. Published 2017 by John Wiley & Sons, Ltd.